Pneumonia

Editor

MICHAEL S. NIEDERMAN

CLINICS IN
CHEST MEDICINE

www.chestmed.theclinics.com

December 2018 • Volume 39 • Number 4

ELSEVIER

1600 John F. Kennedy Boulevard • Suite 1800 • Philadelphia, Pennsylvania, 19103-2899

http://www.theclinics.com

CLINICS IN CHEST MEDICINE Volume 39, Number 4
December 2018 ISSN 0272-5231, ISBN-13: 978-0-323-64320-7

Editor: Colleen Dietzler
Developmental Editor: Casey Potter

Clinics in Chest Medicine (ISSN 0272-5231) is published quarterly by Elsevier Inc., 360 Park Avenue South, New York, NY 10010-1710. Months of issue are March, June, September, and December. Periodicals postage paid at New York, NY and additional mailing offices. Subscription prices are $366.00 per year (domestic individuals), $691.00 per year (domestic institutions), $100.00 per year (domestic students/residents), $419.00 per year (Canadian individuals), $858.00 per year (Canadian institutions), $479.00 per year (international individuals), $858.00 per year (international institutions), and $230.00 per year (international and Canadian students/residents). International air speed delivery is included in all Clinics subscription prices. All prices are subject to change without notice. **POSTMASTER:** Send address changes to Clinics in Chest Medicine, Elsevier Health Sciences Division, Subscription Customer Service, 3251 Riverport Lane, Maryland Heights, MO 63043. **Customer Service: Telephone: 1-800-654-2452** (U.S. and Canada); **1-314-447-8871** (outside U.S. and Canada). **Fax: 1-314-447-8029. E-mail: journalscustomerservice-usa@elsevier.com (for print support); journalsonlinesupport-usa@elsevier.com (for online support).**

Reprints. For copies of 100 or more of articles in this publication, please contact the Commercial Reprints Department, Elsevier Inc., 360 Park Avenue South, New York, NY 10010-1710. Tel.: 212-633-3874; Fax: 212-633-3820; E-mail: reprints@elsevier.com.

Clinics in Chest Medicine is covered in *MEDLINE/PubMed (Index Medicus), Current Contents/Clinical Medicine, EMBASE/Excerpta Medica, Science Citation Index,* and *ISI/BIOMED.*

Contributors

EDITOR

MICHAEL S. NIEDERMAN, MD
Professor of Clinical Medicine, Clinical Director
and Associate Chief, Pulmonary and Critical
Care Medicine, NewYork-Presbyterian/Weill
Cornell Medical College, New York, New York,
USA

AUTHORS

ROBERT A. BALK, MD
Professor of Medicine, Division of Pulmonary,
Critical Care, and Sleep Medicine, Rush
University Medical Center, Rush Medical
College, Chicago, Illinois, USA

ENRIC BARBETA, MD
Pneumology Department, Respiratory Institute
(ICR), Hospital Clinic of Barcelona, Institut
d'Investigacions Biomèdiques August Pi i
Sunyer (IDIBAPS), University of Barcelona
(UB), SGR 911 - Ciber de Entermedades
Respiratorias (CIBERES), ICREA Academia,
Barcelona, Spain

MATTEO BASSETTI, MD, PhD
Infectious Diseases Clinic, Department of
Medicine, University of Udine, Azienda
Sanitaria Universitaria, Presidio Ospedaliero
Universitario Santa Maria della Misericordia,
Udine, Italy

NICOLAS BRÉCHOT, MD, PhD
Service de Réanimation Médicale, Institut de
Cardiologie, Groupe Hospitalier Pitié–Salpêtrière,
Assistance Publique–Hôpitaux de Paris, Paris,
France

ALESSIA CARNELUTTI, MD
Infectious Diseases Clinic, Department of
Medicine, University of Udine, Azienda
Sanitaria Universitaria, Presidio Ospedaliero
Universitario Santa Maria della Misericordia,
Udine, Italy

RODRIGO CAVALLAZZI, MD
Associate Professor of Medicine, Division of
Pulmonary, Critical Care, and Sleep Disorders,
University of Louisville, Louisville, Kentucky, USA

ADRIAN CECCATO, MD
Pneumology Department, Respiratory Institute
(ICR), Hospital Clinic of Barcelona, Institut
d'Investigacions Biomèdiques August Pi i
Sunyer (IDIBAPS), University of Barcelona (UB),
SGR 911 - Ciber de Enfermedades Respiratorias
(CIBERES), ICREA Academia, Barcelona, Spain

JEAN CHASTRE, MD
Service de Réanimation Médicale, Institut de
Cardiologie, Groupe Hospitalier Pitié–Salpêtrière,
Assistance Publique–Hôpitaux de Paris,
Sorbonne Universités, UPMC Université Paris 06,
INSERM, UMRS_1166-ICAN Institute of
Cardiometabolism and Nutrition, Paris, France

CHARLES S. DELA CRUZ, MD, PhD
Associate Professor, Pulmonary Critical Care
and Sleep Medicine, Center for Pulmonary
Infection Research and Treatment, Yale
University, New Haven, Connecticut, USA

MIQUEL FERRER, MD, PhD
Pneumology Department, Respiratory Institute
(ICR), Hospital Clinic of Barcelona, Institut
d'Investigacions Biomèdiques August Pi i
Sunyer (IDIBAPS), University of Barcelona (UB),
SGR 911 - Ciber de Enfermedades Respiratorias
(CIBERES), ICREA Academia, Barcelona, Spain

SAMIR GAUTAM, MD, PhD
Clinical Fellow, Pulmonary Critical Care and Sleep Medicine, Center for Pulmonary Infection Research and Treatment, Yale University, New Haven, Connecticut, USA

GUILLAUME HÉKIMIAN, MD
Service de Réanimation Médicale, Institut de Cardiologie, Groupe Hospitalier Pitié–Salpêtrière, Assistance Publique–Hôpitaux de Paris, Paris, France

SUSANNE M. HUIJTS, MD, PhD
Department of Respiratory Medicine, University Medical Center Utrecht, Utrecht, The Netherlands

ANDRE C. KALIL, MD, MPH
Professor of Medicine, Department of Internal Medicine, Division of Infectious Diseases, University of Nebraska Medical Center, Omaha, Nebraska, USA

SEAN KEANE, MD
Department of Anaesthesia and Critical Care Medicine, St. James's Hospital, Dublin 8, Ireland

JAMES M. KIDD, PharmD
Center for Anti-Infective Research and Development, Hartford Hospital, Hartford, Connecticut, USA

MARIN H. KOLLEF, MD
Division of Pulmonary and Critical Care Medicine, Washington University School of Medicine in St. Louis, St Louis, Missouri, USA

CHARLES-EDOUARD LUYT, MD, PhD
Service de Réanimation Médicale, Institut de Cardiologie, Groupe Hospitalier Pitié–Salpêtrière, Assistance Publique–Hôpitaux de Paris, Paris, France

IGNACIO MARTIN-LOECHES, MD, PhD
Department of Anaesthesia and Critical Care Medicine, Multidisciplinary Intensive Care Research Organization (MICRO), Department of Clinical Medicine, Trinity College, Wellcome Trust-HRB Clinical Research Facility, Trinity Centre for Health Sciences, St James's Hospital, Dublin 8, Ireland

MARK L. METERSKY, MD
Professor of Medicine, Division of Pulmonary, Critical Care and Sleep Medicine, University of Connecticut School of Medicine, UConn Health, Farmington, Connecticut, USA

JOSEPH P. MIZGERD, ScD
Professor of Medicine, Microbiology, and Biochemistry, Pulmonary Center, Boston University School of Medicine, Boston, Massachusetts, USA

ANA MOTOS, MSc
Center for Anti-Infective Research and Development, Hartford Hospital, Hartford, Connecticut, USA; Division of Animal Experimentation, Department of Pulmonary and Critical Care, Hospital Clinic, Barcelona, Spain

DAVID P. NICOLAU, PharmD, FCCP, FIDSA
Center for Anti-Infective Research and Development, Division of Infectious Diseases, Hartford Hospital, Hartford, Connecticut, USA

SAAD NSEIR, MD, PhD
Professor, CHU Lille, Centre de Réanimation, Critical Care Center, Lille University, Faculté de Médecine, Lille, France

JULIO A. RAMIREZ, MD
Professor of Medicine, Division of Infectious Diseases, University of Louisville, Louisville, Kentucky, USA

ELDA RIGHI, MD, PhD
Infectious Diseases Clinic, Department of Medicine, University of Udine, Azienda Sanitaria Universitaria, Presidio Ospedaliero Universitario Santa Maria della Misericordia, Udine, Italy

ANAHITA ROUZÉ, MD
CHU Lille, Critical Care Center, Lille, France

ALESSANDRO RUSSO, MD
Infectious Diseases Clinic, Department of Medicine, University of Udine, Azienda Sanitaria Universitaria, Presidio Ospedaliero Universitario Santa Maria della Misericordia, Udine, Italy

LEOPOLDO N. SEGAL, MD, MSc
Division of Pulmonary, Critical Care, and Sleep Medicine, Department of Medicine, NYU Human Microbiome Program, NYU School of Medicine, New York, New York, USA

LOKESH SHARMA, PhD
Post-Doctoral Associate, Pulmonary Critical Care and Sleep Medicine, Center for Pulmonary Infection Research and Treatment, Yale University, New Haven, Connecticut, USA

SARAH SUNGURLU, DO
Assistant Professor of Medicine, Division of
Pulmonary, Critical Care, and Sleep Medicine,
Rush University Medical Center, Rush Medical
College, Chicago, Illinois, USA

ANTONI TORRES, MD, PhD
Professor, Pneumology Department,
Respiratory Institute (ICR), Hospital Clinic of
Barcelona, Institut d'Investigacions
Biomèdiques August Pi i Sunyer (IDIBAPS),
University of Barcelona (UB), SGR 911 - Ciber
de Enfermedades Respiratorias (CIBERES),
ICREA Academia, Barcelona, Spain

MARIA SOLE VALLECOCCIA, MD
Department of Anaesthesia and Critical Care
Medicine, St. James's Hospital, Dublin 8,
Ireland; Department of Anesthesia and
Intensive Care Medicine, Università Cattolica
del Sacro Cuore—Fondazione Policlinico
Universitario A.Gemelli, Rome, Italy

CORNELIS H. VAN WERKHOVEN, MD, PhD
Julius Center for Health Sciences and Primary
Care, University Medical Center Utrecht,
Utrecht, The Netherlands

CRISTINA VAZQUEZ GUILLAMET, MD
Divisions of Pulmonary, Critical Care, and
Sleep Medicine, and Infectious Diseases,
University of New Mexico School of
Medicine, Albuquerque, New Mexico,
USA

GRANT W. WATERER, MBBS, PhD
Professor of Medicine, University of Western
Australia, Royal Perth Hospital, Perth,
Australia; Adjunct Professor of Medicine,
Northwestern University, Chicago, Illinois,
USA

BENJAMIN G. WU, MD, MSc
Division of Pulmonary, Critical Care, and Sleep
Medicine, Department of Medicine, NYU
Human Microbiome Program, NYU
School of Medicine, New York, New York,
USA

RICHARD G. WUNDERINK, MD
Professor, Department of Medicine, Pulmonary
and Critical Care, Northwestern University
Feinberg School of Medicine, Chicago, Illinois,
USA

Contributors

SARAH SUNGURLU, DO

ANTONI TORRES, MD, PhD

CRISTINA VÁZQUEZ-GUILLAMET, MD

GRANT W. WATERER, MBBS, PhD

BENJAMIN G. WU, MSc

Contents

Preface: Respiratory Infections: An Ongoing Challenge with a Promising Future   xv

Michael S. Niederman

Inflammation and Pneumonia: Why Are Some More Susceptible than Others?   669

Joseph P. Mizgerd

Pneumonia is an important cause of morbidity and mortality. However, pneumonia is an unusual outcome of respiratory infection. Most of the time, microbes in the lung can be controlled by a combination of constitutive and recruited defense mechanisms. Inflammation is a key component of recruited defenses. Variations in inflammation that influence pneumonia susceptibility and severity are considered here.

The Lung Microbiome and Its Role in Pneumonia   677

Benjamin G. Wu and Leopoldo N. Segal

The use of next-generation sequencing and multiomic analysis reveals new insights on the identity of microbes in the lower airways blurring the lines between commensals and pathogens. Microbes are not found in isolation; rather they form complex metacommunities where microbe-host and microbe-microbe interactions play important roles on the host susceptibility to pathogens. In addition, the lower airway microbiota exert significant effects on host immune tone. Thus, this review highlights the roles that microbes in the respiratory tract play in the development of pneumonia.

The Role of Biomarkers in the Diagnosis and Management of Pneumonia   691

Sarah Sungurlu and Robert A. Balk

Biomarkers are used in the diagnosis, severity determination, and prognosis for patients with community-acquired pneumonia (CAP). Selected biomarkers may indicate a bacterial infection and need for antibiotic therapy (C-reactive protein, procalcitonin, soluble triggering receptor expressed on myeloid cells). Biomarkers can differentiate CAP patients who require hospital admission and severe CAP requiring intensive care unit admission. Biomarker-guided antibiotic therapy may limit antibiotic exposure without compromising outcome and thus improve antibiotic stewardship. The authors discuss the role of biomarkers in diagnosing, determining severity, defining the prognosis, and limiting antibiotic exposure in CAP and ventilator-associated pneumonia patients.

Influenza and Viral Pneumonia   703

Rodrigo Cavallazzi and Julio A. Ramirez

Influenza and other respiratory viruses are commonly identified in patients with community-acquired pneumonia, hospital-acquired pneumonia, and in immunocompromised patients with pneumonia. Clinically, it is difficult to differentiate viral from bacterial pneumonia. Similarly, the radiological findings of viral infection are nonspecific. The advent of polymerase chain reaction testing has enormously facilitated the identification of respiratory viruses, which has important implications for infection control measures and treatment. Currently, treatment options for patients with viral infection are limited, but there is ongoing research on the development and clinical testing of new treatment regimens and strategies.

Guidelines to Manage Community-Acquired Pneumonia
723

Richard G. Wunderink

Few guidelines have greater acceptance than that for management of community-acquired pneumonia (CAP). Despite this, areas remain controversial, and new challenges continue to emerge. Current guidelines differ from those of northern European countries predominantly in need for macrolide combination with β-lactams for hospitalized, non–intensive care unit patients. A preponderance of evidence favors combination therapy. Challenges for current and future CAP guidelines include new antibiotic classes, emergence of viruses as major causes for CAP, new diagnostic modalities, alternative risk stratification for pathogens resistant to usual CAP antibiotics, and evidence-based management of severe CAP, including immunomodulatory therapy such as corticosteroids.

Vaccines to Prevent Pneumococcal Community-Acquired Pneumonia
733

Cornelis H. van Werkhoven and Susanne M. Huijts

Streptococcus pneumoniae is the most frequent pathogen in community-acquired pneumonia and also causes invasive diseases like bacteremia and meningitis. Young children and elderly are especially at risk for pneumococcal diseases and are, therefore, eligible for pneumococcal vaccination in most countries. This reviews provides an overview of the current epidemiology of pneumococcal infections, history and evidence of available pneumococcal polysaccharide and conjugate vaccines, and current recommendations.

Adjunctive Therapies for Community-Acquired Pneumonia
753

Adrian Ceccato, Miquel Ferrer, Enric Barbeta, and Antoni Torres

The use of adjuvant therapies for community-acquired pneumonia is still in development. Combinations of antibiotics with macrolides seem to be the best option when there is no risk of resistance. The use of corticosteroids is the treatment of choice in patients with severe pneumonia and a high inflammatory response who do not present contraindications for these drugs. Other drugs await confirmation of their benefit and should be used only on exceptional occasions at this time.

Health Care–Associated Pneumonia: Is It Still a Useful Concept?
765

Grant W. Waterer

"Health care–associated pneumonia (HCAP) was introduced into guidelines because of concerns about the increasing prevalence of drug-resistant pathogens (DRPs) not covered by standard empirical therapy. We now know that DRPs are very localized phenomena with low rates in most sites. Although HCAP risk factors are associated with a higher mortality, this is driven by comorbidities rather than the pathogens. Empirical coverage of DRPs has generally not resulted in better patient outcomes. A far more nuanced approach must be taken for patients with risk factors for DRPs taking into account the local cause and severity of disease.

Airway Devices in Ventilator-Associated Pneumonia Pathogenesis and Prevention
775

Anahita Rouzé, Ignacio Martin-Loeches, and Saad Nseir

Airway devices play a major role in the pathogenesis of microaspiration of contaminated oropharyngeal and gastric secretions, tracheobronchial colonization, and ventilator-associated pneumonia (VAP) occurrence. Subglottic secretion drainage is an effective measure for VAP prevention, and no routine change of ventilator circuit. Continuous control of cuff pressure, silver-coated tracheal tubes, low-volume low-pressure tracheal tubes, and the mucus shaver are promising devices that should be further evaluated by large randomized controlled trials. Polyurethane-cuffed, conical-shaped cuff, and closed tracheal suctioning system are not effective and should not be used for VAP prevention.

How Can We Distinguish Ventilator-Associated Tracheobronchitis from Pneumonia?   785

Sean Keane, Maria Sole Vallecoccia, Saad Nseir, and Ignacio Martin-Loeches

Ventilator-associated tracheobronchitis (VAT) might represent an intermediate process between lower respiratory tract colonization and ventilator-associated pneumonia (VAP), or even a less severe spectrum of VAP. There is an urgent need for new concepts in the arena of ventilator-associated lower respiratory tract infections. Ideally, the gold standard of care is based on prevention rather than treatment of respiratory infection. However, despite numerous and sometimes imaginative efforts to validate the benefit of these measures, most clinicians now accept that currently available measures have failed to eradicate VAP. Stopping the progression from VAT to VAP could improve patient outcomes.

Management of Ventilator-Associated Pneumonia: Guidelines   797

Mark L. Metersky and Andre C. Kalil

Two recent major guidelines on diagnosis and treatment of ventilator-associated pneumonia (VAP) recommend consideration of local antibiotic resistance patterns and individual patient risks for resistant pathogens when formulating an initial empiric antibiotic regimen. One recommends against invasive diagnostic techniques with quantitative cultures to determine the cause of VAP; the other recommends either invasive or noninvasive techniques. Both guidelines recommend short-course therapy be used for most patients with VAP. Although neither guideline recommends use of procalcitonin as an adjunct to clinical judgment when diagnosing VAP, they differ with respect to use of serial procalcitonin to shorten the length of antibiotic treatment.

Is Zero Ventilator-Associated Pneumonia Achievable?: Practical Approaches to Ventilator-Associated Pneumonia Prevention   809

Cristina Vazquez Guillamet and Marin H. Kollef

Ventilator-associated pneumonia (VAP) remains a significant clinical entity with reported incidence rates of 7% to 15%. Given the considerable adverse consequences associated with this infection, VAP prevention became a core measure required in most US hospitals. Many institutions implemented effective VAP prevention bundles that combined head of bed elevation, hand hygiene, chlorhexidine oral care, and subglottic drainage. More recently, spontaneous breathing and awakening trials have consistently been shown to shorten the duration of mechanical ventilation and secondarily reduce the occurrence of VAP. More recent data question the overall positive impact of prevention bundles, including some of their core component interventions.

Aerosol Therapy for Pneumonia in the Intensive Care Unit   823

Charles-Edouard Luyt, Guillaume Hékimian, Nicolas Bréchot, and Jean Chastre

Antibiotic aerosolization in patients with ventilator-associated pneumonia (VAP) allows very high concentrations of antimicrobial agents in the respiratory secretions, far more than those achievable using the intravenous route. However, data in critically ill patients with pneumonia are limited. Administration of aerosolized antibiotics might increase the likelihood of clinical resolution, but no significant improvements in important outcomes have been consistently documented. Thus, aerosolized antibiotics should be restricted to the treatment of extensively resistant gram-negative pneumonia. In these cases, the use of a vibrating-mesh nebulizer seems to be more efficient, but specific settings and conditions are required to improve lung delivery.

Optimizing Antibiotic Administration for Pneumonia   837

Ana Motos, James M. Kidd, and David P. Nicolau

Pneumonia, including community-acquired bacterial pneumonia, hospital-acquired bacterial pneumonia, and ventilator-acquired bacterial pneumonia, carries unacceptably high morbidity and mortality. Despite advances in antimicrobial therapy, emergence of multidrug resistance and high rates of treatment failure have made optimization of antibiotic efficacy a priority. This review focuses on pharmacokinetic and pharmacodynamic approaches to antibacterial optimization within the lung environment and in the setting of critical illness. Strategies for including these approaches in drug development programs as well as clinical practice are described and reviewed.

New Antibiotics for Pneumonia   853

Matteo Bassetti, Elda Righi, Alessandro Russo, and Alessia Carnelutti

Delayed antimicrobial prescriptions and inappropriate treatment can lead to poor outcomes in pneumonia. In nosocomial infections, especially in countries reporting high rates of antimicrobial resistance, the presence of multidrug-resistant gram-negative and gam-positive bacteria can limit options for adequate antimicrobial treatment. New antibiotics, belonging to known classes of antimicrobials or characterized by novel mechanisms of actions, have recently been approved or are under development. Advantages of the new compounds include enhanced spectrum of activity against resistant bacteria, high lung penetration, good tolerability, and possibility for intravenous to oral sequential therapy. This article reviews characteristics of newly approved and investigational compounds.

Personalizing the Management of Pneumonia   871

Samir Gautam, Lokesh Sharma, and Charles S. Dela Cruz

Pneumonia is a highly prevalent disease with considerable morbidity and mortality. However, diagnosis and therapy still rely on antiquated methods, leading to the vast overuse of antimicrobials, which carries risks for both society and the individual. Furthermore, outcomes in severe pneumonia remain poor. Genomic techniques have the potential to transform the management of pneumonia through deep characterization of pathogens as well as the host response to infection. This characterization will enable the delivery of selective antimicrobials and immunomodulatory therapy that will help to offset the disorder associated with overexuberant immune responses.

PROGRAM OBJECTIVE

The goal of the *Clinics in Chest Medicine* is to provide provide practitioners with state-of-the-art information that is clinically useful, concise, well referenced, and comprehensive.

TARGET AUDIENCE

All practicing physicians and healthcare professionals who provide patient care utilizing findings from *Chest Medicine Clinics of North America*.

LEARNING OBJECTIVES

Upon completion of this activity, participants will be able to:

1. Review the current epidemiology of pneumococcal infections, history and evidence of available vaccines, and current recommendations
2. Discuss currently available and potential future options for the treatment of respiratory tract infections.
3. Recognize the role of biomarkers in the diagnoses and management of Pneumonia.

ACCREDITATION

The Elsevier Office of Continuing Medical Education (EOCME) is accredited by the Accreditation Council for Continuing Medical Education (ACCME) to provide continuing medical education for physicians.

The EOCME designates this enduring material for a maximum of 15 *AMA PRA Category 1 Credit*(s)™. Physicians should claim only the credit commensurate with the extent of their participation in the activity.

All other health care professionals requesting continuing education credit for this enduring material will be issued a certificate of participation.

DISCLOSURE OF CONFLICTS OF INTEREST

The EOCME assesses conflict of interest with its instructors, faculty, planners, and other individuals who are in a position to control the content of CME activities. All relevant conflicts of interest that are identified are thoroughly vetted by EOCME for fair balance, scientific objectivity, and patient care recommendations. EOCME is committed to providing its learners with CME activities that promote improvements or quality in healthcare and not a specific proprietary business or a commercial interest.

The planning committee, staff, authors and editors listed below have identified no financial relationships or relationships to products or devices they or their spouse/life partner have with commercial interest related to the content of this CME activity:

Enric Barbeta, MD; Matteo Bassetti, MD, PhD; Nicolas Bréchot, MD, PhD; Alessia Carnelutti, MD; Dietzler Colleen; Adrian Ceccato, MD; Charles S. Dela Cruz, MD, PhD; Miquel Ferrer, MD, PhD; Samir Gautam, MD, PhD; Cristina Vazquez Guillamet, MD; Guillaume Hékimian, MD; Andre C. Kalil, MD, MPH; Sean Keane, MD, Alison Kemp; Jamoo M. Kidd, PharmD; Marin H. Kollef, MD; Ignacio Martin-Loeches, MD, PhD; Mark L. Metersky, MD; Joseph P. Mizgerd, ScD; Ana Motos, MSc; Julio A. Ramirez, MD; Elda Righi, MD, PhD; Anahita Rouzé, MD; Alessandro Russo, MD; Leopoldo N. Segal, MD; Lokesh Sharma, PhD; Sarah Sungurlu, DO; Antoni Torres, MD, PhD; Maria Sole Vallecoccia, MD; Grant W. Waterer, MBBS, PhD; Benjamin G. Wu, MD.

The planning committee, staff, authors and editors listed below have identified financial relationships or relationships to products or devices they or their spouse/life partner have with commercial interest related to the content of this CME activity:

Robert A. Balk, MD: has received research support, honoraria, and participated in advisory boards for bioMérieux, Inc., F. Hoffmann-La Roche Ltd, and Thermo Fisher Scientific Inc.

Rodrigo Cavallazzi, MD: has acted as a consultant/advisor for Gilead and GlaxoSmithKline plc.

Jean Chastre, MD: has participated on an advisory board and received research support from Bayer AG

Susanne M. Huijts, MD, PhD: has received research support from Pfizer, Inc.

Charles-Edouard Luyt, MD, PhD: has participated on an advisory board and received research support from Bayer AG

David P. Nicolau, PharmD, FCCP, FIDSA: has participated on an advisory board, acted as a consultant/advisor, and received research support from Achaogen, Inc., Bayer AG, Cepheid, Merck & Co., Inc., Melinta Thereapeutics, Inc., Pfizer, Inc., and Shionogi Inc.

Michael S. Niederman, MD: has been a consultant/advisor for Pfizer, Inc., Shionogi, Inc., Paratek Pharmaceuticals, Inc., Melinta Therapeutics, Inc., and Nabriva Therapeutics plc. He has been a consultant/advisor and received research support from Merck & Co., Inc.

Saad Nseir, MD, PhD: has participated on a speaker's bureau for Merck & Co., Inc. and has acted as a consultant/advisor for Ciel Medical, Inc.

Cornelis H. van Werkhoven, MD, PhD: has received research support and has participated on advisory boards for Pfizer, Inc. and Merck & Co., Inc.

Richard G. Wunderink, MD: has acted as a consultant/advisor for Accelerate Diagnostics, Inc., Arsanis, Inc., Biotest Pharmaceuticals Corporation, Curetis GmbH, GenMark Diagnostics, Inc., GlaxoSmithKline plc, InflaRx N.V., KBP BioSciences Co., Ltd., Merck & Co., Inc., Nabriva Thera

UNAPPROVED/OFF-LABEL USE DISCLOSURE

The EOCME requires CME faculty to disclose to the participants:

1. When products or procedures being discussed are off-label, unlabelled, experimental, and/or investigational (not US Food and Drug Administration [FDA] approved); and
2. Any limitations on the information presented, such as data that are preliminary or that represent ongoing research, interim analyses, and/or unsupported opinions. Faculty may discuss information about pharmaceutical agents that is outside of FDA-approved labelling. This information is intended solely for CME and is not intended to promote off-label use of these medications. If you have any questions, contact the medical affairs department of the manufacturer for the most recent prescribing information.

TO ENROLL

To enroll in the *Chest Medicine Clinics* Continuing Medical Education program, call customer service at 1-800-654-2452 or sign up online at http://www.theclinics.com/home/cme. The CME program is available to subscribers for an additional annual fee of USD $225.

METHOD OF PARTICIPATION

In order to claim credit, participants must complete the following:

1. Complete enrolment as indicated above.
2. Read the activity.
3. Complete the CME Test and Evaluation. Participants must achieve a score of 70% on the test. All CME Tests and Evaluations must be completed online.

CME INQUIRIES/SPECIAL NEEDS

For all CME inquiries or special needs, please contact elsevierCME@elsevier.com.

CLINICS IN CHEST MEDICINE

FORTHCOMING ISSUES

March 2019
Asthma
Serpil Erzurum and Sumita Khatri, *Editors*

June 2019
Clinical Respiratory Physiology
Denis O'Donnell and Alberto Neder, *Editors*

September 2019
Tuberculosis
Charles L. Daley and David Lewinsohn, *Editors*

RECENT ISSUES

September 2018
Pulmonary Embolism
Peter Marshall and Wassim Fares, *Editors*

June 2018
Respiratory Manifestations of Neuromuscular and Chest Wall Disorders
F. Dennis McCool and Joshua O. Benditt, *Editors*

March 2018
Interventional Pulmonology
Ali I. Musani, *Editor*

RELATED INTEREST

Infectious Disease Clinics, Volume 31, Issue 1 (March 2017)
Legionnaire's Disease
Cheston B. Cunha and Burke A. Cunha, *Editors*

THE CLINICS ARE AVAILABLE ONLINE!
Access your subscription at:
www.theclinics.com

Preface
Respiratory Infections: An Ongoing Challenge with a Promising Future

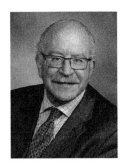

Michael S. Niederman, MD
Editor

Respiratory tract infections remain an important source of morbidity and mortality with pneumonia and influenza serving as the eighth leading cause of death in the United States and the number one cause of death from infectious diseases. Advances in medicine have led to more complex patient populations than in the past, with the advent of novel chemotherapies, immune modulating interventions, and transplantation all creating unique types of immune impairment. Our understanding of the pathogenesis of lung infections had led to the possibility of a uniquely personalized approach to each patient, recognizing the specific pathogens that they may be infected by, and designing therapeutic management that is tailored to their specific needs.

This issue of *Clinics in Chest Medicine* explores these subjects through the efforts of world leaders in the management of Respiratory Infections. Included in this issue is an exploration of specific immune impairments that can help explain why certain patients are more commonly afflicted with specific respiratory infections than others. Our understanding of bacterial pathogenesis is also evolving, and key among new concepts is the Lung Microbiome, a field of investigation that challenges the previous concept that the lower respiratory tract is sterile in healthy individuals and now helps us understand respiratory infection from the perspective of emergence of a preexisting flora. Early recognition of infection has been enhanced with new biomarkers, which are also discussed here.

Pneumonia management has been greatly impacted by the advent of guidelines. Our expert authors discuss influenza and community-acquired pneumonia (CAP) management, drawing on new concepts of therapy and disease recognition. CAP has patient subsets, including those with severe illness, who need a unique approach to care, and all at-risk patients can now benefit from new vaccines, which are discussed in detail. One controversial subset of pneumonia patients, those with health care–associated pneumonia, is also discussed, examining whether patients with contact with the health care environment prior to pneumonia onset are best regarded as a form of CAP or hospital-acquired pneumonia (HAP).

Our understanding of HAP has been evolving, but an important pathogenetic concept is the role played by airway devices that are used to assist in the management of respiratory failure. Another important concept that is discussed is that of ventilator-associated tracheobronchitis, a putative predecessor to ventilator-associated pneumonia (VAP), which can be managed by new guidelines that have been developed in both the Unites States and Europe. VAP prevention is

Clin Chest Med 39 (2018) xv–xvi
https://doi.org/10.1016/j.ccm.2018.09.001
0272-5231/18/© 2018 Published by Elsevier Inc.

certainly possible, and simple bundles may have a huge impact, but may not be able to reduce VAP rates to zero.

The therapy of respiratory infections remains in evolution as we look for the most effective ways to use our current armamentarium to eradicate lung infection. The approaches discussed here include the use of aerosolized antibiotics and optimizing drug delivery by exploiting pharmacokinetic and pharmacodynamics principles. While these approaches make the most of our existing therapeutic options, fortunately, a number of new antibiotics, including agents in new classes of drugs with new mechanisms of action, are in development and can potentially improve and simplify our care of patients with HAP and CAP.

Finally, to unveil the future, the issue concludes with an examination of how all this information can be synthesized to develop a personalized approach to care. For me, this is the most exciting prospect for the future, and one that demonstrates the integration of all the new information that our expert authors have discussed.

Once again, I am hopeful that this issue of *Clinics in Chest Medicine* will serve as a summary of existing knowledge, but also as a roadmap for future research and a catalyst for using our current knowledge to improve the care of a wide range of patients with respiratory infections.

I want to thank our expert authors for all of their hard work and their desire to synthesize and share new information with our readers.

Michael S. Niederman, MD
Pulmonary and Critical Care Medicine
New York Presbyterian/
Weill Cornell Medical College
425 East 61st Street
4th Floor
New York, NY 10065, USA

E-mail address:
msn9004@med.cornell.edu

Inflammation and Pneumonia
Why Are Some More Susceptible than Others?

Joseph P. Mizgerd, ScD

KEYWORDS

- Cytokines • Epithelial cells • Innate lymphocytes • Macrophages • Neutrophils • NF-κB
- Pneumococcus • Resident memory cells

KEY POINTS

- The respiratory pathogens that cause pneumonia are ubiquitous and unavoidable, but pneumonia is an unusual outcome of infection.
- When microbes are particularly numerous or virulent, then inflammation is essential to lung defense.
- The quantity and quality of inflammation are key determinants of pneumonia susceptibility.
- Acute pulmonary inflammation is influenced by prior infections, which remodel the lung immune system in ways that help prevent pneumonia.
- Acute pulmonary inflammation is influenced by chronic diseases and conditions, compromising lung defense and increasing pneumonia susceptibility.

INTRODUCTION

Pneumonia is a very unusual outcome of very common host-microbe interactions. Pneumonias are caused by a large variety of ubiquitous and unavoidable microbes, such as rhinovirus, influenza virus, pneumococcus, and *Staphylococcus aureus*.[1–3] These microbes are encountered frequently by most people, but pneumonia occurs only rarely. What differences in host-microbe interactions determine whether pneumonia ensues?

Some people tend to be more prone to pneumonia, including the very young, the elderly, and those with diverse conditions or diseases, such as stress, poverty, poor air quality, obesity, diabetes, and atherosclerosis.[4] Mechanisms responsible for rendering these individuals more susceptible to pneumonia are largely speculative.[4] Multiple factors are involved, including variations in the inflammatory response during respiratory infection.

THE MICROBES

No single species of microbe is responsible for more than a small fraction of pneumonia cases.[1–3] Although the microbe may be less pivotal than the host response to the microbe,[4] the biology of the microbe does matter. Properties of microbes can influence pneumonia likelihood and severity.[5–9] Some of the microbial variations related to pneumonia pathogenesis center on how microbes interact with host inflammatory pathways. As one example of this, pneumococci that are less stimulatory of inflammatory responses in macrophages are more virulent and likely to cause pneumonia.[10] Pneumococcus is the most common bacterial

Disclosure: No conflicts to declare. Funding was provided by the US NIH (R35 HL135756, R01 AI115053, R56 AI122763, R61 HL137081).
Pulmonary Center, Boston University School of Medicine, 72 East Concord Street, Boston, MA 02115, USA
E-mail address: jmizgerd@bu.edu

Clin Chest Med 39 (2018) 669–676
https://doi.org/10.1016/j.ccm.2018.07.002
0272-5231/18/
© 2018 Elsevier Inc. All rights reserved.

cause of community-acquired pneumonia in both children and adults in the United States.[1,2] Analyses of pneumococcal isolates found in children, collected from blood or empyema fluid of patients or from nasal passages of carriers without pneumococcal disease, revealed a marked variation in macrophage nuclear factor κB (NF-κB) activation.[10] NF-κB is a transcription factor essential to induction of diverse proinflammatory cytokines.[11] Pneumococcal isolates collected from children with complicated pneumonia are more likely to be low NF-κB activators, compared with isolates from other children.[10] These pneumococci induce lower and slower proinflammatory cytokine expression from macrophages in vitro and in vivo, and they are cleared less effectively from the lungs of mice during experimental infection.[10] These findings suggest that avoiding inflammatory triggering is a virulence property for pneumococcus,[12] supporting the concept that the degree to which inflammation is rapidly and effectively triggered in the lungs is one important determinant of whether pneumonia results from a lower respiratory infection.

CONSTITUTIVE IMMUNE DEFENSE OF THE LUNG

The respiratory tract is protected by many continuously functioning defenses that work together.[4] The branching system of conducting airways favors impaction of inhaled organisms before they reach the deep lung. The mucociliary escalator throughout the conducting airways traps impacted microbes and impels them toward the glottis, where they are swallowed for digestion and/or elimination. The surface lining fluids of the respiratory tract are inhospitable to microbes, from nose to alveoli, by limiting essential nutrients and including factors noxious to microbes. Alveolar macrophages patrol the lung surface and phagocytose microbes that manage to evade these defenses. When microbes reaching the lungs are sparse and not highly virulent, these constitutive defenses are often sufficient to prevent clinically relevant microbial accumulations. Although the lungs are not sterile and contain a dynamic microbiome,[13] they typically remain free of infection despite extensive microbial exposure.

Defects in these constitutive defenses can render individuals susceptible to pneumonia. Although beyond the scope of this article focusing on inflammation specifically, it is relevant to recognize that there are many instances in which airway structural changes (eg, in chronic respiratory diseases), mucociliary escalator dysfunction (eg, primary ciliary dyskinesia), altered surface lining characteristics (eg, changes in salts, carbohydrates, or other metabolites), or other defects in constitutive lung defenses contribute to pneumonia risk.[4]

INFLAMMATION FOR RECRUITED DEFENSE OF THE LUNG

When constitutive defenses are overwhelmed by numerous or virulent microbes, recruitment of additional defense (ie, inflammation) becomes necessary. Rapid neutrophil accumulation is especially key to effective microbe elimination. These inflammatory cells kill microbes by phagocytosis, degranulation, and the release of neutrophil extracellular traps.[14] In addition to neutrophils, other leukocytes recruited to aid in antimicrobial lung defense include monocytes, dendritic cells, natural killer (NK) cells, invariant NK T (iNKT) cells, γδ-T cells, mucosa-associated invariant T (MAIT) cells, and innate lymphoid cells (ILCs) of various types.[4] Beyond these cell accumulations, there is an accumulation of extravascular plasma, which results in the radiological infiltrate that is used in pneumonia diagnosis. Although pulmonary edema contributes directly to lung injury, this fluid exudate is also important to immune defense because it includes antimicrobial factors such as complement and antibodies. The coordination of these inflammatory processes helps eliminate virulent and/or numerous microbes in the lungs.

Although rapidly ramping up inflammation helps fight infection, brakes on the inflammatory response also are critical.[4] Multiple activities function to slow or reverse inflammation in the infected or previously infected lung. Alveolar macrophages calm the inflammatory responses of epithelial cells using gap junction connections.[15] Removal of inflammatory exudate fluid is accomplished by ion transport proteins in epithelial cells,[16] pumping fluid from the air spaces into the interstitial spaces from where it can be cleared by lymphatics. Dead and dying inflammatory cells, such as apoptotic neutrophils, are removed via efferocytosis, stimulated by specialized proresolving mediators such as Lipoxin A4 and Resolvin D1.[17] Cells specialized for limiting inflammation and injury, such as regulatory T cells[18,19] and myeloid-derived suppressor cells,[20] are recruited to the infected lung to govern the resolution of inflammation. The coordinated actions of these antiinflammatory and inflammation-resolving processes help prevent and limit the clinical severity of pneumonia.

INBORN VARIATIONS IN INFLAMMATORY PATHWAYS AND PNEUMONIA SUSCEPTIBILITY

Carefully controlled studies using genetic engineering in mouse models are empowered to show connections between a gene of interest and pneumonia susceptibility. By comparing groups that differ only in defined genetic elements during a directly comparable exposure to the exact same microbe, unique roles for select gene products in distinct cells can be precisely delineated. Many genes related to inflammation have been shown to be essential to pneumonia defense with such studies.[4] As one example, the NF-κB transcription factor, which induces the expression of myriad inflammatory mediators,[11] is essential to preventing pneumonia,[21] with different but essential roles in many different cell-types.[4] Interrupting 1 NF-κB gene in macrophages or in epithelial cells is sufficient to reduce expression of inflammatory mediators from these cells and slow the recruitment of neutrophils into newly infected air spaces,[22,23] enabling microbes to establish more severe lung infection. In parallel, inflammatory pathways involving interferons and interferon stimulated genes (ISGs) are elicited, which are especially important against respiratory viruses and intracellular bacteria or fungi.[24–26] The ISGs and interferon regulatory factor (IRF) transcription factors are necessary for preventing some pneumonias, such as those caused by influenza or Legionella.[27,28] These animal studies show that the triggering of inflammatory gene expression via NF-κB, IRFs, and other transcription factors initiates and guides the effective elimination of virulent microbes that get into the lung.

Similar concepts are supported by human studies. Rare but serious human mutations in genes involved in inflammation support the roles of these inflammatory processes in protecting against pneumonia. At least 24 different genes have been found to result in neutropenia when mutated, and these patients have increased risk of infections, including pneumonia.[29] Related to NF-κB activity, patients with mutations in signaling intermediates upstream of this transcription factor, such as in the MYD88 or IRAK4 genes, are profoundly susceptible to infections by respiratory pathogens such as pneumococcus.[30] Invasive pneumococcal disease, but not pneumonia, is commonly diagnosed in such patients, likely because the inflammatory exudate essential to a pneumonia diagnosis is blunted in the absence of MyD88 or IRAK4 function. In contrast, mutations in which an exudate is not diminished but inflammatory functions are compromised predispose to infections that are readily diagnosed as pneumonia. For example, defective NADPH (nicotinamide adenine dinucleotide phosphate, reduced form) oxidase components in chronic granulomatous disease lead to fungal and bacterial pneumonias,[31] and defective IFN-α expression caused by

IRF7 deficiency leads to influenza pneumonias.[32] Although such genetic diseases are rare, they reveal essential roles of inflammatory components in human lung defense against respiratory pathogens.

More common genetic polymorphisms in components of inflammation have been observed, but their connections to pneumonia are less firmly established.[33] The significance of such polymorphisms on regulation and function of a gene is often unclear or modest. Furthermore, human studies are generally less well suited than mouse studies to connecting genetic variation to pneumonia defense. Virtually all such human studies involve genomes and also environments and comorbidities that are very far from uniform across subjects, confounding analyses. Most, but not all, such human studies are observational and associative by design, involving noncontrolled and highly varying exposures to disparate types of respiratory pathogens. The vagaries of pneumonia diagnosis, including the subjective assessment of the diagnosis itself as well as typically uncertain cause and inconsistently quantified severity, coupled with the rare and seemingly stochastic nature of this disease even in susceptible populations, further complicate such research. Although the net contributions remain largely unclear, it is plausible that genetic variations in inflammatory and other pathways contribute to many cases of pneumonia.

ACQUIRED VARIATIONS IN INFLAMMATORY PATHWAYS: IMPROVEMENTS CAUSED BY INFECTION HISTORY

The U-shaped curve of pneumonia incidence over the age spectrum is well established.[4] The youngest children and older adults have much higher annual incidences of pneumonia than do older children and young adults. The mechanisms protecting older children and young adults against pneumonia are becoming elucidated, and variations in these pathways may influence who does or does not get pneumonia.[4]

The successful resolution of prior respiratory infections results in a substantial improvement in pulmonary defense, conferred by local changes in lung cells (**Fig. 1**). Respiratory infections are inevitable throughout the life course, and recovery from these infections is a guiding force in reshaping pulmonary inflammation to more effectively prevent pneumonia. Such experienced lungs respond more quickly and more effectively on subsequent infections, whether microbes are similar to or different from those that infected the lungs previously.

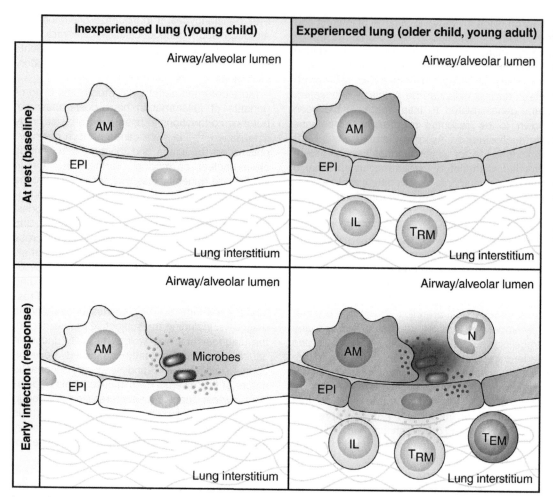

Fig. 1. Changes in lung cells and inflammatory responses caused by resolution of prior respiratory infections. The cells in the resting uninfected lung differ in early life and after the experience of multiple prior respiratory infections (*upper 2 panels*). Alveolar macrophages (AM) and epithelial cells (EPI) are present in both cases, but can be preprogrammed to respond differently because of trained immunity in experienced lungs (noted by color changes in upper panels). Furthermore, numerous additional cells are present in the experienced lung (*upper right*), including innate immunity cells such as innate lymphocytes (IL), NK cells, iNKT cells, γδ-T cells, mucosa-associated invariant T cells, and ILCs, as well as adaptive immunity cells, in particular resident memory T cells (T_RM). The lung responds differently to infection based on such changes (*bottom panels*). Because of the epigenetic and metabolic changes of trained immunity plus the newly derived signals coming from IL and T_RM cells, the AM and EPI cells elaborate different patterns of mediators with altered kinetics, altogether accelerating the recruitment of immune defense cells such as neutrophils (N) and effector memory T cells (T_EM) to improve antimicrobial lung defense.

One aspect of this inflammatory remodeling is immunologic memory, including both memory T cells and B cells, some of which (such as resident memory T cells) persist exclusively in the lung tissue to mediate localized protection (see **Fig. 1**), whereas other components (such as central memory T cells) circulate to offer more systemic protection.[4] This memory provides new effector mechanisms that are unavailable in naive individuals, including neutralizing antibodies and cytotoxic T cells (CTLs). Beyond these antigen-specific immune effector mechanisms, memory lymphocytes confer protection by altering inflammatory processes in the lung.[4] Adaptive immune memory cells help lung immunity by changing the kinetics and amplitudes of inflammatory cytokines and chemokines in the tissue,[34,35] accelerating and bolstering the antimicrobial defenses that would traditionally be characterized as components of innate immunity (see **Fig. 1**). The immunity protecting the lungs against pneumonia must extend across multiple serotypes/subtypes of a given bacteria (such as pneumococcus) or virus (such as influenza). Such heterotypic immunity is mediated by the rewiring of inflammatory responses by adaptive immunologic memory, more than by antigen-targeted immune effector actions such as neutralizing antibodies and CTLs.[4]

In addition to adaptive immune memory, innate immunity itself has some capacity for memory. At least 2 components of innate immune memory are relevant to pneumonia and inflammatory responses elicited by microbes in the lung, and both result from the resolution of prior respiratory infections: new types of inflammatory cell types populating the lung, and altered inflammatory responses from the cells already present in the lung.

The resolution of pulmonary infection in mice leaves behind many types of innate lymphocytes in lung tissue (see **Fig. 1**), reflecting the diverse types of innate lymphocytes in adult human lungs,[4] including γδ-T cells, MAIT cells, iNKT cells, NK cells, and various ILCs. Some of these cells have specialized receptors allowing them to recognize select types of signals from microbial pathogens. All of them elaborate immunomodulating cytokines that reshape inflammatory responses during lung infection, similar to the adaptive immune memory cells described earlier. Innate lymphocytes in the lung contribute to pneumonia prevention by steering the local inflammatory responses to respiratory pathogens.

Beyond being under new direction from newly present adaptive and innate lymphocytes in the lung, the constituent cells of the lungs behave intrinsically differently after resolution of prior respiratory infections, making different types and amounts of inflammatory mediators (see **Fig. 1**). Often referred to as trained immunity, this intracellular remodeling involves a combination of epigenetic and metabolic changes,[36] causing lung cells to respond differently to microbes in the respiratory tract based on prior experiences of that tissue.[4] This applies to alveolar macrophages and likely many other cells in the lung as well, which generate different types and amounts of inflammatory mediators, depending on prior experience. Typically, these trained immune responses are far more effective at controlling and eliminating microbes.

ACQUIRED VARIATIONS IN INFLAMMATORY PATHWAYS: IMPAIRMENTS CAUSED BY EXPOSURES AND CONDITIONS

Many exposures (**Fig. 2**) can interfere with the inflammatory responses described earlier as essential to preventing pneumonia. A profound defect related to inflammation is neutropenia, which is more commonly iatrogenic (such as from bone marrow suppressive treatments for cancer or organ transplant) than genetic. Pneumonia is a major concern in such neutropenic patients, and efforts to reverse neutropenia with granulocyte-colony stimulating factor can diminish pneumonia incidence during myeloablative treatments.[37] Other drugs that suppress components of inflammation less profoundly than neutropenia, such as corticosteroids or biologics that inhibit tumor necrosis factor (TNF) or interleukin (IL)-1 signaling, also increase the risk of infections including pneumonia.

Inflammatory dysregulations may play causative roles in many of the risk factors recognized to associate with pneumonia. Multiple risk factors

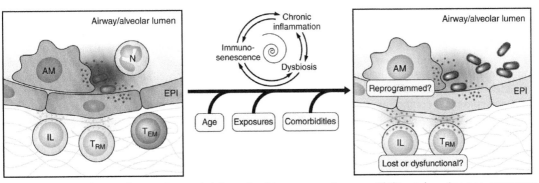

Fig. 2. Changes in lung inflammation and defense lead to pneumonia susceptibility. Advancing age, exposures (such as cigarette smoke, air pollution, alcohol, resolving viral infection, and sepsis), and comorbidities (diseases or conditions such as neutropenia, obesity, diabetes, chronic respiratory disease) all increase pneumonia risk. Many of these factors involve chronic or acute inflammatory dysregulation, which drives susceptibility. Furthermore, chronic low-level systemic inflammation exists in a feed-forward loop with immunosenescence and dysbiosis to perpetuate a vicious cycle of decline in pulmonary defense. The specific cellular, molecular, or other changes that are caused by these risk factors and physiologic changes and then increase pneumonia susceptibility are mostly speculative at present but may involve loss of training and reprogramming of AM or EPI, as well as loss or dysfunction among lung immune cells such as IL and T_{RM}.

for pneumonia have effects on the inflammatory pathways that defend the lungs against infection.[4] Exposures (see **Fig. 2**) that associate with pneumonia, such as cigarette smoking, air pollution, and alcohol abuse, have deleterious effects on neutrophils, macrophages, cytokine signaling, and other components of inflammation.[4] Similarly, many of the comorbidities (see **Fig. 2**) that associate with pneumonia, such as advanced age, chronic diseases (of respiratory, cardiovascular, renal, hepatic, or other systems), diabetes, and obesity, include impairments in inflammatory cells and mediators.[4] It is likely that some of these inflammatory dysfunctions are responsible for increasing pneumonia susceptibility, implying that reversing such inflammatory alterations could help sever the link between pneumonia and its risk factors. However, most of these associations remain correlative at present.

Local alterations in pulmonary inflammation can have adverse consequences on lung defense. A prominent example of this is secondary bacterial pneumonia (eg, caused by pneumococcus) after a preceding respiratory virus infection (such as influenza). Many mechanisms contribute to this acute pneumonia susceptibility, most of which include dysregulations of inflammation.[4] For example, viral infections cause a local surge in interferon activity, and abundant type I or type II interferons can inhibit subsequent elicitation of neutrophil recruitment and macrophage antimicrobial activities.[38,39] Stimulating inflammation using polyinosinic-polycytidylic acid molecules to mimic viral double-stranded RNA without causing any infection is sufficient to render lungs susceptible to bacterial pneumonia, dependent on the same interferon pathways that were responsible in influenza infections.[40] Thus, inflammatory responses to a respiratory viral infection are a clear example of an exposure that renders lungs more susceptible to bacterial pneumonia (see **Fig. 2**).

Inflammatory responses outside the lung are also important. Excessive and/or prolonged systemic inflammation compromises lung defense. This finding applies to acute hyperstimulation of systemic inflammation, such as with extrapulmonary sepsis, which increases pneumonia risk in human patients and decreases lung defense in animal experiments.[41] Triggering systemic inflammation in the absence of infection, such as via intravenous injection of endotoxin or cytokines, is sufficient to compromise local defenses in the lung. Thus, extrapulmonary inflammation is an exposure that can be detrimental and predispose to pneumonia (see **Fig. 2**).

This general principle may apply more broadly to chronic smoldering levels of systemic inflammation. Many of the diseases and conditions that are risk factors for pneumonia associate with chronic systemic inflammation, including aging, obesity, diabetes, and cardiovascular disease. Patients with the recognized pneumonia risk factors tend to have higher circulating levels of inflammatory markers than those without, and those with more advanced stages of the disease or condition tend to have yet higher levels.[42] After accounting for confounding factors such as age and comorbidities, those patients with higher concentrations of inflammatory markers such as TNF, IL-6, and C-reactive protein in their blood are more likely to develop pneumonia in ensuing years.[43] Because systemic inflammation is sufficient to compromise lung defense, associates with diverse acute and chronic conditions that predispose to pneumonia, and associates independently with the risk of pneumonia, it may contribute to the increased pneumonia risk caused by comorbidities. Systemic chronic inflammation may be a common mechanism linking diverse risk factors to pneumonia (see **Fig. 2**).

In addition to chronic inflammation, the elderly and others with increased pneumonia susceptibility have changes in their microbiota (dysbiosis) and immune activities (immunosenescence), which may contribute to inflammatory dysfunction and impaired pulmonary defense.[4,44,45] Because chronic inflammation, immunosenescence, and dysbiosis all can influence each other,[45] these factors can form a vicious cycle leading to a downward spiral of ever-worsening lung defense (see **Fig. 2**).

If systemic inflammation predisposes to pneumonia, then diminishing systemic inflammation might decrease pneumonia risk. Blunting chronic inflammation is a goal for arthritis, inflammatory bowel disease, cardiovascular disease, and other chronic inflammatory diseases. Diminishing inflammation can slow the progression of these diseases. However, because strategies for limiting chronic inflammation (eg, TNF or IL-1 inhibitors) often compromise pathways essential to inflammatory antimicrobial defense, such agents instead pose an increased risk for serious infections, including pneumonia. Preventing pneumonia susceptibility by targeting inflammation in persons at risk may require selectively targeting mechanisms underlying the chronic systemic inflammatory processes but not themselves essential to acute pulmonary inflammation and lung antimicrobial defense.

SUMMARY

The biological mechanisms responsible for making some individuals more susceptible to pneumonia need to be better defined. This specific recommendation was forwarded by a group of investigators convened by the United States National Heart, Lung, and Blood Institute to discuss priority areas for pneumonia research.[46] Variations in the inflammatory response are a major component of interindividual variability in pneumonia risk. However, which specific changes in inflammatory processes in any given individual substantially affect that individual's pneumonia susceptibility demands greater attention from the biomedical research community. The kinetics, quantity, and quality of inflammation help determine whether and when a given microbe in the lung results in pneumonia.

REFERENCES

1. Jain S, Self WH, Wunderink RG, et al. Community-acquired pneumonia requiring hospitalization among U.S. adults. N Engl J Med 2015;373(5):415–27.

2. Jain S, Williams DJ, Arnold SR, et al. Community-acquired pneumonia requiring hospitalization among U.S. children. N Engl J Med 2015;372(9):835–45.

3. Anand N, Kollef MH. The alphabet soup of pneumonia: CAP, HAP, HCAP, NHAP, and VAP. Semin Respir Crit Care Med 2009;30(1):3–9.

4. Quinton LJ, Walkey AJ, Mizgerd JP. Integrative physiology of pneumonia. Physiol Rev 2018;98(3):1417–64

5. Feldman C, Anderson R. Epidemiology, virulence factors and management of the pneumococcus. F1000Res 2016;5:2320.

6. Moore ML, Stokes KL, Hartert TV. The impact of viral genotype on pathogenesis and disease severity: respiratory syncytial virus and human rhinoviruses. Curr Opin Immunol 2013;25(6):761–8.

7. Palavecino CE, Cespedes PF, Lay MK, et al. Understanding lung immunopathology caused by the human metapneumovirus: implications for rational vaccine design. Crit Rev Immunol 2015;35(3):185–202.

8. Parker D, Ahn D, Cohen T, et al. Innate immune signaling activated by MDR bacteria in the airway. Physiol Rev 2016;96(1):19–53.

9. Schrauwen EJ, de Graaf M, Herfst S, et al. Determinants of virulence of influenza A virus. Eur J Clin Microbiol Infect Dis 2014;33(4):479–90.

10. Coleman FT, Blahna MT, Kamata H, et al. Capacity of pneumococci to activate macrophage nuclear factor κB: influence on necroptosis and pneumonia severity. J Infect Dis 2017;216(4):425–35.

11. Ghosh S, Hayden MS. Celebrating 25 years of NF-κB research. Immunol Rev 2012;246(1):5–13.

12. Hakansson AP, Bergenfelz C. Low NF-κB activation and necroptosis in alveolar macrophages: a new virulence property of Streptococcus pneumoniae. J Infect Dis 2017;216(4):402–4.

13. Dickson RP, Erb-Downward JR, Martinez FJ, et al. The microbiome and the respiratory tract. Annu Rev Physiol 2016;78:481–504.

14. Kaufmann SHE, Dorhoi A. Molecular determinants in phagocyte-bacteria interactions. Immunity 2016;44(3):476–91.

15. Westphalen K, Gusarova GA, Islam MN, et al. Sessile alveolar macrophages communicate with alveolar epithelium to modulate immunity. Nature 2014;506(7489):503–6.

16. Peteranderl C, Morales-Nebreda L, Selvakumar B, et al. Macrophage-epithelial paracrine crosstalk inhibits lung edema clearance during influenza infection. J Clin Invest 2016;126(4):1566–80.

17. Basil MC, Levy BD. Specialized pro-resolving mediators: endogenous regulators of infection and inflammation. Nat Rev Immunol 2016;16(1):51–67.

18. Braciale TJ, Sun J, Kim TS. Regulating the adaptive immune response to respiratory virus infection. Nat Rev Immunol 2012;12(4):295–305.

19. D'Alessio FR, Tsushima K, Aggarwal NR, et al. CD4+CD25+Foxp3+ Tregs resolve experimental lung injury in mice and are present in humans with acute lung injury. J Clin Invest 2009;119(10):2898–913.

20. Poe SL, Arora M, Oriss TB, et al. STAT1-regulated lung MDSC-like cells produce IL-10 and efferocytose apoptotic neutrophils with relevance in resolution of bacterial pneumonia. Mucosal Immunol 2013;6(1):189–99.

21. Alcamo EA, Mizgerd JP, Horwitz BH, et al. Targeted mutation of tumor necrosis factor 1 rescues the RelA-deficient mouse and reveals a critical role for NF-κB in leukocyte recruitment. J Immunol 2001;167:1592–600.

22. Pittet JF, Mackersie RC, Martin TR, et al. Biological markers of acute lung injury: prognostic and pathogenetic significance. Am J Respir Crit Care Med 1997;155(4):1187–205.

23. Yamamoto K, Ahyi AN, Pepper-Cunningham ZA, et al. Roles of lung epithelium in neutrophil recruitment during pneumococcal pneumonia. Am J Respir Cell Mol Biol 2014;50(2):253–62.

24. Billiau A, Matthys P. Interferon-gamma: a historical perspective. Cytokine Growth Factor Rev 2009;20(2):97–113.

25. Boxx GM, Cheng G. The roles of type I interferon in bacterial infection. Cell Host Microbe 2016;19(6):760–9.

26. Lazear HM, Nice TJ, Diamond MS. Interferon-λ: immune functions at barrier surfaces and beyond. Immunity 2015;43(1):15–28.

27. Hatesuer B, Hoang HT, Riese P, et al. Deletion of Irf3 and Irf7 genes in mice results in altered interferon pathway activation and granulocyte-dominated

inflammatory responses to influenza A infection. J Innate Immun 2017;9(2):145–61.

28. Majoros A, Platanitis E, Szappanos D, et al. Response to interferons and antibacterial innate immunity in the absence of tyrosine-phosphorylated STAT1. EMBO Rep 2016;17(3):367–82.

29. Donadieu J, Beaupain B, Fenneteau O, et al. Congenital neutropenia in the era of genomics: classification, diagnosis, and natural history. Br J Haematol 2017;179(4):557–74.

30. Casanova JL. Severe infectious diseases of childhood as monogenic inborn errors of immunity. Proc Natl Acad Sci U S A 2015;112(51):E7128–37.

31. Marciano BE, Spalding C, Fitzgerald A, et al. Common severe infections in chronic granulomatous disease. Clin Infect Dis 2015;60(8):1176–83.

32. Ciancanelli MJ, Huang SX, Luthra P, et al. Infectious disease. Life-threatening influenza and impaired interferon amplification in human IRF7 deficiency. Science 2015;348(6233):448–53.

33. Patarcic I, Gelemanovic A, Kirin M, et al. The role of host genetic factors in respiratory tract infectious diseases: systematic review, meta-analyses and field synopsis. Sci Rep 2015;5:16119.

34. Smith NMS, Wasserman GA, Coleman FT, et al. Regionally compartmentalized resident memory T cells mediate naturally acquired protection against pneumococcal pneumonia. Mucosal Immunol 2017;11(1):220–35.

35. Strutt TM, McKinstry KK, Dibble JP, et al. Memory CD4+ T cells induce innate responses independently of pathogen. Nat Med 2010;16(5):558–64, 1p following 564.

36. Netea MG, Joosten LA, Latz E, et al. Trained immunity: a program of innate immune memory in health and disease. Science 2016;352(6284):aaf1098.

37. Mehta HM, Malandra M, Corey SJ. G-CSF and GM-CSF in neutropenia. J Immunol 2015;195(4):1341–9.

38. Shahangian A, Chow EK, Tian X, et al. Type I IFNs mediate development of postinfluenza bacterial pneumonia in mice. J Clin Invest 2009;119(7):1910–20.

39. Sun K, Metzger DW. Inhibition of pulmonary antibacterial defense by interferon-gamma during recovery from influenza infection. Nat Med 2008;14(5):558–64.

40. Tian X, Xu F, Lung WY, et al. Poly I:C enhances susceptibility to secondary pulmonary infections by gram-positive bacteria. PLoS One 2012;7(9):e41879.

41. Delano MJ, Ward PA. The immune system's role in sepsis progression, resolution, and long-term outcome. Immunol Rev 2016;274(1):330–53.

42. Bektas A, Schurman SH, Sen R, et al. Aging, inflammation and the environment. Exp Gerontol 2018;105:10–8.

43. Yende S, Tuomanen EI, Wunderink R, et al. Preinfection systemic inflammatory markers and risk of hospitalization due to pneumonia. Am J Respir Crit Care Med 2005;172(11):1440–6.

44. Nikolich-Zugich J. The twilight of immunity: emerging concepts in aging of the immune system. Nat Immunol 2018;19(1):10–9.

45. Thevaranjan N, Puchta A, Schulz C, et al. Age-associated microbial dysbiosis promotes intestinal permeability, systemic inflammation, and macrophage dysfunction. Cell Host Microbe 2017;21(4):455–66.e4.

46. Dela Cruz CS, Wunderink RG, Christiani DC, et al. Future research directions in pneumonia: NHLBI working group report. Am J Respir Crit Care Med 2018;198(2):256–63.

The Lung Microbiome and Its Role in Pneumonia

Benjamin G. Wu, MD, MSc, Leopoldo N. Segal, MD, MSc*

KEYWORDS

• Lung • Microbiome • Antibiotics • Immune responses • Inflammation • Bacterial taxa

KEY POINTS

- A significant research gap exists in the study of the lung microbiome and pneumonia.
- Complex microbial communities exist in the upper and lower airway.
- Microbe-host and microbe-microbe interactions blur the line between pathogen and commensal.
- The use of next-generation sequencing with reference microorganism databases allows for an unbiased approach to identifying large communities of microbes and potential pathogens.
- The microbial community of the lung may play an important role in pneumonia impacting susceptibility and the natural history of disease.

Until recently, the purpose of studying microbes in pneumonia was the identification of an organism that could assume the role of "pathogen" in disease. Common findings, using culture techniques designed to isolate these possible pathogens, often identify these microbes as "confounders." An example is the frequent identification of oral flora in lower airway samples from clinical cultures obtained in patients with pneumonia.[1] This finding is frequently disregarded as contamination. However, with recent advances in sequencing techniques, new insights on the role of these oral flora are being discovered. Indeed, the lower airways of healthy individuals are not sterile but rather frequently visited by varying degrees of these microbes, predominantly from sources in the upper airways (**Fig. 1**).

Exposure of the lower airways to microbes commonly occurs among healthy individuals, such as microaspiration of oral secretions containing high concentrations of microbes or inhalation of airborne microbes (low biomass but constant exposure). In many airway diseases, epidemiologic evidence suggests that some of these events occur more often in illness than in health. Examples include the association between gastroesophageal reflux disease (GERD) and microaspiration with chronic obstructive pulmonary disease (COPD), bronchiectasis, asthma, and cystic fibrosis.[2–4] With the use of culture-independent approaches to study the lower airway microbiota (the collection of microbes present in the lower airways), new insights have been gained about the complex microbial community that exists in the pulmonary environment. In this review, the authors highlight the existing evidence that supports a potentially critical role for the lower airway microbiota in patients with pneumonia as well as in chronic respiratory diseases with an increased prevalence of pneumonia.

Sources of Support: This work was supported by K23 AI102970 (L.N. Segal) Flight Attendant Medical Research Institute Young Clinical Scientist Award (B.G. Wu), Stony Wold-Herbert Fund Fellowship (B.G. Wu), T32 CA193111 (B.G. Wu), and UL1TR001445 (B.G. Wu).
Financial Disclosure: None.
Division of Pulmonary, Critical Care, and Sleep Medicine, Department of Medicine, NYU Human Microbiome Program, New York University School of Medicine, New York, NY 10028, USA
* Corresponding author. New York University School of Medicine, 462 First Avenue 7W54, New York, NY 10016.
E-mail address: Leopoldo.Segal@nyumc.org

Clin Chest Med 39 (2018) 677–689
https://doi.org/10.1016/j.ccm.2018.07.003

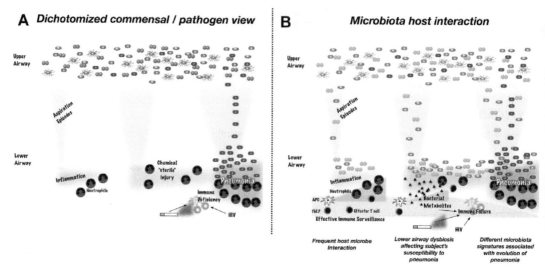

Fig. 1. Schema of the change in pathophysiologic view of pneumonia in the era of culture-independent approaches used to study microbial communities. (*A*) Previous conceptualization of pneumonia stratified microbes into commensals (*gray bacteria*) and pathogens (*red bacteria*). Identification of a commensal in the lower airways was deemed a contaminant. Aspiration episodes were recognized as cause of lower airway injury thought to be "sterile" chemical noxious stimuli. Aspiration of "pathogens" was the key event leading to the development of pneumonia. (*B*) A more complex view of microbes in the upper airways where multiple different types of bacteria coexist. Aspiration events bring microbes to the lower airways that may be cleared by the host immune response or may persist leading to lower airway dysbiosis (bacterial seeding). Effector T cells, Th17 cells, and antigen-presenting cells (APC) will be determinants of the effectiveness of the immune surveillance. These host immune cells are likely affected by frequent interactions with microbes. Some of the bacterial products have significant effects on the inflammatory tone, such as SCFAs. The dynamics of the aspiration events, lower airway microbiota, and lower airway immune tone will be determinants of the conditions that may favor the development of pneumonia.

WHY SHOULD CULTURE-INDEPENDENT TECHNIQUES BE CONSIDERED IN THE SETTING OF PNEUMONIA?

The paradigmatic view of microorganisms in pneumonia focuses on microbes preassigned to a pathogenic role. Typical pathogens associated with pneumonia include *Streptococcus pneumoniae*, *Staphylococcus aureus*, *Klebsiella pneumoniae*, and *Hemophilus influenzae*, whereas atypical microbes include *Chlamydophila psittaci*, *Mycoplasma pneumoniae*, and *Legionella pneumophilia* (see **Fig. 1**A). However, culture-based methods identify positive cultures in approximately half of patients with community-acquired pneumonia (CAP).[5,6] Rates of identification of microorganisms in hospital-associated pneumonia (HAP) and Ventilator-associated pneumonia (VAP) can also vary greatly.[7–11] A major limitation of pathogen identification is related to difficulties growing microorganisms using culture-dependent techniques, such as *Legionella* and *Mycobacterium* that require specialized media and conditions.[12,13] In addition, misidentification of pathogens may have significant effects on treatment, such as the selection of inappropriate antibiotics,[14–17] leading to increased morbidity and mortality.[12,18,19]

Moreover, subjects with culture-negative pneumonia may represent a different group of patients than those with positive culture pneumonia. In a study of patients with culture-negative pneumonia, subjects had lower mortality and less severity of illness than their culture-positive counterparts.[8] These findings suggest that culture-negative pneumonia may be a "milder" form of local and systemic injury. Another example of commonly considered culture-negative lung injury is aspiration pneumonitis. In subjects who suffer aspiration, the dogma has been that the nature of the lung injury present in this condition is related to "sterile" chemical injury (see **Fig. 1**A), despite the large number of bacteria present in the upper airways and the upper gastrointestinal tract. Thus, therapeutic recommendations do not include the use of antibiotics except for (a) presence of poor dentition, (b) alcohol use, and (c) evidence of abscess on chest imaging. Most microbes responsible for pneumonia come from the upper airway. Thus, periodic exposure of the lower airways to upper airway microorganisms represents an important seeding mechanism that may influence microbial selection in the lower airways. As an example of this selection pressure,

S pneumoniae, a minor component of both the upper and the lower airway microbiomes, causes more than half of all cases of CAP (see **Fig. 1**A).

Among the cases of pneumonia with a pathogen identified by culture, institution of accurate antimicrobial therapy results in favorable clinical outcomes.[18] Data from these cultures have shown frequent isolation of oral microorganisms in samples from the lower airways.[1,20–23] However, the techniques used to sample the lower airways require passage through the upper airways, and sterile surgical lung biopsies are often not feasible. Thus, contamination of samples with oral flora is commonly blamed for these results.[24–26] Other factors that limit the use of culture-based techniques include (a) the time required to grow organisms; (b) low bacterial burden in the lungs; (c) difficulties growing fastidious bacteria; and (d) the inability to describe complex microbial communities.[27–29]

New culture-independent techniques may hold the advantage of earlier identification without the need to grow microbes.[30,31] Some of these techniques are not new, and targeted culture-independent techniques have been used to identify specific microbes suspected of having a pathogenic role in the lung. Examples of this include (a) the screening for *Streptococcus* antigens in oral swabs, (b) the search for Legionella antibodies in serum, and (c) the identification of DNA from mycobacteria using polymerase chain reaction.[32–34] These techniques are based on approaches biased toward a suspected agent and aim to provide an expedited diagnosis of a possible pathogenic microbe.

Newer sequencing technology takes advantage of the ability to identify multiple microbial products in a high-throughput approach and to process large amounts of data. These bioinformatic tools allow for the identification of microbes using an "unbiased" approach. For example, a technique widely used in research is the amplification and sequencing of the 16S ribosomal RNA (rRNA) gene.[35] The 16S rRNA gene, a constituent gene of the bacteria domain, contains genomic signatures (defined by hypervariable regions) and allows for specific taxonomic identification and description of complex mixtures of microbes. In addition, it provides semi-quantitative data about each microbe present in the sample expressed as relative abundance. The presence of microbial DNA of an organism with a potential pathogenic role, especially if present in high relative abundance, can be seen as supporting a causative role in the correct clinical context.[30] Culture-independent methods, including next-generation sequencing coupled with microbial reference databases, represent a powerful new technology that may have significant clinical impact on the identification of microbes in pneumonia.

The use of high throughput approaches provides a view of the intricate landscape of microbes present in the lower airways without an a priori bias toward specific pathogen identification. Our new view is changing the understanding of the complex mixture of microbes in the lower airways and poses new scientific dilemmas to consider for the pathogenesis of pneumonia: (a) How does a microbe become a pathogen? (b) What are the main sources of microbes in the lower airways? (c) How does host and microbe interaction affect the immunologic tone of the lower airways? (d) How does upper and lower airway dysbiosis increase susceptibility to pneumonia? and (e) How do distinct microbiota signatures in pneumonia affect the natural history of this disease?

HOW DOES A MICROBE BECOME A PATHOGEN IN THE NEW ERA OF THE LUNG MICROBIOME?

Classifying microbes as commensals or pathogens has been the foundation of a dichotomized view of infection (see **Fig. 1**A). In recent years, an evolution from this view occurred suggesting that pathogenicity and commensalism may fall across a spectrum based on host-microbial interactions. Several tenets describe the pathogenic role of microbes: (1) pathogenesis is the result of both host and microbe; (2) the pathologic or clinical outcome is determined by the damage to the host; and (3) this damage can result from the host immune response and/or the effects of virulence factors from the microbe.[36,37] Therefore, microorganisms frequently considered commensals can have a major role in the pathogenesis of pneumonia. For example, *Staphylococcus epidermidis* is a common inhabitant of the upper airways, but can cause disease under certain conditions.[37,38] Complex interactions between microorganisms and the host are determined by multiple factors, likely noncanonical, that will define the pathogenic role, a clear evolution from the classical Koch's postulates.[39]

The current understanding of the lung microbiome has contributed to the complexity of the host-microbe interactions, introducing another factor in the debate: what is the role of the complex microbial community that exists in the lower airway? Many studies of the lung microbiota now show that multiple species of oral commensals in the lower airways can be frequently found, and the implications for the host may further obscure the distinction between pathogens and commensals.[40] The presence of these bacteria frequently regarded as commensals from the oral cavity in the lower airways impacts how other cooccurring microbes respond to the environment and host.[41] In the schematic in **Fig. 1**B, the complex community of microbes in the lower airway may increase or hinder a microorganism's ability to cause infection. Microorganisms that regularly inhabit certain mucosae (eg, oral) may contribute to the pathogenic process by inducing inflammation when found in other sites (eg, lung mucosa).

The presence of oral commensals in the lung microbiome allows one to ask: what is the role of these microorganisms in the lower airways? Do these microbes affect other microbes, especially those classically identified as the responsible pathogen? **Fig. 1**B depicts a more complex cross-pollination of microbes between the upper and lower airway leading to dysbiosis of the lower airway microbiota and affecting not only microbial-host interaction but also *microbe-microbe interaction*, both of which may contribute to the pathogenic process. It is reasonable to postulate that in the healthy lower airway microbiota some microbes outcompete others with greater pathogenic potential. Microbial strategies may include sequestering vital nutrients and by-products necessary for growth and promoting the host immune defense to enhance recognition and killing of pathogens. Alternatively, some of these host immune mechanisms may be impaired due to lower airway dysbiosis, increasing an individual's susceptibility to pneumonia.

WHAT ARE THE SOURCES OF MICROBES TO THE LOWER AIRWAYS?

Culture data in subjects with acute lung infections and chronic airway inflammatory conditions, such as COPD and cystic fibrosis, have shown that the upper airway is the most common contributor of microbes to the lower airways.[42–45] Culture-independent data also suggest that "microaspiration" is frequently observed in normal subjects, leading to episodic seeding of oral microbes into the lower airways,[2,3,46] and with a higher prevalence in several lung diseases, including COPD, asthma, obstructive sleep apnea, cystic fibrosis, and lung infections.[3,4,47–50] Microaspiration occurs more frequently while sleeping due to reduced coordination of breathing with swallowing and GERD.[2–4,47]

Several chronic pulmonary diseases are characterized by impairment of airway clearance, such as in COPD and cystic fibrosis, which likely favors the seeding of microaspirated organisms.[51,52] Environmental exposures, frequent antibiotic and/or anti-inflammatory use, or diet may also contribute

to the selection pressure on the lower airway microbiome.[53] The current understanding of the dynamics that determine the lung microbiota is best explained by an adapted island model and complex adaptive lung ecosystem, processes present in both health and disease.[40] It is now known that when the airway microbiota is characterized topographically, the greatest similarity with the upper airway microbiota occurs in areas with the greatest potential for deposition of microaspiration (eg, carina and main stem bronchi and alveolar spaces), evidence that supports that the main route of enrichment for the lower airways remains microaspiration of oropharyngeal secretions.[40] The rate of elimination of the aspirated microorganisms will depend on the environment present in the lower airways (eg, protein and nutrients available, pH, oxygen tension, biofilms) and active immune clearance.

THE ROLE OF HOST-MICROBE INTERACTION IN THE MUCOSAL IMMUNOLOGIC TONE

Humans evolved to coexist with microorganisms. Since the discovery of single-celled organisms by Antoni van Leeuwenhoek, multiple mucosae within the human body were found to be colonized with microorganisms. However, the lungs were thought to be sterile despite being in direct communication with other mucosae with very high bacterial burden.[54] In the past 10 years, with the utilization of culture-independent techniques, a complex community of microorganisms has been identified on multiple mucosal surfaces that coexist in the body.[55] Indeed, the sum of these microbes that inhabit our bodies can be considered a subject-specific superorganism that carries genetic information more diverse than our own human DNA.[55–58]

In mucosal surfaces other than the lungs, examples of the coevolution of microbes and host include the intricate functions performed by microbes that are needed for immune modulation[59,60] and immune maturation and host homeostasis.[61–65] It is now known that there are microbes in the lower airways of humans[40] and experimental models,[66] challenging the anachronistic dogma that the lower airways are sterile. 16S rRNA gene sequencing techniques revealed complex microbial communities in the lower airways associated with distinct host immune tone. The distinct immunologic homeostasis of the lung mucosa may be from either viable and metabolically active bacteria or from exposure to bacterial by-products.[67]

Multiple studies demonstrated that the bronchoalveolar lavage (BAL) and lung tissue of healthy subjects and smokers frequently contain an enrichment with bacteria commonly considered oral commensals.[40,67–69] The enrichment of the lower airway microbiota with oral commensals, such as *Prevotella*, *Streptococcus*, *Fusobacterium*, *Rothia*, and *Veillonella*, is associated with subclinical inflammation.[40,67] The inflammatory signal is characterized by an increase in neutrophils and lymphocytes. Further endotyping of the lower airway inflammatory tone supports that exposure to these microbes is associated with a Th17 phenotype, characterized by increase in $CD4^+$ $IL-17^+$ lymphocytes, increased STAT3 expression, Fractalkine, and $IL-1\alpha$.[67,69] Again, it is unclear if the inflammatory signal is due to viable and metabolically active bacteria, dead bacteria, or by-products of bacterial metabolism.[67]

It is also likely that microorganisms shape the immune system as much as the immune system shapes the microbiome. Studies done in large European cohorts show that the exposure to diverse microbes during childhood, such as growing up on a farm, is protective against asthma and allergies.[70–72] House dust mite exposure from households with large canines attenuates Th2 cytokine production, decreases activated T cells, and leads to an enrichment with *Lactobacillus johnsonii* in the nasal microbiome.[73] This observation is coincident with gut microbiota data whereby early exposure to bacteria is needed for immune maturation in early life.[65,74] These data is supportive of what's commonly referred to as the "hygiene hypothesis," under which restricted microbial exposure in early life may lead to inadequate "priming" of the immune system during maturation, resulting in Th1/Th2 cell subset imbalances,[75] Treg cell deficiency,[76] and innate immune abnormalities.[77]

Changes in diet, improved sanitary conditions, and use of antibiotics may limit the exposure to environmental microbes and be responsible for the increase in autoimmune diseases observed in recent decades.[70,78–83] In childhood asthma, 2 observations about the microbial exposure in early life highlight the importance of the microbiome in the development of the immune system. First, childhood exposure to a diverse microbial environment, by either farm habitation or pet exposure, is protective and reduces the risk of asthma.[70,84] Second, the acquisition of airway microbiota enrichment with pathogenic microorganisms (eg, *S pneumoniae*, *Moraxella catarrhalis*, *H influenzae*) in infancy increases susceptibility to asthma.[85] More recently, nasal carriage with *Streptococcus* was found to be a strong asthma predictor.[33] Importantly, although the proinflammatory role pathogenic bacteria such as *S pneumoniae*, *M catarrhalis*, and *H influenzae* are well defined,

less is known about "healthy" microbial exposure responsible for an anti-inflammatory role suggested by the "hygiene hypothesis." In mouse models, nasal inhalation of an innocuous strain of *Escherichia coli* leads to reprogramming dendritic cells and macrophages in the lungs and results in protection against allergic responses.[86] This model suggests that direct exposure of the airways to certain bacteria is sufficient to elicit a protective effect.

In addition, gastrointestinal microbiota trigger immunologic cross-talk between the gut and lung.[73] For example, children colonized in the stomach with *Helicobacter pylori* are 40% to 60% less likely to develop asthma than children who are not carriers.[87,88] Lessons from animal models show that disruption of the gastrointestinal microbiota may lead to abnormal immune responses that affect the airway mucosa.[89–93] Ultimately, both the gut and the lung mucosa may function as a single aerodigestive immune system and share the physiologic role of immune surveillance that shapes the host immune tone locally and systemically.

HOW DOES UPPER AND LOWER AIRWAY DYSBIOSIS INCREASE SUSCEPTIBILITY TO PNEUMONIA?

The upper airways are a microbial reservoir and the main source of microbes to the lower airways. It is not unexpected that the composition of the upper airway microbiota has direct effects on an individual's risks for pneumonia. Recent data using culture-independent approaches suggest that reduction in nasal microbiome diversity and domination by *Rothia*, *Lactobacillus*, and *Streptococcus* increased the risk of pneumonia.[94] Among neonates, nasal colonization with *S pneumoniae*, *H influenzae*, *M catarrhalis*, and *S aureus* occurs frequently.[95] Importantly, enrichment of the nasal microbiota with *Moraxella*, *Streptococcus*, and *Haemophilus* was associated with an increase of acute respiratory infections.[33]

The composition of the lower airway microbiota may also affect a subject's susceptibility to pneumonia. The lung microbiome of advanced human immunodeficiency virus (HIV) subjects shows dysbiosis with increasing *Prevotella* and *Veillonella* that persists for years despite treatment.[96] These treatment-naive participants also have decreased diversity and greater intersample diversity than those subjects uninfected by HIV. Thus, this dysbiotic signature may be associated with increased pneumonia susceptibility seen in HIV patients.[97]

The lower airway microbiota may also affect a subject's susceptibility to pneumonia through immunologic regulation mediated by bacterially derived metabolites. For example, short chain fatty acids (SCFAs), an end-product of bacterial anaerobic metabolism, is associated with an increase of an individual's susceptibility to tuberculosis in an HIV cohort.[98] One possible mechanism is that SCFAs, such as butyrate, have direct inhibitory effects on T-cell function by suppressing INF-γ and IL-17 production.[98]

In cystic fibrosis and COPD, a decrease in α diversity (a measure of within sample diversity or how many different types of taxa are in a sample) of the lower airway microbiota is associated the severity of disease.[45] Considering that advanced-stage cystic fibrosis and COPD are associated with increased risk of developing pneumonia and that the prognosis of pneumonia is worse in these conditions than in healthier population,[99,100] it is possible that changes to the lung microbiota may impact the natural course of pneumonia in these diseases.[101,102] It is also possible that the associated changes to the lung microbiome may assist to evaluate the prognosis in these patients. Those patients who have a lower α diversity may have worse outcomes and an accelerated declination in their disease.

The changes to the upper or lower airway microbiome may modulate the immune response, increasing host susceptibility to the development of pneumonia (see **Fig. 1**B). For example, the presence of anaerobic taxa in the nasal microbiome was correlated with increased nasal IgA against the influenza virus in the nasal microbiome after inoculation with live-attenuated influenza vaccine. *Prevotella melaninogenica* positively correlated with increased influenza-specific IgA antibodies.[103] In a cohort of asthmatic subjects with clinically stable but suboptimally controlled asthma, bronchial hyperresponsiveness was associated with increased bacterial burden and microbial diversity in airway brush samples. Perturbations of the commensal microbial community may influence the clinical phenotype in asthma and highlight the potential "pathogenic" role of commensal bacteria possibly resulting in increased risk for lower airway infections.

In advanced COPD, increased bacterial colonization and recurrent infections are associated with increased risk of exacerbations and accelerated loss of lung function.[104] In moderate to advanced COPD, there is reduced bacterial diversity as compared with healthy or mild COPD.[105] Exacerbations often occur after infection with a new bacterial strain or change in bacterial load,[106] and dysbiosis of the microbiome has been associated with increased inflammation.[107] In severe COPD exacerbations requiring mechanical ventilation, there is a diverse bacterial community suggesting a polymicrobial cause.[108] These data highlight the potential for ecological interaction of different bacterial strains during exacerbations. The core of this bacterial community may be composed of previously unrecognized lung pathogens such as oropharyngeal bacterial species that are part of the lung microbiome during health, but in periods of dysbiosis with microbe-microbe interaction may result in increased frequency of COPD exacerbations and risk of pneumonia (see **Fig. 1**B).

In cystic fibrosis, reduction in bacterial diversity is associated with disease progression and colonization with pathogens.[45] Low microbiota diversity also precedes the development of cystic fibrosis exacerbations.[42] It is likely that dynamic changes of airway microbiota occur over time, where a change from a "healthy" well-balanced polymicrobial microbiome to an "unhealthy" restricted, less-diverse airway microbiota renders the airway susceptible to a dominant pathogen (eg, *Pseudomonas* or *Burkholderia*) and consequent lung injury.

The risk for developing HAP increases with the recent use of antibiotics.[109] Differences in exposures, environments, fomites, colonization, host factors, host-microbe interactions, and hospital antibiotic nomograms influence patients' susceptibility to pneumonia.[109] It is plausible that some of the increased risk is due to the selection pressure by antibiotics, leading to upper/lower airway dysbiosis once a subject is admitted to a hospital and increases the chance for a "pathogen" to bloom. These selection pressures may affect healthy microbes in the upper and lower airways, interrupt immune surveillance, and encourage development of a lower airway microenvironment supportive for pathogens (see **Fig. 1**B).

Host immune characteristics are obviously determinants of the selection pressure to the microbiota. In subjects with immunodeficiency due to HIV and no lung disease, the lung microbiome is enriched with *Tropheryma whipplei* as compared with controls.[110] The increased relative abundance of this taxon in the lung, as compared with paired upper airway samples, suggests that the lung may constitute a true niche of *T whipplei*. In addition, antiretroviral medication leads to changes in the lung microbiome with enrichment with *Prevotella* and *Veillonella*.[96] The persistence of the dysbiosis despite the use of anti-retroviral medications may be responsible for the increased susceptibility to inflammatory lung diseases as well as to pneumonia among HIV subjects fully reconstituted with normal CD4 counts.

Although this article focuses on changes observed in either the upper or lower airway microbiota that might be linked to increased risk for pneumonia, there are data suggesting that the microbiota of distant mucosal sites may impact pneumonia. For example, in allogenic hematopoietic cell transplantation patients, changes in gut microbiota are associated with pulmonary complications.[111] Pulmonary complications, defined in that study as abnormal parenchymal findings on chest imaging with respiratory symptoms, were found in most participants. The use of antibiotics, low baseline gut microbiome diversity, and gammaproteobacteria enrichment in the gut microbiome predicted pulmonary complications.[111] It is possible that changes in gut microbiota may affect systemic immune tone. Moreover, the epithelial barrier in these subjects is frequently disrupted due to intensive immunosuppressive treatment allowing for bacterial translocation to the lung. Future investigations must consider evaluating interactions between different mucosae by carefully sampling the involved mucosae and the systemic compartments.

Even less is known about the roles of viruses or fungi on the susceptibility to pneumonia. Nonbacterial microbes are mostly neglected from current lung microbiome studies due to technical difficulties but should receive further attention. Viruses play a major role in chronic inflammatory diseases of the lung, such as asthma, COPD, and cystic fibrosis. However, few studies have evaluated the airway virome.[112,113] Infection with rhinovirus in COPD patients has been shown to be associated with increased bacterial load and change in microbiota composition.[114] Rhinovirus infection leads to a change in the relative abundances of many pathogenic and nonpathogenic bacteria with an increase in Hemophilus and Neisseriaceae species at day 15. These data support that interkingdom interactions (in this case, viruses with bacteria) may affect subjects' susceptibility to acquire microbes with potential pathogenic relevance and could explain the propensity to develop pneumonia among patients with chronic inflammatory airway diseases, such as COPD or cystic fibrosis.

HOW DISTINCT MICROBIOTA SIGNATURES IN PNEUMONIA AFFECT THE NATURAL HISTORY OF THE DISEASE

For the last 50 years, research has focused on pathogen-host interactions that occur when patients develop pneumonia. The current understanding of the complex microbial communities existing in the lower airways invites a broadening of this view to uncover the role of microbiota-host interactions during pneumonia. Studies in HIV-

infected patients in Uganda and the United States[115] demonstrate that the oral and lung microbiome in HIV-infected patients treated with antimicrobials changes during acute pneumonia.[116] The lower airway microbiota exhibited significantly higher relative abundance of multiple members of the Proteobacteria phyla, including several pathogens such as K pneumoniae and Pseudomonas species, and these distinct microbiota signatures may contribute to the natural history of the disease. In another study performed with the Ugandan cohort of HIV subjects admitted to a local hospital for pneumonia, distinct lung microbiota signatures were associated with disease progression.[117] Using a clustering approach on the 16S rRNA gene sequencing data, the lower airway samples from HIV subjects with pneumonia organized into distinct groups. One group was dominated by Pseudomonaceae (group MCS1). The second group was subdivided into 2 subclusters enriched with Streptococcaeae (MCS2A) or Prevotellaceae (MCS2B).[117] Enrichment with Prevotellaceae trended toward an increase in mortality at 1 week after bronchoscopy (MSC1 0.0% mortality vs MSC2B 7.4%) and 70 days after bronchoscopy (MSC1 13% mortality compared with MSC2A 16%, and MSC2B 22%).[117] The clusters were also associated with distinct immune profiles based on metabolomics.[117] These data suggest that lung microbiota signatures among subjects with pneumonia may play a role in the pathogenesis and may help one understand differences in outcomes when patients develop pneumonia. It is possible that a "healthier" microbiome enriched with Pseudomonaceae may suppress virulence of potential pathogens and promote the restoration of a "healthy" lung microbiome. Conversely, a lower airway microbiota enriched with Streptococcacceae or Prevotellaceae may favor a more proinflammatory endotype that may promote the persistence and blooming of pathogens by driving nutrients to the alveolar space or promote virulence factors (see **Fig. 1**B).[118] In transplant, the lung microbiota of subjects diagnosed with pneumonia was found to have decreased diversity and was dominated with Pseudomonas, Staphylococcus, and Streptococcus.[119]

Difficulties obtaining samples before the development of pneumonia are a significant limitation for studying the lung microbiome during CAP. Although confounded by multiple issues, insight can be gained by studying intubated patients before the development of VAP. In a small study wherein samples were obtained longitudinally from the upper and lower respiratory tract, there was a significant decrease over time in α diversity of their upper airways (although not in lower respiratory samples) associated with the development of pneumonia.[16] The reduction in diversity before the development of pneumonia may be an important step reflecting dysbiosis along the airway microbiome.

LUNG MICROBIOME: WHAT CAN BE EXPECTED FROM FUTURE INVESTIGATIONS?

A better understanding of the lung microbiota in pneumonia is needed to uncover important microbiota-host and microbe-microbe interactions that will likely yield improvements in prevention, diagnosis, and treatment of pneumonia. The microbial dynamics across mucosal membranes (ie, upper/lower airways and gut) in different disease states likely affects an individual's susceptibility to pneumonia. Defining the pathways that dictate microbe-microbe interactions, microbe-host interactions, and selection pressure differences using unbiased, culture-independent methods allows one to characterize the complex microbial community dynamics of the lower airways. The gut microbiota may also shape the immune system, and "spillover" affecting the lower airway deserves careful consideration. In addition, other mucosal locations and/or specific timing (eg, early childhood) may shape the immune tone and will be critical to the understanding of an individual's susceptibility to pneumonia. By studying the microbial reservoirs to the lower airways (eg, oropharynx and nasopharynx), one may be able to identify potentially more accessible therapeutic targets that will indirectly affect the lower airway microbiota. Existing examples of this already exist, such as decontamination of nasal carriage with methicillin-resistant S aureus with mupirocin,[120] oral hygiene to prevent HAP,[121] and oral decontamination with chlorhexidine for intubated patients.[122] These decontamination strategies have been based on culture-based understanding of microbes, and the approach has been targeting specific pathogens or a "sledgehammer" antimicrobial approach. Better understanding of the complexity of the existing microbial communities will likely lead to a more targeted approach tailored to multiple microbes and keystone species personalized for each individual patient.

Currently, there is no unbiased, high-throughput culture-independent technique widely available to guide individualized patient care. This area is an area of active research and relevant to the care of patients at the bedside. As sequencers become smaller and even attachable to a USB port on a laptop, major limitations and challenges for these approaches remain the bioinformatic power and time needed to perform analysis. As these techniques are entering the phase of possible clinical bedside application, it will be important to start testing these approaches in large cohort studies, whereby reproducibility and feasibility can be best assessed.[30]

Among the potential therapeutic options for either prevention or treatment of pneumonia, a better understanding of the lung microbiota may shift current "pathogen-killing" focus to include the use of probiotics (eg, living bacteria intended to benefit health), prebiotics (eg, diet ingredients that confer specific changes in the microbiome and lead to beneficial effects in the host), or selective antibiotics (eg, eradication of specific strains of bacteria not necessarily identified as pathogen but may augment the pathogenic process).[123] Other therapies attempting to modify the composition of the airway microbiota may include the use of antibacterial conjugate vaccines or focused bacteriophages eliminating individual strains of a single species[124,125] and replacing the entire community with a new intact airway microbiota (following the example of fecal transplantation in Clostridium difficile colitis). Similar to the rationale for using probiotics in diet, it might be feasible to nurture and promote a "healthier" airway microbiota by inhaling a specific mixture of microbial species or microbial metabolites tailored to an individual's microbiota to restore or promote airways health.

As research of the microbiota in pneumonia grows, the following major challenges have been identified: (a) lack of animal models developed to study microbe-host and microbe-microbe interactions that account for the complexities of microbial communities existing in humans; (b) difficulties examining virome and mycobiome due to limitation with current gene marker approaches and reference libraries; (c) limited access to lower airway samples; (d) difficulties studying the events that occur at early time points of pneumonia or preclinical disease; (e) heterogeneity of pneumonia as a pathogenic condition and clinical diagnosis; and (f) multiple confounders present at the time of diagnosis, such as comorbidities, environmental factors, and effect of different treatments.

Preclinical models have been key to the mechanistic understanding of pneumonia. However, these models have been tailored to study the acquisition of a single organism without considering resident or microbial communities (beyond the use of either germ-free or pathogen-free models). Future investigations will need to design how to study complex microbial interactions in these models of disease. Experiments using longitudinal, prospective cohorts may give insight into the changes in the upper and lower airway that predict the development of pneumonia. CAP, HAP, and VAP may share some common pathophysiologic events but are fundamentally different clinical entities that will require different study designs and approaches.

In summary, high-throughput sequencing enables more comprehensive characterization of airway microbial community composition and has the potential to detect more difficult to culture microbes that have significant relevance in the pathogenesis of pneumonia. The line between what is understood as a commensal and a pathogen has become more blurred with the discovery of the lung microbiome. The use of culture-independent techniques to study the lung microbiome challenges the belief that the healthy lung is sterile and provides new insights into the importance of the microbiome for mucosal immune maturation and response that is relevant to the development and natural history of pneumonia.

Rather than prescribing antibiotics, the evaluation of the airway microbiota and its immune interactions may allow for better-targeted and individualized approaches with antimicrobials as well as other nonantibiotic therapies intended to regulate microbial community composition and microbial metabolism or enhance the efficacy of the immune response. The paradigm will move away from a sole pathogen causing disease, to that of a disrupted community of microorganisms that may enhance the pathogenic potential of each other (see **Fig. 1D**). The research efforts to understand the role of the lung microbiota in pneumonia require both preclinical models and rigorous and well-designed prospective cohort studies that the field currently lacks to understand the interactions between the host and the community of microorganisms in the airway to contribute to the understanding of the pathogenesis of pneumonia.

REFERENCES

1. Yamasaki K, Kawanami T, Yatera K, et al. Significance of anaerobes and oral bacteria in community-acquired pneumonia. PLoS One 2013; 8(5):e63103.
2. Rascon-Aguilar IE, Pamer M, Wludyka P, et al. Role of gastroesophageal reflux symptoms in exacerbations of COPD. Chest 2006;130(4):1096–101.
3. Cvejic L, Harding R, Churchward T, et al. Laryngeal penetration and aspiration in individuals with stable COPD. Respirology 2011;16(2):269–75.
4. Morse CA, Quan SF, Mays MZ, et al. Is there a relationship between obstructive sleep apnea and gastroesophageal reflux disease? Clin Gastroenterol Hepatol 2004;2(9):761–8.
5. Jain S, Self WH, Wunderink RG, et al. Community-acquired pneumonia requiring hospitalization among U.S. Adults. N Engl J Med 2015;373(5): 415–27.
6. Gadsby NJ, Russell CD, McHugh MP, et al. Comprehensive molecular testing for respiratory pathogens in community-acquired pneumonia. Clin Infect Dis 2016;62(7):817–23.
7. Schlueter M, James C, Dominguez A, et al. Practice patterns for antibiotic de-escalation in culture-negative healthcare-associated pneumonia. Infection 2010;38(5):357–62.
8. Labelle AJ, Arnold H, Reichley RM, et al. A comparison of culture-positive and culture-negative health-care-associated pneumonia. Chest 2010;137(5):1130–7.
9. Webb BJ, Dangerfield BS, Pasha JS, et al. Guideline-concordant antibiotic therapy and clinical outcomes in healthcare-associated pneumonia. Respir Med 2012;106(11):1606–12.
10. Sanchez-Nieto JM, Torres A, Garcia-Cordoba F, et al. Impact of invasive and noninvasive quantitative culture sampling on outcome of ventilator-associated pneumonia: a pilot study. Am J Respir Crit Care Med 1998;157(2):371–6.
11. Hayon J, Figliolini C, Combes A, et al. Role of serial routine microbiologic culture results in the initial management of ventilator-associated pneumonia. Am J Respir Crit Care Med 2002;165(1):41–6.
12. Kumar A, Haery C, Paladugu B, et al. The duration of hypotension before the initiation of antibiotic treatment is a critical determinant of survival in a murine model of Escherichia coli septic shock: association with serum lactate and inflammatory cytokine levels. J Infect Dis 2006;193(2):251–8.
13. Kumar R, Maynard CL, Eipers P, et al. Colonization potential to reconstitute a microbe community in patients detected early after fecal microbe transplant for recurrent C. difficile. BMC Microbiol 2016;16:5.
14. Dortet L, Legrand P, Soussy CJ, et al. Bacterial identification, clinical significance, and antimicrobial susceptibilities of Acinetobacter ursingii and Acinetobacter schindleri, two frequently misidentified opportunistic pathogens. J Clin Microbiol 2006;44(12):4471–8.
15. Seki M, Gotoh K, Nakamura S, et al. Fatal sepsis caused by an unusual Klebsiella species that was misidentified by an automated identification system. J Med Microbiol 2013;62(Pt 5):801–3.
16. Kelly BJ, Imai I, Bittinger K, et al. Composition and dynamics of the respiratory tract microbiome in intubated patients. Microbiome 2016;4:7.
17. Horvat RT, El Atrouni W, Hammoud K, et al. Ribosomal RNA sequence analysis of Brucella infection misidentified as Ochrobactrum anthropi infection. J Clin Microbiol 2011;49(3):1165–8.

18. Kumar A, Roberts D, Wood KE, et al. Duration of hypotension before initiation of effective antimicrobial therapy is the critical determinant of survival in human septic shock. Crit Care Med 2006;34(6): 1589–96.

19. McMenamin JD, Zaccone TM, Coenye T, et al. Misidentification of Burkholderia cepacia in US cystic fibrosis treatment centers: an analysis of 1,051 recent sputum isolates. Chest 2000;117(6): 1661–5.

20. Monso E, Ruiz J, Rosell A, et al. Bacterial infection in chronic obstructive pulmonary disease. A study of stable and exacerbated outpatients using the protected specimen brush. Am J Respir Crit Care Med 1995;152(4 Pt 1):1316–20.

21. Goldstein EJ, Citron DM, Goldman PJ, et al. National hospital survey of anaerobic culture and susceptibility methods: III. Anaerobe 2008;14(2):68–72.

22. Lagier JC, Edouard S, Pagnier I, et al. Current and past strategies for bacterial culture in clinical microbiology. Clin Microbiol Rev 2015;28(1): 208–36.

23. Lagier JC, Hugon P, Khelaifia S, et al. The rebirth of culture in microbiology through the example of culturomics to study human gut microbiota. Clin Microbiol Rev 2015;28(1):237–64.

24. Chastre J, Fagon JY, Bornet-Lecso M, et al. Evaluation of bronchoscopic techniques for the diagnosis of nosocomial pneumonia. Am J Respir Crit Care Med 1995;152(1):231–40.

25. Fagon JY, Chastre J, Trouillet JL, et al. Characterization of distal bronchial microflora during acute exacerbation of chronic bronchitis. Use of the protected specimen brush technique in 54 mechanically ventilated patients. Am Rev Respir Dis 1990; 142(5):1004–8.

26. Sethi S. Bacteria in exacerbations of chronic obstructive pulmonary disease: phenomenon or epiphenomenon? Proc Am Thorac Soc 2004;1(2): 109–14.

27. Cabello H, Torres A, Celis R, et al. Bacterial colonization of distal airways in healthy subjects and chronic lung disease: a bronchoscopic study. Eur Respir J 1997;10(5):1137–44.

28. Monso E, Rosell A, Bonet G, et al. Risk factors for lower airway bacterial colonization in chronic bronchitis. Eur Respir J 1999;13(2):338–42.

29. Riise GC, Andersson B, Ahlstedt S, et al. Bronchial brush biopsies for studies of epithelial inflammation in stable asthma and nonobstructive chronic bronchitis. Eur Respir J 1996;9(8):1665–71.

30. Pendleton KM, Erb-Downward JR, Bao Y, et al. Rapid pathogen identification in bacterial pneumonia using real-time metagenomics. Am J Respir Crit Care Med 2017;196(12):1610–2.

31. Yan Q, Cui S, Chen C, et al. Metagenomic analysis of sputum microbiome as a tool toward culture-independent pathogen detection of patients with ventilator-associated pneumonia. Am J Respir Crit Care Med 2016;194(5):636–9.

32. Xu L, Zhu Y, Ren L, et al. Characterization of the nasopharyngeal viral microbiome from children with community-acquired pneumonia but negative for Luminex xTAG respiratory viral panel assay detection. J Med Virol 2017;89(12):2098–107.

33. Teo SM, Mok D, Pham K, et al. The infant nasopharyngeal microbiome impacts severity of lower respiratory infection and risk of asthma development. Cell Host Microbe 2015;17(5):704–15.

34. von Eiff C, Becker K, Machka K, et al. Nasal carriage as a source of Staphylococcus aureus bacteremia. Study group. N Engl J Med 2001; 344(1):11–6.

35. Turnbaugh PJ, Ley RE, Hamady M, et al. The human microbiome project. Nature 2007;449(7164):804–10.

36. Casadevall A, Pirofski LA. The damage-response framework of microbial pathogenesis. Nat Rev Microbiol 2003;1(1):17–24.

37. Casadevall A, Pirofski LA. What is a pathogen? Ann Med 2002;34(1):2–4.

38. Otto M. Staphylococcus epidermidis–the 'accidental' pathogen. Nat Rev Microbiol 2009;7(8): 555–67.

39. Byrd AL, Segre JA. Infectious disease. Adapting Koch's postulates. Science 2016;351(6270):224–6.

40. Dickson RP, Erb-Downward JR, Freeman CM, et al. Bacterial topography of the healthy human lower respiratory tract. MBio 2017;8(1) [pii:e02287-16].

41. Pustelny C, Komor U, Pawar V, et al. Contribution of Veillonella parvula to Pseudomonas aeruginosa-mediated pathogenicity in a murine tumor model system. Infect Immun 2015;83(1):417–29.

42. Carmody LA, Zhao J, Schloss PD, et al. Changes in cystic fibrosis airway microbiota at pulmonary exacerbation. Ann Am Thorac Soc 2013;10(3):179–87.

43. Huang YJ, LiPuma JJ. The microbiome in cystic fibrosis. Clin Chest Med 2016;37(1):59–67.

44. Lipuma JJ. The changing microbial epidemiology in cystic fibrosis. Clin Microbiol Rev 2010;23(2): 299–323.

45. Zhao J, Schloss PD, Kalikin LM, et al. Decade-long bacterial community dynamics in cystic fibrosis airways. Proc Natl Acad Sci U S A 2012;109(15): 5809–14.

46. Gleeson K, Eggli DF, Maxwell SL. Quantitative aspiration during sleep in normal subjects. Chest 1997; 111(5):1266–72.

47. Teramoto S, Ohga E, Matsui H, et al. Obstructive sleep apnea syndrome may be a significant cause of gastroesophageal reflux disease in older people. J Am Geriatr Soc 1999;47(10):1273–4.

48. Field SK, Underwood M, Brant R, et al. Prevalence of gastroesophageal reflux symptoms in asthma. Chest 1996;109(2):316–22.

49. Scott RB, O'Loughlin EV, Gall DG. Gastroesophageal reflux in patients with cystic fibrosis. J Pediatr 1985;106(2):223–7.

50. Koh WJ, Lee JH, Kwon YS, et al. Prevalence of gastroesophageal reflux disease in patients with nontuberculous mycobacterial lung disease. Chest 2007;131(6):1825–30.

51. Randell SH, Boucher RC. Effective mucus clearance is essential for respiratory health. Am J Respir Cell Mol Biol 2006;35(1):20–8.

52. Taylor AE, Finney-Hayward TK, Quint JK, et al. Defective macrophage phagocytosis of bacteria in COPD. Eur Respir J 2010;35(5):1039–47.

53. Pragman AA, Kim HB, Reilly CS, et al. The lung microbiome in moderate and severe chronic obstructive pulmonary disease. PLoS One 2012;7(10): e47305.

54. Dickson RP, Huffnagle GB. The lung microbiome: new principles for respiratory bacteriology in health and disease. Plos Pathog 2015;11(7):e1004923.

55. Aagaard K, Petrosino J, Keitel W, et al. The Human Microbiome Project strategy for comprehensive sampling of the human microbiome and why it matters. FASEB J 2013;27(3):1012–22.

56. Grice EA, Kong HH, Conlan S, et al. Topographical and temporal diversity of the human skin microbiome. Science 2009;324(5931):1190–2.

57. Group NHW, Peterson J, Garges S, et al. The NIH human microbiome project. Genome Res 2009; 19(12):2317–23.

58. Grice EA, Segre JA. The human microbiome: our second genome. Annu Rev Genomics Hum Genet 2012;13:151–70.

59. Zaiss MM, Rapin A, Lebon L, et al. The intestinal microbiota contributes to the ability of helminths to modulate allergic inflammation. Immunity 2015; 43(5):998–1010.

60. Fonseca DM, Hand TW, Han SJ, et al. Microbiota-dependent sequelae of acute infection compromise tissue-specific immunity. Cell 2015;163(2):354–66.

61. Sawa S, Lochner M, Satoh-Takayama N, et al. RORgammat+ innate lymphoid cells regulate intestinal homeostasis by integrating negative signals from the symbiotic microbiota. Nat Immunol 2011;12(4):320–6.

62. Satoh-Takayama N, Vosshenrich CA, Lesjean-Pottier S, et al. Microbial flora drives interleukin 22 production in intestinal NKp46+ cells that provide innate mucosal immune defense. Immunity 2008;29(6):958–70.

63. Farkas AM, Panea C, Goto Y, et al. Induction of Th17 cells by segmented filamentous bacteria in the murine intestine. J Immunol Methods 2015; 421:104–11.

64. Ivanov II, Atarashi K, Manel N, et al. Induction of intestinal Th17 cells by segmented filamentous bacteria. Cell 2009;139(3):485–98.

65. Ivanov II, Frutos Rde L, Manel N, et al. Specific microbiota direct the differentiation of IL-17-producing T-helper cells in the mucosa of the small intestine. Cell Host Microbe 2008;4(4):337–49.

66. Pezzulo AA, Kelly PH, Nassar BS, et al. Abundant DNase I-sensitive bacterial DNA in healthy porcine lungs and its implications for the lung microbiome. Appl Environ Microbiol 2013;79(19):5936–41.

67. Segal LN, Clemente JC, Tsay J-CJ, et al. Enrichment of the lung microbiome with oral taxa is associated with lung inflammation of a Th17 phenotype. Nature Microbiology 2016;1:16031.

68. Charlson ES, Bittinger K, Haas AR, et al. Topographical continuity of bacterial populations in the healthy human respiratory tract. Am J Respir Crit Care Med 2011;184(8):957–63.

69. Segal LN, Alekseyenko AV, Clemente JC, et al. Enrichment of lung microbiome with supraglottic taxa is associated with increased pulmonary inflammation. Microbiome 2013;1(1):19.

70. Ege MJ, Mayer M, Normand AC, et al. Exposure to environmental microorganisms and childhood asthma. N Engl J Med 2011;364(8):701–9.

71. Ege MJ, Bieli C, Frei R, et al. Prenatal farm exposure is related to the expression of receptors of the innate immunity and to atopic sensitization in school-age children. J Allergy Clin Immunol 2006;117(4):817–23.

72. Roduit C, Wohlgensinger J, Frei R, et al. Prenatal animal contact and gene expression of innate immunity receptors at birth are associated with atopic dermatitis. J Allergy Clin Immunol 2011;127(1): 179–85, 185.e1.

73. Fujimura KE, Demoor T, Rauch M, et al. House dust exposure mediates gut microbiome Lactobacillus enrichment and airway immune defense against allergens and virus infection. Proc Natl Acad Sci U S A 2014;111(2):805–10.

74. Atarashi K, Tanoue T, Shima T, et al. Induction of colonic regulatory T cells by indigenous Clostridium species. Science 2011;331(6015):337–41.

75. Dimmitt RA, Staley EM, Chuang G, et al. Role of postnatal acquisition of the intestinal microbiome in the early development of immune function. J Pediatr Gastroenterol Nutr 2010;51(3):262–73.

76. Smith PM, Howitt MR, Panikov N, et al. The microbial metabolites, short-chain fatty acids, regulate colonic Treg cell homeostasis. Science 2013; 341(6145):569–73.

77. Thaiss CA, Zmora N, Levy M, et al. The microbiome and innate immunity. Nature 2016;535(7610):65–74.

78. van Nimwegen FA, Penders J, Stobberingh EE, et al. Mode and place of delivery, gastrointestinal microbiota, and their influence on asthma and atopy. J Allergy Clin Immunol 2011;128(5):948–55.e1-3.

79. Bager P, Melbye M, Rostgaard K, et al. Mode of delivery and risk of allergic rhinitis and asthma. J Allergy Clin Immunol 2003;111(1):51–6.

80. Marra F, Marra CA, Richardson K, et al. Antibiotic use in children is associated with increased risk of asthma. Pediatrics 2009;123(3):1003–10.

81. Murk W, Risnes KR, Bracken MB. Prenatal or early-life exposure to antibiotics and risk of childhood asthma: a systematic review. Pediatrics 2011; 127(6):1125–38.

82. Depner M, Ege MJ, Genuneit J, et al. Atopic sensitization in the first year of life. J Allergy Clin Immunol 2013;131(3):781–8.

83. Eder W, Ege MJ, von Mutius E. The asthma epidemic. N Engl J Med 2006;355(21):2226–35.

84. Fujimura KE, Johnson CC, Ownby DR, et al. Man's best friend? The effect of pet ownership on house dust microbial communities. J Allergy Clin Immunol 2010;126(2):410–2, 412.e1–3.

85. Bisgaard H, Hermansen MN, Buchvald F, et al. Childhood asthma after bacterial colonization of the airway in neonates. N Engl J Med 2007; 357(15):1487–95.

86. Nembrini C, Sichelstiel A, Kisielow J, et al. Bacterial-induced protection against allergic inflammation through a multicomponent immunoregulatory mechanism. Thorax 2011;66(9):755–63.

87. Chen Y, Blaser MJ. Inverse associations of Helicobacter pylori with asthma and allergy. Arch Intern Med 2007;167(8):821–7.

88. Reibman J, Marmor M, Filner J, et al. Asthma is inversely associated with Helicobacter pylori status in an urban population. PLoS One 2008;3(12): e4060.

89. Noverr MC, Falkowski NR, McDonald RA, et al. Development of allergic airway disease in mice following antibiotic therapy and fungal microbiota increase: role of host genetics, antigen, and interleukin-13. Infect Immun 2005;73(1):30–8.

90. Noverr MC, Noggle RM, Toews GB, et al. Role of antibiotics and fungal microbiota in driving pulmonary allergic responses. Infect Immun 2004;72(9): 4996–5003.

91. Forsythe P, Inman MD, Bienenstock J. Oral treatment with live Lactobacillus reuteri inhibits the allergic airway response in mice. Am J Respir Crit Care Med 2007;175(6):561–9.

92. Ezendam J, van Loveren H. Lactobacillus casei Shirota administered during lactation increases the duration of autoimmunity in rats and enhances lung inflammation in mice. Br J Nutr 2008;99(1): 83–90.

93. Kitagaki K, Businga TR, Kline JN. Oral administration of CpG-ODNs suppresses antigen-induced asthma in mice. Clin Exp Immunol 2006;143(2): 249–59.

94. de Steenhuijsen Piters WA, Huijskens EG, Wyllie AL, et al. Dysbiosis of upper respiratory tract microbiota in elderly pneumonia patients. ISME J 2016;10(1):97–108.

95. Vissing NH, Chawes BL, Bisgaard H. Increased risk of pneumonia and bronchiolitis after bacterial colonization of the airways as neonates. Am J Respir Crit Care Med 2013;188(10):1246–52.

96. Twigg HL Iii, Knox KS, Zhou J, et al. Effect of advanced HIV infection on the respiratory microbiome. Am J Respir Crit Care Med 2016;194(2): 226–35.

97. Selwyn PA, Feingold AR, Hartel D, et al. Increased risk of bacterial pneumonia in HIV-infected intravenous drug users without AIDS. AIDS 1988;2(4): 267–72.

98. Segal LN, Clemente JC, Li Y, et al. Anaerobic bacterial fermentation products increase tuberculosis risk in antiretroviral-drug-treated HIV patients. Cell Host Microbe 2017;21(4):530–7.e4.

99. Ledson MJ, Gallagher MJ, Jackson M, et al. Outcome of Burkholderia cepacia colonisation in an adult cystic fibrosis centre. Thorax 2002;57(2): 142–5.

100. Restrepo MI, Mortensen EM, Pugh JA, et al. COPD is associated with increased mortality in patients with community-acquired pneumonia. Eur Respir J 2006;28(2):346–51.

101. Mullerova H, Chigbo C, Hagan GW, et al. The natural history of community-acquired pneumonia in COPD patients: a population database analysis. Respir Med 2012;106(8):1124–33.

102. Flume PA, Mogayzel PJ Jr, Robinson KA, et al. Cystic fibrosis pulmonary guidelines: treatment of pulmonary exacerbations. Am J Respir Crit Care Med 2009;180(9):802–8.

103. Salk HM, Simon WL, Lambert ND, et al. Taxa of the nasal microbiome are associated with influenza-specific IgA response to live attenuated influenza vaccine. PLoS One 2016;11(9):e0162803.

104. Sethi S, Murphy TF. Infection in the pathogenesis and course of chronic obstructive pulmonary disease. N Engl J Med 2008;359(22):2355–65.

105. Erb-Downward JR, Thompson DL, Han MK, et al. Analysis of the lung microbiome in the "healthy" smoker and in COPD. PLoS One 2011;6(2):e16384.

106. Sethi S, Evans N, Grant BJ, et al. New strains of bacteria and exacerbations of chronic obstructive pulmonary disease. N Engl J Med 2002;347(7): 465–71.

107. Sze MA, Dimitriu PA, Suzuki M, et al. Host response to the lung microbiome in chronic obstructive pulmonary disease. Am J Respir Crit Care Med 2015;192(4):438–45.

108. Huang YJ, Kim E, Cox MJ, et al. A persistent and diverse airway microbiota present during chronic obstructive pulmonary disease exacerbations. OMICS 2010;14(1):9–59.

109. Kalil AC, Metersky ML, Klompas M, et al. Executive summary: management of adults with hospital-acquired and ventilator-associated pneumonia:

2016 clinical practice guidelines by the Infectious Diseases Society of America and the American Thoracic Society. Clin Infect Dis 2016;63(5): 575–82.

110. Lozupone C, Cota-Gomez A, Palmer BE, et al. Widespread colonization of the lung by tropheryma whipplei in HIV infection. Am J Respir Crit Care Med 2013;187(10):1110–7.

111. Harris B, Morjaria SM, Littmann ER, et al. Gut microbiota predict pulmonary infiltrates after allogeneic hematopoietic cell transplantation. Am J Respir Crit Care Med 2016;194(4):450–63.

112. Willner D, Haynes MR, Furlan M, et al. Case studies of the spatial heterogeneity of DNA viruses in the cystic fibrosis lung. Am J Respir Cell Mol Biol 2012;46(2):127–31.

113. Willner D, Furlan M, Schmieder R, et al. Metagenomic detection of phage-encoded platelet-binding factors in the human oral cavity. Proc Natl Acad Sci U S A 2011;108(Suppl 1):4547–53.

114. Molyneaux PL, Mallia P, Cox MJ, et al. Outgrowth of the bacterial airway microbiome after rhinovirus exacerbation of chronic obstructive pulmonary disease. Am J Respir Crit Care Med 2013;188(10): 1224–31.

115. Iwai S, Huang D, Fong S, et al. The lung microbiome of Ugandan HIV-infected pneumonia patients is compositionally and functionally distinct from that of San Franciscan patients. PLoS One 2014;9(4):e95726.

116. Iwai S, Fei M, Huang D, et al. Oral and airway microbiota in HIV-infected pneumonia patients. J Clin Microbiol 2012;50(9):2995–3002.

117. Shenoy MK, Iwai S, Lin DL, et al. Immune response and mortality risk relate to distinct lung microbiomes in patients with HIV and pneumonia. Am J Respir Crit Care Med 2017;195(1):104–14.

118. Dickson RP, Erb-Downward JR, Huffnagle GB. Towards an ecology of the lung: new conceptual models of pulmonary microbiology and pneumonia pathogenesis. Lancet Respir Med 2014;2(3): 238–46.

119. Shankar J, Nguyen MH, Crespo MM, et al. Looking beyond respiratory cultures: microbiome-cytokine signatures of bacterial pneumonia and tracheobronchitis in lung transplant recipients. Am J Transplant 2016;16(6):1766–78.

120. Perl TM, Cullen JJ, Wenzel RP, et al. Intranasal mupirocin to prevent postoperative Staphylococcus aureus infections. N Engl J Med 2002;346(24): 1871–7.

121. Baker D, Quinn B. Hospital acquired pneumonia prevention initiative-2: incidence of nonventilator hospital-acquired pneumonia in the United States. Am J Infect Control 2018;46(1):2–7.

122. Genuit T, Bochicchio G, Napolitano LM, et al. Prophylactic chlorhexidine oral rinse decreases ventilator-associated pneumonia in surgical ICU patients. Surg Infect (Larchmt) 2001;2(1):5–18.

123. Bowater RJ, Stirling SA, Lilford RJ. Is antibiotic prophylaxis in surgery a generally effective intervention? Testing a generic hypothesis over a set of meta-analyses. Ann Surg 2009;249(4):551–6.

124. Schooley RT, Biswas B, Gill JJ, et al. Development and use of personalized bacteriophage-based therapeutic cocktails to treat a patient with a disseminated resistant acinetobacter baumannii infection. Antimicrob Agents Chemother 2017; 61(10) [pii:e00954-17].

125. Mitsi E, Roche AM, Reine J, et al. Agglutination by anti-capsular polysaccharide antibody is associated with protection against experimental human pneumococcal carriage. Mucosal Immunol 2017; 10(2):385–94.

The Role of Biomarkers in the Diagnosis and Management of Pneumonia

Sarah Sungurlu, DO, Robert A. Balk, MD*

KEYWORDS

- Biomarkers • Pneumonia diagnosis • Procalcitonin • Scoring systems • Prognosis

KEY POINTS

- Objective criteria and severity scoring system should be supplemented by clinical judgment and evaluation of outside factors, including patient resources, in the diagnosis and management of pneumonia.
- Presently, the diagnosis of pneumonia and the initiation of antibiotics are based on chest radiograph, clinical judgment with guideline-directed antibiotic management not based on the presence or absence of a biomarker.
- Antibiotic stewardship may be enhanced by using biomarkers, specifically procalcitonin, to limit duration of therapy.
- When procalcitonin level is less than 80% of the first peak concentration, or if it reaches an absolute concentration of less than 0.5 ng/mL, a physician is encouraged to stop antibiotics in the treatment of pneumonia as long as this decision is also supported by patient improvement and clinical judgment.
- Biomarkers such as the neutrophil-to-lymphocyte ratio, lactate, and serial procalcitonin clearance, along with severity scoring systems, may be useful in the prognostication of pneumonia.

INTRODUCTION

According to the US Centers for Disease Control and Prevention in 2014, pneumonia and influenza were the eighth leading cause of death in the United States accounting for 15.9 deaths per 100,000 population. Community-acquired pneumonia (CAP) is diagnosed in approximately 4 million adults in the United States annually and accounts for $10 billion in costs in the United States and €10 billion in Europe.[1] Hospital-acquired pneumonia (HAP) and ventilator-associated pneumonia (VAP) have been associated with increased mortalities, length of hospital stay, and cost of care.[2] Pneumonia is also a frequent cause of sepsis, and sepsis guidelines have emphasized the importance of early initiation of the "correct" antibiotic in order to produce improved outcomes.[3] Guidelines have been published and are widely used to aid the clinician in the initiation of antibiotic treatment of CAP, HAP, and VAP.[2] However, a consequence of early initiation of potent antibiotic treatment to patients suspected of having pneumonia is the potential overtreatment of some non-bacterial-infected patients in order to prevent delayed antibiotic administration to those who do have a bacterial pulmonary infection.

Disclosure Statement: Dr S. Sungurlu has no conflicts of interest to disclose. Dr R.A. Balk has received research support and honoraria and participated in advisory boards for BioMerieux, Roche Scientific, and ThermoFisher. He also represented the American College of Chest Physicians in the Multi-Society Panel to the CDC on the definition of Ventilator-Associated Events and Ventilator-Associated Pneumonia.

Division of Pulmonary, Critical Care, and Sleep Medicine, Rush University Medical Center, Rush Medical College, 1725 West Harrison Street Suite 054, Chicago, IL 60612, USA
* Corresponding author.
E-mail address: robert_balk@rush.edu

Clin Chest Med 39 (2018) 691–701
https://doi.org/10.1016/j.ccm.2018.07.004

Overtreatment with antibiotics and unnecessary antibiotic treatment can give rise to selected pressure on bacteria, result in multidrug-resistant organisms, and give rise to resistant infections, such as *Clostridium difficile*, methicillin-resistant *Staphylococcus aureus*, and fungal superinfections.[4] Balancing appropriate antibiotic use is part of antibiotic stewardship. This process has been aided by rapid assays to detect resistant organisms and sensitivity patterns as well as by the proposed use of biomarkers to help identify selected populations of pneumonia patients who may have more severe disease requiring intensive care unit (ICU) treatment and/or those who more likely have a bacterial pathogen as the cause of the pneumonia.

As defined by the World Health Organization, a biomarker is "any substance, structure, or process that can be measured in the body and influence or predict the incidence or outcome of disease."[5] Several investigations have sought to identify a biomarker or group of biomarkers that can be easily and reliably measured and that will have a high sensitivity, specificity, positive and negative predictive value and demonstrate benefit in the management of patients with pneumonia. Biomarkers have been used to aid in the diagnosis, decision to start antibiotic therapy, assist with triage decisions, determine the duration of antibiotic treatment, and assist with prognostication for patients with pneumonia. Some biomarkers have had greater acceptance compared with others. This article reviews some of the common biomarkers (**Box 1**) used in the diagnosis, management, and treatment of patients with both CAP and HAP. **Box 2** describes some of the ways various biomarkers may be used to assist in the management of patients with pneumonia. The list includes using biomarkers to assist with the diagnosis of pneumonia, severity of illness scoring, risk stratification and triage decisions, initiation of antibiotic therapy, continuation of antibiotic therapy, duration, and/or discontinuation of antibiotic therapy, and with determining the prognosis of patients with suspected pneumonia.

BIOMARKER DIAGNOSIS OF PNEUMONIA

Presently, the diagnosis of pneumonia remains a clinical one and includes an abnormal chest radiograph or chest computed tomographic (CT) scan coupled with clinical criteria that include fever, cough, purulent sputum, chest pain, and often evidence of decrease in oxygen saturation.[4,6] VAP can include similar criteria, but can be more difficult to diagnose because the patients often have preexisting pulmonary infiltrates that

---

Box 1
Common biomarkers used in the diagnosis, management, and treatment of community and/or hospital-acquired pneumonia

Severity scoring systems for severe community-acquired pneumonia

British Thoracic Society (BTS) guideline

CURB-65

CUROX-80

Pneumonia Severity Index (PSI)

IDSA/ATS major and minor criteria to define SCAP

Clinical Pulmonary Infection Score (CPIS)

Selected blood biomarkers

Procalcitonin

C-reactive protein

White blood cell count

Lactate

Soluble triggering receptor expressed on myeloid cells (sTREM)

Pro-adrenomedullin (Pro-ADM)

B-natriuretic peptide (BNP)

Troponin I

Thrombocytopenia

---

account for the reason the patient was on a ventilator in the first place.[2] To aid in the surveillance diagnosis of VAP, a multisociety task force has recently proposed a new diagnostic strategy that includes ventilator-associated events, ventilator-associated conditions, infectious ventilator-associated complications, and possible or probableVAP.[7,8] Several investigators have proposed the use of biomarkers to help establish a diagnosis of VAP and distinguish it

---

Box 2
Biomarker use in pneumonia

Diagnosis of pneumonia

Determining severity of pneumonia with scoring systems

Risk stratification and triage of pneumonia

Initiation of antibiotic therapy

Continuation of antibiotic therapy

Duration/discontinuation of antibiotic therapy (antibiotic stewardship)

Determining prognosis

rom airway colonization or ventilator-associated tracheobronchitis.[9–12] Unfortunately, as of this time, there is no uniformly agreed on biomarker or diagnostic test that on its own will establish the diagnosis of VAP or CAP.

SEVERITY SCORING SYSTEMS

There are several scoring systems to identify patients appropriate for outpatient versus inpatient care, to prognosticate risk of death, and to potentially aid in the decision of initiating antibiotics. The Infectious Disease Society of America (IDSA)/American Thoracic Society (ATS) guidelines suggest that objective criteria or scores should always be supplemented with physician judgment and factors including the ability to take medications and access support resources.[4] Proper triage of CAP patients has been associated with improved survival in comparison to those patients who are initially admitted to a general medical floor and then require transfer to an ICU.[13,14] To aid in the decision of hospital admission as well as the classification of SCAP, there have been several severity of illness scoring systems, some of which are easier to use than others. The authors describe some of the more common severity of pneumonia scoring systems in use today.

British Thoracic Society Guidelines

The original British Thoracic Society (BTS) guidelines, developed in 1987, were based on the finding that the risk of death was increased 21-fold if a patient had 2 of the following 3 criteria on admission: tachypnea (respiratory rate ≥30 breaths per minute), diastolic hypotension (diastolic blood pressure ≤60 mm Hg), elevated blood urea nitrogen (BUN >7 mmol/L).[4] The BTS tool stratified patients into a severe or nonsevere category and had an overall sensitivity and specificity in predicting death of approximately 80%. Lim and colleagues[15] performed a multivariate analysis of 1068 patients in 2003, which expanded on the BTS guidelines and led to the concept of CURB-65 as a tool to define SCAP.

CURB-65

The CURB-65 pneumonia severity score incorporates the BTS guidelines (respiratory rate, hypotension, and BUN) with mental status and age to create a scoring system to aid patient disposition when diagnosed with pneumonia.[15] One point per category is assigned for confusion (based on mental test score <8 or disorientation to person, place or time), urea >7 mmol/L (20 mg/dL), respiratory rate ≥30 breaths per minute, hypotension

(systolic blood pressure <90 mm Hg or diastolic ≤60 mm Hg), and age ≥65 years. If the score is 0 to 1, mortality is 1.5%, and therefore, the patient is suitable for home treatment. If the score is 2, the mortality is 9.2% and the physician should consider hospital-supervised treatment (short-stay inpatient or intensive in-home health care services). Finally, if score is ≥3, then mortality is approximately 22%, and in-hospital management for severe pneumonia is recommended with the additional recommendation of assessment for ICU admission (especially if score is >3).[15] This scoring system is rated as a moderate recommendation (level III evidence) in the updated IDSA recommendations based on a validation study, which found that a score of 4 had a mortality of 40% and a score of 5 had a mortality of 57%.[4,16] Of note, for community physicians who do not have access to rapid blood work to obtain a BUN, the simplified CRB-65 was found to also correlate with risk of mortality and need for ventilatory support. For this system, a score of 0 is associated with low mortality (1.2%) and therefore suitable for home; a score of 1 to 2 is intermediate mortality (8.15%) and should have hospital referral and assessment, and a score of ≥3 has a high mortality (31%) and needs urgent hospitalization.[15,16]

CUROX-80

Spanish investigators have developed a severe community-acquired pneumonia (SCAP) prediction rule to aid patient disposition and triage.[17] In their study, 1057 emergency room patients with presumed pneumonia underwent multivariate analyses of 8 predictive factors for SCAP. They included 2 major criteria (1 needed): arterial pH less than 7.30 or systolic blood pressure less than 90 mm Hg, and 6 minor criteria abbreviated CUROX-80 (>2 needed): confusion/altered mental status, urea (BUN >30 mg/dL), respiratory rate greater than 30 breaths per minute, partial pressure of oxygen in arterial blood (P_aO_2) less than 54 mm Hg, or ratio of arterial oxygen tension to fraction of inspired oxygen (P_aO_2/F_iO_2) less than 250, multilobar/bilateral infiltrates on chest radiograph, and age ≥80 years old. The SCAP prediction score had a sensitivity and specificity for predicting SCAP of 92.1% and 73.8%, respectively. In comparison, the sensitivity and specificity for CURB-65 in diagnosing SCAP were 68.4% and 86.4%, and Pneumonia Severity Index (PSI) were 94.7% and 68.1%, respectively. The investigators concluded that the SCAP prediction score was more sensitive than CURB-65, but less than PSI, in identifying severe pneumonia.[17]

Pneumonia Severity Index

The PSI is another prognostic model that is based on weighting several comorbidities, clinical findings, and age rather than solely the severity of illness.[4] It has been used as a mortality prediction model and to help determine the need for inpatient admission versus outpatient management as well as to identify the population with a high risk for mortality that should be cared for in the ICU.[4,13] The prediction rule was derived from data on 14,199 adult inpatients with CAP and validated with data on 38,039 inpatients and 2287 mixed inpatients and outpatients with CAP. Patients are stratified into 5 mortality classes according to total points from 20 different variables, including age, presence of coexisting disease, abnormal physical findings (respiratory rate, temperature), and abnormal laboratory findings (pH, BUN, sodium) on presentation. Based on the associated mortality, class I and II should be considered for treatment as an outpatient, class III as a short hospitalization, and class IV and V as an inpatient admission.[4] There are several limitations to PSI, primarily related to the complexity of the tool that necessitates the use of scoring sheets, thereby creating a time constraint and limiting its practice utility.

Infectious Disease Society of America/ American Thoracic Society Definition for Severe versus Nonsevere Pneumonia

The 2007 IDSA/ATS CAP guideline established major and minor criteria to diagnose SCAP that required ICU admission with a goal to avoid delayed admission to the ICU.[4] The investigators recognized that there is increased mortality (up to 45%) for patients with CAP that have such delayed transfers to the ICU. A retrospective study of CAP patients admitted to the ICU who were categorized by CURB-65 and PSI led to the observation that both were overly sensitive and nonspecific in comparison to clinical decision, which prompted the IDSA/ATS guideline committee to suggest the following major and minor criteria to define SCAP that should be cared for in the ICU.[13] Both of the 2 major criteria (need for invasive mechanical ventilation or septic shock with need for vasopressors) are absolute indications for admission to the ICU, independently. The presence of 3 or more of the minor criteria is a moderate recommendation for admission to the ICU. The minor criteria include respiratory rate of greater than 30 breaths per minute, P_aO_2/F_iO_2 ratio of less than 250 (or need for noninvasive ventilation), multilobar infiltrates, confusion/disorientation, uremia (BUN >20 mg/dL), leukopenia (<4000 cells/mm^3 caused by infection), thrombocytopenia (<100,000 cells/mm^3),

hypothermia (<36°C), and hypotension requiring aggressive fluid resuscitation.[4]

Clinical Pulmonary Infection Score

Unlike the other scoring systems, the Clinical Pulmonary Infection Score (CPIS) was developed as a diagnostic tool for VAP. The score is calculated based on several clinical factors (temperature, white blood cell [WBC] count, oxygenation [P_aO_2/F_iO_2 ratio], radiographic findings, radiographic progression, tracheal secretions, and culture of tracheal aspirate). Each factor can be scored from 0 to 2 points. If the total is >6 points, this is suggestive of VAP. The 2016 IDSA/ATS guidelines recommend not using the CPIS to aid in the decision to initiate antibiotics based on a meta-analysis of 13 studies, which found a sensitivity of 65% and specificity of 64% to confirm or exclude VAP. Likewise, the IDSA/ATS guidelines do not recommend for the CPIS to be used as an aid in discontinuation of antibiotics after a review of 3 studies had inconsistent evidence, suggesting it does not reliably discriminate patients who can have their antibiotics safely discontinued.[2]

SELECTED BIOMARKERS AND THEIR ROLE
Procalcitonin

Arguably, the most commonly used biomarker in the diagnosis and management of pneumonia is procalcitonin (PCT), which is a 116-amino-acid peptide produced by the liver as an acute phase reactant as well as by thyroid C cells and lung K cells.[11,18] PCT is then cleaved into the hormone calcitonin, katacalcin, and an N-terminal fragment. Bacterium-specific proinflammatory cytokines (interleukin-1beta [IL-1β], tumor necrosis factor-alpha [TNF-α], IL6) as well as microbial toxins (endotoxins) stimulate nonneuroendocrine calcitonin gene expression and release of PCT from parenchymal tissue, such as the liver. For this reason, the circulating PCT level elevates without a corresponding increase in the circulating calcitonin level during this inflammatory response. In contrast, viral infections stimulate release of interferon-γ, which along with other cytokines downregulates this pathway. Therefore, although PCT may have some increase in response to sterile inflammation or viral infection, it is less profound than other biomarkers.[11] However, PCT can be falsely low in some localized infections, such as abscesses or empyema.[19] Because the cleavage of PCT occurs before release of calcitonin, healthy individuals normally have a very low circulating level (<0.1 ng/mL).[11] It is released into the circulation within 6 to 12 hours of infection, and the half-life is approximately 25 to 30 hours.[20]

C-Reactive Protein

C-reactive protein (CRP) is a pentameric protein, with 5 identical noncovalently bound subunits, synthesized by hepatocytes (molecular mass 118,000 Da). Infection or inflammation can generate cytokine release (IL-6, IL-1, and TNF-α), which then stimulates CRP synthesis. As a nonspecific acute phase reactant, it cannot accurately differentiate potential sources of tissue destruction.[21] However, there is a reasonable correlation between the severity of sepsis and degree of organ failure with CRP concentrations.[22]

White Blood Cell

Both the elevation and the depression of white blood cell (WBC) count are used to aid in the diagnosis of infection. In addition, the differential of WBCs (neutrophil to lymphocyte count ratio) can provide information on the type of response. For example, leukopenia has been associated with an increased mortality.[20]

Lactate

Normal healthy patients have a circulating blood lactate level of 0.5 to 1 mmol/L, and patients with critical illness can have normal concentrations up to 2 mmol/L. Lactate production by anaerobic metabolism (type A lactic acidosis) is used as a marker for tissue hypoperfusion and sepsis. It is clinically necessary to distinguish type B lactic acidosis (B1, liver failure; B2, drug or toxins; B3, errors of metabolism). In addition, decreased lactate clearance (primarily liver and to some extent kidney) can contribute to increased concentration of lactate not correlated with tissue hypoxia.[23]

Soluble Triggering Receptor Expressed on Myeloid Cells

An activating receptor that is expressed on the surface of neutrophils, mature monocytes, and macrophages, which amplifies the inflammatory response synergistically with the toll-like receptor signaling pathway when stimulated by bacteria or fungi.[5,24] As opposed to the membranous form, soluble triggering receptor expressed on myeloid cells (sTREM) is known to be specifically released during infectious processes.[25]

Pro-Adrenomedullin

Adrenomedullin is also a member of the calcitonin family. It acts as a vasodilating agent with immune modulating, metabolic, and bactericidal activity. However, with its rapid degradation and clearance, it is not stable, and therefore, for improved reliability, the midregional fragment

Pro-Adrenomedullin (Pro-ADM) is measured.[19] The midregional fragment Pro-ADM seems to correlate with the severity of pneumonia and the intensity of the inflammatory cytokine response to the infection, but may also be elevated in heart failure and/or renal dysfunction (**Box 3**).[26]

USE OF BIOMARKERS FOR DIAGNOSIS

The diagnosis of pneumonia is predominantly based on an abnormal chest radiograph or chest CT scan coupled with clinical manifestations of cough, fever, purulent sputum, elevated WBC

Box 3
Use of selected biomarkers in pneumonia management

Procalcitonin (PCT)

Diagnosis of bacterial versus nonbacterial infection

Need for antibiotic therapy

Prediction of severity of CAP (ICU admission/triaging emergency room patients)

Prognosis of pneumonia patients

Duration of antibiotic treatment

C-reactive protein (CRP)

Prediction of severity of CAP

Diagnosis of bacterial versus nonbacterial infection

Pro-adrenomedullin (Pro-ADM)

Severity of CAP

B-natriuretic peptide (BNP)

Severity of CAP

Troponin I

Degree of hypoxemia: severity of illness

Soluble triggering receptor expressed on myeloid cells (sTREM)

Diagnosis of VAP

Lactate

Severity of pneumonia

Prognosis and mortality prediction

White blood cells

Severity of pneumonia

Thrombocytopenia

Severity of pneumonia

P_aO_2/F_iO_2 Ratio

Degree of oxygenation abnormality

count, in addition to absence of another likely explanation for the clinical findings and radiographic abnormalities.[4,6] With the recognition that most of the time the cause of CAP is undetermined or viral, it has been advocated that use of biomarkers specific for bacterial infection would be beneficial in defining the patient population that would benefit from antibiotic administration.[4,27,28] In the era of rapidly advancing antibiotic resistance and a greater number of infections with multiple drug-resistant organisms, it would be beneficial to have either rapid determination of the causative organism and/or the availability of a biomarker or biomarkers that would signify a bacterial infection that requires antibiotic treatment. Of the currently used biomarkers, PCT has shown the most promise in aiding in the diagnosis of bacterial infections, including pneumonia.[19] However, there still are several limitations. Localized infections, such as empyema, may have no systemic release of PCT (only localized synthesis). ICU patients often suffer from sepsis, shock, or multiorgan failure, or can have the systemic inflammatory response syndrome (SIRS) from surgery and/or trauma, all of which can raise the PCT without the presence of a bacterial infection. Finally, a time lag of 24 to 48 hours can exist between bacterial infection onset and peak PCT, and therefore, at the time of diagnosis, there may be a false low PCT level.[11] PCT levels were helpful in diagnosing bacterial infection in immunosuppressed organ transplant recipients, even in the setting of acute rejection.[29–31] The PCT elevations in the setting of infection are not influenced by the use of corticosteroids, immunosuppressants, or leukopenia.[29–31] In a prospective study of postoperative infections in adult patients who underwent vascular surgery, significant elevations in PCT levels were found in those patients who had renal dysfunction in comparison to normal renal function.[32] Although the diagnostic accuracy of PCT to detect bacterial infection was still present, the threshold for determining bacterial infection needed to be adjusted upward.[32]

Most of the data in support of using initial PCT levels to determine which patients with a presumed lower respiratory tract infection (LRTI) require antibiotic treatment has come from European studies, predominantly conducted in Switzerland and Germany.[33–35] ProHosp, a large multicenter trial conducted in Switzerland with 1825 patients, found that in patients with LRTI PCT guidance compared with standard guidelines reduced antibiotic exposure and adverse effects associated with antibiotic use without adversely affecting patient outcomes.[35] Schuetz and colleagues[27] included acute bronchitis, acute exacerbations of chronic obstructive pulmonary disease, and pneumonia in their definition of LRTI, noting that 75% of LRTIs are treated with antibiotics despite a predominant viral cause. However, for the creation of the IDSA/ATS guideline, a meta-analysis looking at 6 studies (665 participants) found a low sensitivity of 67% and specificity of 83% for PCT in the diagnosis of HAP/VAP. Therefore, the IDSA/ATS guideline has a strong recommendation against use of PCT with clinical criteria to decide when to initiate antibiotics.[2]

Many of the previously mentioned biomarkers have been studied as potential tools for the diagnosis of pneumonia, but have thus far failed to show reproducible benefit. Systemic sTREM levels, along with the presence of 2 of the SIRS criteria, have been used to help differentiate patients with and without underlying infection.[24] However, there have been contradictory findings for measuring sTREM in bronchoalveolar lavage (BAL) fluid for the diagnosis of VAP.[12,36] In a meta-analysis of 6 studies, including 2008 patients with clinically suspected pneumonia, the sensitivity for sTREM was 84% and specificity was 49% for the diagnosis of HAP/VAP. Therefore, The IDSA/ATS guidelines give a strong recommendation against use of BAL fluid sTREM level plus clinical criteria to decide when to start antibiotic therapy.[2]

In a study of 48 patients, using the CRP threshold level of greater than 9.6 mg/dL, the sensitivity was 87.5% and the specificity was 86.1% for the diagnosis of VAP.[22] In addition, a meta-analysis of 3 studies found that in critically ill patients with and without pneumonia, the CRP levels were the same. Therefore, like sTREM, the IDSA/ATS guidelines give a strong recommendation against use of serum CRP plus clinical criteria to decide when to start antibiotics.[2]

USE OF BIOMARKERS FOR RISK STRATIFICATION

Another role for biomarkers is to aid in risk stratification for patients with pneumonia, including inpatient versus outpatient treatment and ICU versus general medical floor (GMF) admission.[4,13,15] As previously discussed, many of the severity scoring indices are used for this purpose. A systematic review and meta-analysis compared the performance of PSI, CURB-65, CRB-65, and CURB. The sensitivity and specificity for differentiating survivors versus nonsurvivors were 90% and 53% for PSI, 62% and 79% for CURB-65, 33% and 92% for CRB-65, and 63% and 77% for CURB, respectively.[37] For the identification of

SCAP, the SCAP prediction score (CUROX-80) had a sensitivity and specificity of 92.1% and 73.8%, compared with 68.4% and 86.4% for CURB-65, and 94.7% and 68.1% for PSI.[17] The IDSA/ATS guidelines created severe versus non-severe pneumonia major and minor criteria due to concerns that the PSI and CURB-65 were overly sensitive and not specific enough for clinical decision making.[13] The accuracy of the minor severity criteria of the IDSA/ATS guidelines was better than biomarkers alone in predicting ICU admission. In a secondary analysis of 453 CAP patients admitted to the ICU within 3 days of emergency room presentation, there was a decreased mortality (11.7% versus 23.4% [odds ratio, OR, 2.31, confidence interval, CI, 1.11–4.77, P<.02]) and shorter length of stay (7 versus 13 days [OR 0.55, CI 0.40–0.76, P<.001]) when the patient was initially admitted to the ICU compared with delayed ICU admission.[14] Biomarkers and scoring systems can improve clinical decision-making and triaging ability so that patients are admitted to the best unit for care. For example, a patient who has severe pneumonia, defined by the IDSA/ATS minor criteria, but a low level of PCT may be safely admitted to GMF.[38] The addition of biomarkers, such as CRP or PCT, to pneumonia severity scores will assist with the identification of those patients with greater need for hospital or even ICU management.[26] Much of the focus on the addition of biomarkers to pneumonia severity scores has been directed toward determining which patients will benefit from antibiotic therapy and which patients do not require antibiotic therapy. In the United States, antibiotic decisions are primarily based on guidelines that classify patients based on clinical presentation, risk factors, and assessment of severity of their clinical illness. All agree that serum PCT or CRP levels on their own should not be used as a stand-alone tool to identify those patients with bacterial pneumonia or to determine the type of bacterial infection.[39] There are data that suggest that atypical bacteria may not generate the same degree of PCT increase as is seen with other bacterial infections.[39] In a study of 1770 adult CAP patients, the degree of PCT elevation on initial presentation was strongly associated with the risk of requiring invasive respiratory and/or vasopressor support during the ensuing 72 hours.[40]

USE OF BIOMARKERS FOR INITIATION, CONTINUATION, AND DURATION OF ANTIBIOTIC THERAPY

Promoting antibiotic stewardship, and thereby decreasing costs and side effects, is where biomarkers have shown the most promise. The PNEUMA trial compared 401 patients with VAP who received antibiotics for 15 days versus 8 days and found the shorter duration did not have poorer outcomes.[41] They did have a slightly higher rate of recurrent pulmonary infections, however. PCT-guided algorithms for antibiotic stewardship in critically ill patients with VAP had similar mortalities, ICU length of stay, and comparable superinfection and relapsed infection rates.[41] The PRORATA trial looked at a PCT-based algorithm wherein physicians were encouraged to start antibiotics if PCT level was greater than 0.5 ng/mL and discouraged from starting antibiotics if it was less, although their clinical judgment overruled any level. Six hundred twenty-one patients were randomized to receive treatment based on physician judgment versus the PCT level guided algorithm. If a patient did receive antibiotics, a daily PCT was drawn, and when the level was less than 80% of the first peak concentration, or if it reached an absolute concentration of less than 0.5 ng/mL, the physician was encouraged to stop the antibiotics (again physician clinical judgment overruled any level). The PCT-guided algorithm had significantly more antibiotic-free days than the control (absolute difference of 2.7 days) without an increase in adverse outcomes (comparable day 28 and day 60 mortalities).[11]

PCT-guided antibiotic treatment versus usual care for septic patients was evaluated in a prospective, multicenter, randomized, controlled, open-label trial conducted in 15 hospitals in the Netherlands.[42] There was nonbinding advice given to the PCT-guided clinicians when the PCT level decreased by greater than 80% from the peak level or to a level of ≤0.5 μg/L to discontinue antibiotic therapy, whereas the usual care patients were managed according to the local standard of care for antibiotic use and duration. The PCT guidance was associated with a reduction in the duration of antibiotic treatment and decreased daily defined doses of antibiotic therapy. In addition to the reduced antibiotic therapy, the PCT-guided therapy was also associated with a significant decrease in 28-day (20% vs 25% [between group absolute difference 5.4%, 95% CI 1.2–9.5, P = .0122]) and 1-year mortality (36% vs 43% [between groups absolute difference 7.4, 95% CI 1.3-13.8, P = .0188]) rates in comparison to usual care.[42] Schuetz and colleagues[43] reviewed 14 clinical trials involving more than 4200 patients and concluded that using PCT to guide antibiotic discontinuation was not associated with increased mortality or treatment failure. Multiple meta-analyses have also supported a beneficial role for the use of serial PCT to decrease the duration of antibiotic therapy and potentially improve antibiotic stewardship.[27,44,45]

Lam and colleagues[46] conducted a systematic review and meta-analysis of the use of PCT versus usual care to guide the antimicrobial management (initiation, cessation, or mixed approach) in critically ill patients. Their analysis of the 15 studies that met the inclusion and exclusion criteria was that overall PCT guidance did not decrease short-term mortality. However, studies of PCT-guided antibiotic cessation were associated with decreased antibiotic duration and decreased mortality. The use of PCT to guide antibiotic initiation or using PCT in a mixed approach for initiation and cessation did not decrease mortality. There was also no difference in ICU length of stay, hospital length of stay, or recurrent infection.[46] Iankova and coworkers[47] conducted a systematic review and meta-analysis of the efficacy and safety of PCT guidance of antibiotic therapy in patients with suspected or confirmed sepsis. They included 10 randomized controlled trials that included 3489 patients and found that PCT guidance decreased antibiotic duration and there was no adverse impact on mortality or length of stay in the ICU.[47] Presently, there is a weak recommendation by the IDSA/ATS guidelines for the use of PCT levels plus clinical criteria to guide discontinuation of antibiotics in VAP patients. This recommendation is based on a systematic review of 14 randomized trials (4221 patients), which concluded that PCT-based decision making was able decrease the antibiotic exposure (adjusted mean difference of 3.47 days) and was not associated with increased treatment failure or mortality.[2]

USE OF BIOMARKERS FOR PROGNOSIS

The PSI and CURB-65, as previously discussed, are key scoring systems that have demonstrated utility in prognostication of pneumonia. Individual biomarkers have also been studied in their prognostic utility. There has been evidence suggesting that neutrophil to lymphocyte ratio (NTLR) can be used as a prognostic marker. During systemic inflammation, the demargination of neutrophils and stimulation of stem cells by granulocyte colony stimulating factor lead to neutrophilia, whereas accelerated apoptosis and margination and redistribution of lymphocytes cause lymphocytopenia. A prospective study with 195 CAP elderly patients looked at the NTLR as a predictor for mortality. The area under the curve (AUC) for NTLR was 0.95, higher compared with CRP (0.49), WBC count (0.55), PSI (0.87), and CURB-65 (0.61).[48]

In a multicenter prospective cohort study of 1653 emergency department patients, pro-ADM levels increased in correlation with increasing severity of illness and death.[49] The median pro-ADM level in 30-day nonsurvivors was 1.6 mmol/L versus 0.9 mmol/L in survivors. The optimal prognostic cutoff with maximum combined sensitivity and specificity for pro-ADM was determined to be 1.3 mmol/L with a sensitivity of 68% and specificity of 73% for 30-day mortality. However, high pro-ADM levels did not alter PSI risk assessment in most CAP patients and had no additional stratification benefit in high-risk CAP patients.[49]

Lactate and lactate clearance are other commonly used biomarkers for prognostication.[3,50] In normotensive patients with sepsis, lactate is closely monitored because it is independently correlated with a higher mortality if it remains greater than 4 mmol/L.[23] A retrospective observational study of 553 CAP patients calculated a national early warning score-lactate score (NEWS-L score) based on systolic blood pressure, heart rate, respiratory rate, temperature, pulse oximetry, supplemental oxygen use, and lactate level. This study found that the mean lactate level was 1.6 and was significantly higher in nonsurvivors versus survivors (2.5 vs 1.5). In addition, the NEWS-L score was comparable to PSI and CURB-65 in predicting inpatient mortality in adult CAP patients.[51]

PCT levels have been shown to increase with severity of pneumonia, unlike WBC or CRP.[52] In a prospective observational cohort study, looking at 472 patients admitted to the ICU, daily PCT measurements were followed. A high maximum PCT level and a PCT increase for 1 day were found to be independent predictors of 90-day mortality, with a relative risk after 1-day increase of 1.8, after 2-day increase of 2.2, and 3-day increase of 2.8.[52,53] The German multicenter CAPNETZ trial looked at 1671 patients with CAP (66.6% of whom were hospitalized, whereas the remainder were treated as outpatients) and followed their PCT, CRP, WBC, and CRB-65 for 28 days.[33] The PCT level on admission had a similar prognostic accuracy (looking at severity and outcome) to CRB-65 and a higher prognostic accuracy than CRP and leukocyte count. PCT on admission in nonsurvivors (median of 0.88) was significantly higher than that of survivors (median of 0.13). The optimal prognostic accuracy for mortality prediction with PCT was with a cutoff of 0.228 ng/mL (sensitivity of 84.3% and specificity of 66.6%). The AUC for PCT was 0.80, which was not significantly different than CRB-65 (0.79), but significantly higher than CRP (0.62) or WBC (0.61). By combining PCT and CRB-65, the AUC improved to 0.83.[33]

Another large prospective randomized trial by Schuetz and colleagues[53] demonstrated that PCT on admission had only a moderate prognostic ability to predict 30-day mortality, but follow-up PCT measurements did show better prognostic performance. Specifically, the increase in PCT from day 0 to day 3, with a less pronounced PCT decrease thereafter, was identified in nonsurvivors. In addition, the risk of adverse events significantly increased by 3-fold from 6% in the lowest PCT tier to 19% in the highest tier. These data support the idea that a serial PCT increase accurately prognosticates the potential for adverse events associated with CAP, including ICU admission and empyema.[53] Another prospective observational study performed on 63 patients with VAP measured PCT and CRP on days 1 and 7 and likewise found that using a PCT threshold of 0.5 ng/mL on day 7, PCT had a 90% sensitivity and 88% specificity for unfavorable outcomes (including death, VAP recurrence, and extrapulmonary infections).[41]

The MOSES study was a large prospective, multicenter, US trial that evaluated the ability of serial PCT levels to predict mortality in 858 patients admitted to the ICU for treatment of severe sepsis. The patients who were not able to decrease their PCT level by greater than 80% by day 4 were found to have an increase in their 28-day mortality compared with the patients who were able to achieve a greater than 80% reduction in PCT by day 4.[34]

SUMMARY

The use of various biomarkers in the management of pneumonia patients can help identify those patients who should be admitted to the hospital, cared for in the ICU, and may help with decisions related to duration of antibiotic therapy and/or patient prognosis. At this time, there is not a biomarker that on its own will establish a diagnosis of pneumonia. Current US standard of care supports the decision on initiation of antibiotic therapy and the type of antibiotic therapy based on guidelines and a clinical assessment of the patient, which is typically aided by severity guidelines with or without the use of additional biomarkers. As more sensitive and specific biomarkers are found and greater experience is obtained with the use of biomarkers, there may be an expanded use for biomarkers in the diagnosis, management, and treatment of pneumonia in the future.

REFERENCES

1. Fine MJ, Auble TE, Yealy DM, et al. A prediction rule to identify low-risk patients with community-acquired pneumonia. N Engl J Med 1997;336(4):243–50.
2. Kalil AC, Metersky ML, Klompas M, et al. Management of adults with hospital-acquired and ventilator-associated pneumonia: 2016 clinical practice guidelines by the infectious diseases society of America and the American Thoracic Society. Clin Infect Dis 2016;63(5):e61–111.
3. Dellinger RP, Levy MM, Rhodes A, et al. Surviving sepsis campaign: international guidelines for management of severe sepsis and septic shock: 2012. Crit Care Med 2013;41(2):580–637.
4. Mandell LA, Wunderink RG, Anzueto A, et al. Infectious Diseases Society of America/American Thoracic Society consensus guidelines on the management of community-acquired pneumonia in adults. Clin Infect Dis 2007;44(Suppl 2):S27–72.
5. Kaziani K, Sotiriou A, Dimopoulos G. Duration of pneumonia therapy and the role of biomarkers. Curr Opin Infect Dis 2017;30(2):221–5.
6. Musher DM, Thorner AR. Community-acquired pneumonia. N Engl J Med 2014;371(17):1619–28.
7. Klompas M. Ventilator-associated conditions versus ventilator-associated pneumonia: different by design. Curr Infect Dis Rep 2014;16(10):430.
8. Magill SS, Klompas M, Balk R, et al. Developing a new, national approach to surveillance for ventilator-associated events*. Crit Care Med 2013;41(11):2467–75.
9. Craven DE, Chroneou A, Zias N, et al. Ventilator-associated tracheobronchitis: the impact of targeted antibiotic therapy on patient outcomes. Chest 2009;135(2):521–8.
10. Nseir S, Favory R, Jozefowicz E, et al. Antimicrobial treatment for ventilator-associated tracheobronchitis: a randomized, controlled, multicenter study. Crit Care 2008;12(3):R62.
11. Brechot N, Hekimian G, Chastre J, et al. Procalcitonin to guide antibiotic therapy in the ICU. Int J Antimicrob Agents 2015;46(Suppl 1):S19–24.
12. Gibot S, Cravoisy A, Levy B, et al. Soluble triggering receptor expressed on myeloid cells and the diagnosis of pneumonia. N Engl J Med 2004;350(5):451–8.
13. Angus DC, Marrie TJ, Obrosky DS, et al. Severe community-acquired pneumonia: use of intensive care services and evaluation of American and British Thoracic Society Diagnostic criteria. Am J Respir Crit Care Med 2002;166(5):717–23.
14. Renaud B, Santin A, Coma E, et al. Association between timing of intensive care unit admission and outcomes for emergency department patients with community-acquired pneumonia. Crit Care Med 2009;37(11):2867–74.

15. Lim WS, van der Eerden MM, Laing R, et al. Defining community acquired pneumonia severity on presentation to hospital: an international derivation and validation study. Thorax 2003;58(5):377–82.

16. Capelastegui A, Espana PP, Quintana JM, et al. Validation of a predictive rule for the management of community-acquired pneumonia. Eur Respir J 2006;27(1):151–7.

17. Espana PP, Capelastegui A, Gorordo I, et al. Development and validation of a clinical prediction rule for severe community-acquired pneumonia. Am J Respir Crit Care Med 2006;174(11):1249–56.

18. Gilbert DN. Use of plasma procalcitonin levels as an adjunct to clinical microbiology. J Clin Microbiol 2010;48(7):2325–9.

19. Christ-Crain M, Schuetz P, Muller B. Biomarkers in the management of pneumonia. Expert Rev Respir Med 2008;2(5):565–72.

20. Nair GB, Niederman MS. Pneumonia: considerations for the critically ill patient. In: Parrillo JE, Dellinger RP, editors. Critical care medicine: principles of diagnosis and management in the adult. 4h edition. Philadelphia: Elsevier/Saunders; 2013. p. 1. online resource (xx, 1447 pages).

21. Lee JH, Kim J, Kim K, et al. Albumin and C-reactive protein have prognostic significance in patients with community-acquired pneumonia. J Crit Care Jun 2011;26(3):287–94.

22. Povoa P, Coelho L, Almeida E, et al. C-reactive protein as a marker of infection in critically ill patients. Clin Microbiol Infect 2005;11(2):101–8.

23. Suetrong B, Walley KR. Lactic acidosis in sepsis: it's not all anaerobic: implications for diagnosis and management. Chest 2016;149(1):252–61.

24. Ewig S, Welte T. Biomarkers in the diagnosis of pneumonia in the critically ill: don't shoot the piano player. Intensive Care Med 2008;34(6):981–4.

25. Kopterides P, Siempos II, Tsangaris I, et al. Procalcitonin-guided algorithms of antibiotic therapy in the intensive care unit: a systematic review and meta-analysis of randomized controlled trials. Crit Care Med 2010;38(11):2229–41.

26. Schuetz P, Christ-Crain M, Muller B. Biomarkers to improve diagnostic and prognostic accuracy in systemic infections. Curr Opin Crit Care 2007;13: 578–85.

27. Schuetz P, Christ-Crain M, Thomann R, et al. Effect of procalcitonin-based guidelines vs standard guidelines on antibiotic use in lower respiratory tract infections: the ProHOSP randomized controlled trial. JAMA 2009;302(10):1059–66.

28. Schuetz P, Albrich W, Christ-Crain M, et al. Procalcitonin for guidance of antibiotic therapy. Expert Rev Anti Infect Ther 2010;8(5):575–87.

29. Delevaux I, Andre M, Colombier M, et al. Can Procalcitonin measurement help in differentiating between bacterial infection and other kinds of inflammatory processes? Ann Rheum Dis 2003;62: 337–40.

30. Staehler M, Hammer C, Meiser B, et al. Differential Diagnosis of acute rejection and infection with procalcitonin and cytokines. Langenbecks Arch Chir 1997;1:205–9.

31. Al Nawas B, Shah PM. Procalcitonin in patients with and without immunosuppression and sepsis. Infection 1996;24:434–6.

32. Amour J, Birenbaum A, Langeron O, et al. Influence of renal dysfunction on the accuracy of procalcitonin for the diagnosis of postoperative infection after vascular surgery. Crit Care Med 2008;36:1147–54.

33. Kruger S, Ewig S, Marre R, et al. Procalcitonin predicts patients at low risk of death from community-acquired pneumonia across all CRB-65 classes. The Eur Respir J 2008;31(2):349–55.

34. Schuetz P, Birkhahn R, Sherwin R, et al. Serial procalcitonin predicts mortality in severe sepsis patients: results from the multicenter procalcitonin MOnitoring SEpsis (MOSES) study. Crit Care Med 2017;45(5):781–9.

35. Schuetz P, Wirz Y, Sager R, et al. Effect of procalcitonin-guided antibiotic treatment on mortality in acute respiratory infections: a patient level meta-analysis. Lancet Infect Dis 2018;18(1):95–107.

36. Phua J, Koay ES, Zhang D, et al. Soluble triggering receptor expressed on myeloid cells-1 in acute respiratory infections. The Eur Respir J 2006;28(4): 695–702.

37. Loke YK, Kwok CS, Niruban A, et al. Value of severity scales in predicting mortality from community-acquired pneumonia: systematic review and meta-analysis. Thorax 2010;65(10):884–90.

38. Ramirez P, Ferrer M, Marti V, et al. Inflammatory biomarkers and prediction for intensive care unit admission in severe community-acquired pneumonia. Crit Care Med 2011;39(10):2211–7.

39. Schuetz P, Amin DN, Greenwalkd JL. Role of procalcitonin in managing adult patients with respiratory tract infections. Chest 2012;141:1063–73.

40. Self WH, Grijalva CG, Williams DJ, et al. Procalcitonin as an early marker of the need for invasive respiratory or vasopressor support in adults with community-acquired pneumonia. Chest 2016;150: 819–28.

41. Luyt CE, Guerin V, Combes A, et al. Procalcitonin kinetics as a prognostic marker of ventilator-associated pneumonia. Am J Respir Crit Care Med 2005;171(1):48–53.

42. de Jong E, van Oers JA, Beishuizen A, et al. Efficacy and safety of procalcitonin guidance in reducing the duration of antibiotic treatment in critically ill patients: a randomised, controlled, open-label trial. The Lancet Infect Dis 2016;16(7):819–27.

43. Schuetz P, Briel M, Mueller B. Clinical outcomes associated with procalcitonin algorithms to guide

antibiotic therapy in respiratory tract infections. JAMA 2013;309(7):717–8.

44. Huang HB, Peng JM, Weng L, et al. Procalcitonin-guided antibiotic therapy in intensive care unit patients: a systematic review and meta-analysis. Ann Intensive Care 2017;7(1):114.

45. Schuetz P, Wirz Y, Sager R, et al. Procalcitonin to initiate or discontinue antibiotics in acute respiratory tract infections. Cochrane Database Syst Rev 2017;(10):CD007498.

46. Lam SW, Bauer SR, Fowler R, et al. Systematic review and meta-analysis of procalcitonin-guidance versus usual care for antimicrobial management in critically ill patients: focus on subgroups based on antibiotic initiation, cessation, or mixed strategies. Crit Care Med 2018;46:684–90.

47. Iankova I, Thompson-Leduc P, Kirson NY, et al. Efficacy and safety of procalcitonin guidance in patients with suspected or confirmed sepsis: a systematic review and meta-analysis. Crit Care Med 2018;46:691–8.

48. Cataudella E, Giraffa CM, Di Marca S, et al. Neutrophil-to-lymphocyte ratio: an emerging marker predicting prognosis in elderly adults with community-acquired pneumonia. J Am Geriatr Soc 2017;65(8):1796–801.

49. Huang DT, Angus DC, Kellum JA, et al. Midregional proadrenomedullin as a prognostic tool in community-acquired pneumonia. Chest 2009; 136(3):823–31.

50. Gu WJ, Zhang Z, Bakker J. Early lactate clearance-guided therapy in patients with sepsis: a meta-analysis with trial sequential analysis of randomized controlled trials. Intensive Care Med 2015;41(10): 1862–3.

51. Jo S, Jeong T, Lee JB, et al. Validation of modified early warning score using serum lactate level in community-acquired pneumonia patients. The National Early Warning Score-Lactate score. Am J Emerg Med 2016;34(3):536–41.

52. Jensen JU, Heslet L, Jensen TH, et al. Procalcitonin increase in early identification of critically ill patients at high risk of mortality. Crit Care Med 2006;34(10): 2596–602.

53. Schuetz P, Suter-Widmer I, Chaudri A, et al. Prognostic value of procalcitonin in community-acquired pneumonia. Eur Respir J 2011;37(2): 384–92.

Influenza and Viral Pneumonia

Rodrigo Cavallazzi, MD[a],*, Julio A. Ramirez, MD[b]

KEYWORDS

- Influenza • Virus • Pneumonia • Epidemiology • Antiviral • Symptoms • Polymerase chain reaction

KEY POINTS

- Most community-acquired respiratory viruses are RNA viruses except for adenovirus and human bocavirus, which are DNA viruses.
- Using molecular techniques, respiratory viruses are identified in approximately 25% of patients with community-acquired pneumonia.
- In addition to the community-acquired respiratory viruses, immunocompromised patients are particularly susceptible to viruses of the Herpesviridae family.
- It is difficult to diagnose influenza or other viral infection on clinical grounds.
- Patients with influenza pneumonia should be treated with a neuraminidase inhibitor. For other viruses, treatment options are limited.

INTRODUCTION

Respiratory viral infections cause substantial burden. They are prevalent and tend to affect those who are more vulnerable, such as children, elderly, and people living in developing areas, such as sub Saharan Africa and Southeast Asia.[1] The advent of molecular techniques has facilitated the identification of respiratory viruses in patients with pneumonia and has shed a light on how commonly these viruses occur in patients with pneumonia. With the currently available diagnostic tools, viral pathogens are more often identified than bacterial pathogens in community-acquired pneumonia.[2] A large amount of effort is currently being dedicated to elucidate the pathogenicity of respiratory viruses and the interaction between viruses and bacteria in the setting of pneumonia.

Since the last century, a number of devastating pandemics and outbreaks related to respiratory viruses have occurred.[3,4] Recently, there has been a growing interest in the development of new antiviral medications for respiratory infection. In this article, we provide an overview of pneumonia caused by influenza and other respiratory viruses from the practicing clinician perspective and with a focus on the adult population.

MICROBIOLOGY OVERVIEW

Human influenza is an RNA virus that belongs to the Orthomyxoviridae family and is categorized into types A, B, and C based on its nucleoprotein and matrix protein. Influenza A virus is subcategorized into subtypes such as H1N1, H1N2, and H3N2 based on hemagglutinin and neuraminidase.

Conflict of Interest: R. Cavallazzi was a site investigator for a clinical trial investigating a new antiviral for adults with respiratory syncytial virus infection. The study was led by Gilead. R. Cavallazzi was a site investigator for a clinical trial investigating a new drug for influenza. The study was led by GlaxoSmithKline. Funding: None.
[a] Division of Pulmonary, Critical Care, and Sleep Disorders, University of Louisville, 550 South Jackson Street, ACB, A3R27, Louisville, KY 40202, USA; [b] Division of Infectious Diseases, University of Louisville, Med Center One, 501 E. Broadway Suite 100, Louisville, KY 40202, USA
* Corresponding author.
E-mail address: r0cava01@louisville.edu

chestmed.theclinics.com

Influenza B is subcategorized into the B/Yamagata and the B/Victoria lineages.[3,5,6] Most influenza infections are caused by types A and B.[7] The gene mutation that influenza undergoes every year is called antigenic drift and is responsible for seasonal outbreaks. Conversely, influenza pandemics are caused by antigenic shift, which occurs when new hemagglutinin or neuraminidase subtypes are acquired.[7]

Most community-acquired respiratory viruses are RNA viruses except for adenovirus and human bocavirus, which are DNA viruses.[8–15] The Paramyxoviridae family includes respiratory syncytial virus, parainfluenza, and human metapneumovirus. A distinctive feature of the Paramyxoviridae family viruses is the presence of a fusion protein.[9,12,14] The fusion protein, which enables the integration of the virus with the cell membrane, allowing the introduction of the viral genome into the cell cytoplasm, is a potential target for vaccines and antivirals.[16] The Picornaviridae family of virus, which includes enterovirus and human rhinovirus, are characterized by a capsid that contains the viral genome. The capsid has a large cleft (or canyon) that binds to adhesion molecules on the cell surface, leading to the eventual entry of the viral genome into the cell. The capsid and the adhesion molecules are potential targets of antivirals[17,18] (Table 1).

INCIDENCE AND EPIDEMIOLOGY
Epidemiology of Viral Respiratory Infection in Community-Acquired Pneumonia

A systematic review included 31 observational studies that enrolled patients with community-acquired pneumonia who underwent viral polymerase chain reaction testing. The pooled proportion of patients with viral infection was 24.5% (95% confidence interval [CI] 21.5%–27.5%; I^2 = 92.9%).[19] Most of these studies were performed in the inpatient setting and viral polymerase chain reaction was obtained mostly from nasal or oropharyngeal swab. In the only study that was performed in the outpatient setting, the proportion of viral infection was 12.1% (95% CI 7.7%–16.5%; I^2 = 0.0%).[20] The pooled proportion of viral infection was 44.2% (95% CI 35.1%–53.3%; I^2 = 0%) from studies in which a lower respiratory sample was obtained in more than half of the patients.[21,22] The proportion of dual bacterial and viral infection was 10% (95% CI 8%–11%; I^2 = 93.1%). Although the presence of a viral infection did not significantly increase the risk of short-term death, patients with dual bacterial-viral infection had twice the risk of death as compared with patients without dual infection.[19] It is important to

note that the identification of a viral pathogen in a patient with pneumonia does not necessarily mean that the virus has a pathogenic effect, particularly if the identification is via nasopharyngeal swab (**Fig. 1**, **Table 2**).

Epidemiology of Viral Respiratory Infection in Immunocompromised Patients

In immunocompromised patients with pneumonia, infection by respiratory viruses is exceedingly common. Surveillance studies show that a respiratory viral pathogen is identified in close to a third of hospitalized patients with leukemia or hematopoietic stem cell transplantation and respiratory symptoms. Pneumonia occurs in most immunosuppressed patients infected with a respiratory viral pathogen.[23] Immunocompromised patients are commonly infected by the same respiratory viruses that cause infection in immunocompetent patients. However, viruses of the Herpesviridae family also tend to cause infection in immunocompromised patients. As an example, in an early series of patients who underwent allogeneic bone marrow transplantation, cytomegalovirus was the most common viral pathogen.[24] Varicella zoster virus reactivation can occur in patients after hematopoietic stem cell transplantation with early series reporting incidences ranging from 22% to 41%.[25,26] It is not unusual for the infection to present in a disseminated form in these patients, and pneumonia is one of the complications.[25–27]

Epidemiology of Hospital-Acquired Viral Respiratory Infection

Traditionally, hospital-acquired respiratory viral infection has been thought to be limited to immunocompromised patients. However, it is now known that this can also commonly occur in immunocompetent patients. This was highlighted by a prospective cohort study that included 262 patients with hospital-acquired pneumonia. The proportion of viral infection was 36.1% in immunocompromised patients and 11.2% in non-immunocompromised patients. The identified viruses were respiratory syncytial virus (6.1%), parainfluenza virus (6.1%), influenza virus (3.8%), cytomegalovirus (1.9%), human coronavirus (1.5%), bocavirus (0.8%), human metapneumovirus (0.8%), and adenovirus (0.4%).[28] These data underscore the importance of infection control measures in patients with pneumonia.

Pandemics and Outbreaks

Since the past century, there have been 5 influenza pandemics: 1918 to 1919 Spanish influenza, 1957 H2N2 Asian influenza, 1968 H3N2 Hong Kong

Table 1
Characteristics and taxonomy of commonly identified respiratory viruses in patients with community-acquired pneumonia

Virus	Genome	Family	Important Antigenic Structures
Influenza	RNA	Orthomyxoviridae	Surface glycoproteins hemagglutinin (HA) and the neuraminidase (NA).[8]
Respiratory syncytial virus	RNA	Paramyxoviridae	Attachment glycoprotein (G) and fusion (F) glycoprotein.[9]
Human rhinovirus	RNA	Picornaviridae	Viral capsid proteins VP1, VP2, VP3, and VP4.[10]
Adenovirus	DNA	Adenoviridae	Capsid major structures: hexon (the building block of the capsid), penton base, and polypetides.[11]
Parainfluenza	RNA	Paramyxoviridae	Surface glycoproteins hemagglutinin-neuraminidase and fusion protein. Membrane protein.[12]
Coronavirus	RNA	Coronaviridae	Membrane glycoprotein and spike protein.[13]
Human metapneumovirus	RNA	Paramyxoviridae	Virus fusion (F) glycoprotein.[14]
Human bocavirus	DNA	Parvoviridae	Capsid viral proteins (VPs), VP1, and VP2.[15]

influenza, 1977 H1N1 Russian influenza, and the 2009 H1N1 pandemic.[3,4] It is estimated that the 2009 H1N1 pandemic caused 201,200 respiratory deaths and 83,000 cardiovascular deaths. Most of these deaths occurred in patients younger than 65 years old.[29] In 2003, a major outbreak of atypical pneumonia was reported. The cases initially clustered in China but were subsequently reported worldwide. The pneumonia often resulted in acute respiratory failure and was named severe acute respiratory syndrome.[30] Subsequently, the etiologic agent of this disease was identified as a novel coronavirus,[31,32] which was named the Urbani strain of severe acute respiratory syndrome–associated coronavirus.[31] In 2012, another novel coronavirus was isolated from a patient with pneumonia in Saudi Arabia.[33] The virus was subsequently named Middle East respiratory syndrome coronavirus.[34] Infection by this virus causes an illness that is clinically similar to that caused by severe acute respiratory syndrome–associated coronavirus but with higher mortality.[35] Cases of Middle East respiratory syndrome coronavirus were initially reported in Saudi Arabia but were subsequently reported in other countries, including the United States, typically in persons who had traveled from the Arabian Peninsula.[36–38]

Influenza

The incidence of influenza can vary substantially in different seasons. As an example, using online surveillance data, it was estimated that the influenza attack rate for adults aged 20 to 64 years old was 30.5% (95% CI 4.4–49.3) in the 2012 to 2013 season and 7.1 (95% CI −5.1 to 32.5) in the 2013 to 2014 season.[39] The rates of influenza-associated hospitalization per 100,000 persons varied from 4.8 to 18.7 in 3 different seasons in the United States.[40]

Different studies showed that approximately one-third of hospitalized patients with laboratory-confirmed influenza have pneumonia.[41–43] In a study that included 4765 patients hospitalized with influenza, those with pneumonia were older

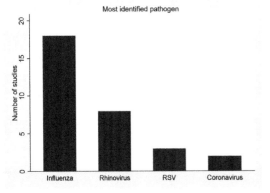

Fig. 1. Number of studies according to most commonly identified viral pathogen. RSV, respiratory syncytial virus. (*Data from* Burk M, El-Kersh K, Saad M, et al. Viral infection in community-acquired pneumonia: a systematic review and meta-analysis. Eur Respir Rev 2016;25(140):178–88.)

Table 2
Different scenarios for the effect of an identified viral pathogen in the setting of pneumonia

Virus is a "bystander" and does not have a pathogenic effect.	Although uncommon in adults, asymptomatic carriage of respiratory viruses occurs.[126]
Virus has a pathogenic effect and is causing pneumonia in isolation.	Potential mechanisms include dysregulation of cytokines and chemokines, infection of epithelial cells in the lungs, and apoptosis.[127]
Virus has a pathogenic effect and is causing pneumonia along with a bacterial pathogen.	A study showed that the mortality for patients with community-acquired pneumonia and bacterial and viral coinfection is higher.[19]
Virus caused a recent infection that prompted a secondary bacterial infection.	This occurs particularly with *Streptococcus pneumoniae* or *Staphylococcus aureus* infection following influenza infection.[128] Lag time of 2–4 wk between the viral and bacterial infection.[129] Polymerase chain reaction test may remain positive for up to 5 wk after a viral infection.[130]

than those without pneumonia (median age of 74 years vs 69 years; $P < .01$). In a multivariate analyses, the following factors were significant predictors of pneumonia in hospitalized patients with influenza: age older than 75 years (odds ratio [OR] 1.27; 95% CI 1.10–1.46), white race (OR 1.24; 95% CI 1.03–1.49), nursing home residence (OR 1.37; 95% CI 1.14–1.66), chronic lung disease (OR 1.37; 95% CI 1.18–1.59), and immunosuppression (OR 1.45; 95% CI 1.19–1.78). Asthma was associated with lower odds of pneumonia (OR 0.76; 95% CI 0.62–0.92).[42] In another study

of 579 adult patients hospitalized with laboratory-confirmed influenza, a multivariate analyses showed that the following factors were significantly associated with pneumonia: older age (OR 1.026; 95% CI 1.013–1.04), higher C-reactive protein, mg/dL (OR 1.128; 95% CI 1.088–1.17), smoking (OR 1.818; 95% CI 1.115–2.965), low albumin level (OR 2.518; 95% CI 1.283–4.9), acute respiratory failure (OR 4.525; 95% CI 2.964–6.907), and productive cough (OR 8.173; 95% CI 3.674–18.182).[43]

During an influenza season, the attributed mortality to pneumonia and influenza in the United States ranges from 5.6% to 11.1%.[44] In a cohort study that included laboratory-confirmed cases of influenza admitted to the hospital, those with pneumonia, as compared with those without pneumonia, were more likely to require intensive care unit (ICU) admission (27% vs 10%) and mechanical ventilation (18% vs 5%), and to die (9% vs 2%)[42] (**Fig. 2**).

Respiratory Syncytial Virus

In older subjects, the burden of respiratory syncytial virus infection is similar to that of influenza. A study prospectively followed 2 outpatient cohorts during 4 seasons: 608 heathy elderly patients and 540 high-risk adults. High-risk status was defined as the presence of congestive heart failure or chronic pulmonary disease. Respiratory syncytial virus infection was diagnosed in 3% to 7% of healthy elderly subjects and 4% to 10% of high-risk subjects. This accounted for 1.5 respiratory syncytial virus infections per 100 person-months in high-risk adults and 0.9 in healthy elderly subjects.[45] In an analysis of hospitalization and viral surveillance data that encompassed several years, it was estimated that the respiratory syncytial virus–associated hospitalization rate per 100,000 person-years in the United States was 12.8 (95% CI 2.4–73.9) for patients age 50 to 64 years old and 86.1 (95% CI 37.3–326.2) for patients aged ≥65 years old. In contrast to influenza-associated hospitalizations, the rates of respiratory syncytial virus–associated hospitalizations were relatively similar across the years.[46] In a cohort of 1388 hospitalized adults older than 65 years or with underlying cardiopulmonary diseases, respiratory syncytial virus infection was diagnosed in 8% to 13% of these patients depending on the year. Of the 132 hospitalized patients with respiratory syncytial virus infection, 41 (31%) had an infiltrate on chest radiograph, 20 (15%) required ICU admission, 17 (13%) required mechanical ventilation, and 10 (8%) died.[45]

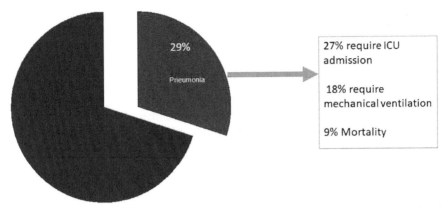

Fig. 2. Proportion of pneumonia and associated outcomes in patients admitted to the hospital with influenza infection. (*Data from* Garg S, Jain S, Dawood FS, et al. Pneumonia among adults hospitalized with laboratory-confirmed seasonal influenza virus infection-United States, 2005-2008. BMC Infect Dis 2015;15:369.)

Epidemiology of Other Respiratory Viruses

Rhinovirus

- Most common cause of common cold, a self-limited acute illness that occurs 2 to 4 times per year in adults.
- This infection is characterized by sneezing, nasal discharge, sore throat, and low-grade fever.[47]
- Rhinovirus tends to occur more often in the early fall or spring.[48]
- Rhinovirus is commonly identified in the upper respiratory tract of patients with community-acquired pneumonia via molecular techniques. In fact, rhinovirus was the most commonly identified pathogen in a large cohort of adult patients hospitalized with community-acquired pneumonia conducted in the United States.[2]

Coronavirus

- Occurs more commonly in the winter and follows a seasonal pattern that resembles that of influenza.[49]
- Coronaviruses HCoV-229E, HCoV-NL63, HCoV-OC43, and HCoV-HKU1 have ubiquitous circulation and are a usual etiology of common cold.[35]
- Coronaviruses have also been commonly associated with lower respiratory tract symptoms.[49]
- Adult hospitalized patients with coronavirus infection are often immunocompromised, and pneumonia is a common occurrence.[50]
- Severe acute respiratory syndrome coronavirus and Middle East respiratory syndrome coronavirus caused outbreaks and pandemics of an acute respiratory illness, often leading to respiratory failure.[35]

Adenovirus

- Adenovirus is a common cause of upper respiratory tract symptoms and conjunctivitis.[51]
- Adult patients with adenovirus pneumonia are relatively young.
- Different studies have reported that patients with community-acquired pneumonia and adenovirus infection have mean age that ranges from 30 to 38 years old.[52,53]
- Adenovirus also causes serious infection in immunocompromised patients. The adenovirus species found in immunocompromised patients are not typically found in the community, which indicates endogenous viral reactivation in those patients.[54]
- No clear seasonality, although cases may spike in some months.[55]
- A number of outbreaks caused by adenovirus have been reported. Some examples include reports of outbreaks in military personnel,[56] psychiatric care facility,[57] and ICU.[58]

Parainfluenza

- Most infections are caused by parainfluenza 1 and 3.[59] Parainfluenza 2 is less commonly identified, and parainfluenza 4 is a rare cause of respiratory infection.
- In adults, influenzalike symptoms are a common manifestation of parainfluenza infection.[60] In children, common presentations are croup and bronchiolitis.[59]
- In a population-based study of adults hospitalized for lower respiratory tract infection in 2 counties in Ohio, parainflueza-1 and parainfluenza-3 were detected in 2.5% to 3.1% of tested patients. Parainfluenza-1 epidemic season spanned the summer-autumn. Parainfluenza-3 epidemic season

spanned the spring-summer. Median age was 61.5 years for parainfluenza-1–infected patients and 77.5 years for parainfluenza-3–infected patients. Of those infected by parainfluenza-3, 59% had an infiltrate on chest radiograph, 23% required ICU stay, and none died.[61]

Metapneumovirus

- It has been identified in 4.5% of acute respiratory illnesses of adults prospectively followed as outpatients.[62]
- It has been identified in 4% of patients with community-acquired pneumonia.[63]
- Among outpatient adults, those of younger age tend to be more commonly infected by metapneumovirus, which has been presumably attributed to their closer contact with children; however, hospitalized patients with metapneumovirus infection are older.[62]
- Mean age in a series of community-acquired pneumonia and metapneumovirus infection: 62 years.[63]
- In the outpatient setting, cough and nasal congestion are the most common symptoms.[62]
- In patients with metapneumovirus infection and pneumonia, common symptoms are cough with sputum production, dyspnea, and fatigue.[63]

Human bocavirus

- Commonly identified in symptomatic and asymptomatic children but it seems to be a less common cause of respiratory symptoms in adults.[64]
- Human bocavirus infection is more common in the winter.[65]
- Common clinical presentations include upper respiratory tract symptoms, bronchiolitis. and pneumonia.[66] Cases of encephalitis have been reported.[67,68]
- It has been detected in acute respiratory illness of adults with immunosuppression and chronic lung disease.[69,70]
- A study showed that it can be often identified in the sinus tissue specimens of adult patients with chronic sinusitis.[71]

CLINICAL PRESENTATION
Clinical Manifestations

Patients with influenza infection in general (not just pneumonia) commonly present with cough, fever, fatigue, myalgia, runny nose, and sweating. Wheezing as a symptom can occur in close to half of the patients.[72] Patients with influenza pneumonia tend to have the same symptoms as patients with nonpneumonic influenza infection but an important distinction is that patients with pneumonia more often have dyspnea.[73] Perhaps the greatest clinical clue for influenza in a patient with acute respiratory symptoms (or pneumonia) is whether the patient is presenting during an influenza epidemic. As an example, the absence of coughing and temperature higher than 37.8°C make influenza very unlikely in patients presenting with influenzalike illness outside an influenza epidemic but has a lesser impact on the likelihood of influenza if the same patient presenting during an epidemic. On the other hand, the presence of these symptoms during an epidemic substantially increases the probability of influenza but has a lesser impact outside of an epidemic.[74]

Studies have assessed the accuracy of clinical manifestations for the diagnosis of influenza in patients with acute respiratory symptoms. Some of the earlier studies were limited by retrospective design, leading to potential classification bias, or by the reliance on clinical manifestations for the final diagnosis of influenza, leading to incorporation bias.[75] More recent studies used a prospective design and viral polymerase chain reaction test as the reference standard. A prospective study enrolled 100 patients with influenzalike illness who presented to 3 different clinics. Viral polymerase chain reaction test was used for the diagnosis of influenza. The accuracy of a number of symptoms was tested. On multivariate analysis, only cough and temperature remained significant predictors of influenza.[76] In a prospective study of 258 patients who presented to the emergency department with acute respiratory symptoms, a symptom inventory and influenza polymerase chain reaction test was applied to the patients. Using polymerase chain reaction test as the reference standard, the accuracy of clinical judgment, decision rule, and rapid influenza test was provided. The presence of cough and fever had a positive likelihood ratio of 5.1 and a negative likelihood ratio of 0.7.[72] In a prospective study of 270 high-risk patients who presented to an emergency department with acute respiratory illness, clinicians were asked whether they thought the patient had influenza. Viral polymerase chain reaction was the reference standard. A clinician diagnosis of influenza had a positive likelihood ratio of 1.63 and negative likelihood ratio of 0.82.[77] Likelihood ratios are an interesting way of providing the accuracy of symptoms or clinical diagnosis because they allow for the estimate of the probability of a disease after taking into account the pre-test probability[78] (**Fig. 3**). See **Table 3** for a summary of these studies.

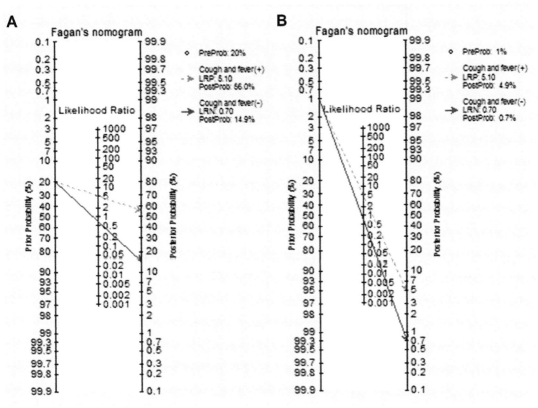

Fig. 3. Probability of influenza according to presence of combined cough and fever in patients presenting during influenza season (*A*) and outside the influenza season (*B*). (*Data for likelihood ratios from* Stein J, Louie J, Flanders S, et al. Performance characteristics of clinical diagnosis, a clinical decision rule, and a rapid influenza test in the detection of influenza infection in a community sample of adults. Ann Emerg Med 2005;46(5):412–9.)

Overall, the previously described studies indicate that the predictive value of symptoms, combination of symptoms, or clinical impression for the diagnosis of influenza is only modest for patients presenting with acute illness. Symptoms or clinical impression are not enough to rule in or rule out influenza. In fact, clinicians failed to clinically diagnose influenza in approximately two-thirds of influenza-confirmed patients in a prospective series.[77] Ultimately, clinicians need to pay close attention to surveillance data, and if there is evidence of influenza activity in the area where they practice, any acute febrile respiratory illness should place influenza as a high possibility in the differential diagnosis. In the United States, the Centers for Disease Control and Prevention provide weekly data on influenza activity according to regions in the country. This is available at https://www.cdc.gov/flu/weekly/index.htm. Other important aspects of clinical history include close contact with persons with acute febrile illness, and recent travel. Additionally, it is important to realize that in some tropical countries, influenza circulates throughout the year.[79]

A hallmark of respiratory syncytial virus infection is the presence of wheezing, which occurs in a higher frequency as compared with patients with influenza. Hospitalized patients with respiratory syncytial virus infection may present with clinical-radiological dissociation, in which patients may appear toxemic despite mild radiological abnormalities. In a cohort of 118 hospitalized patients with respiratory syncytial virus infection, the most common symptoms were cough (97%), dyspnea (95%), wheezing (73%), and nasal congestion (68%). On physical examination, wheezing was present in 82% of the patients. A temperature higher than 39°C was present in only 13% of the patients. It should be noted, however, that these percentages are for all hospitalized patients with respiratory syncytial virus infection. When assessing only those hospitalized patients with respiratory syncytial virus infection and pneumonia, wheezing and nasal congestion were less common.[80] In another study of 57 patients with respiratory syncytial virus infection and clinical diagnosis of pneumonia, the most common symptoms were cough (88%), dyspnea (82%), wheezing (79%),

Table 3
Characteristics of studies that prospectively assessed the accuracy of symptoms for the diagnosis of influenza infection

Author, Year	Design	Setting	Sample	Inclusion Criteria	Reference	Results
Boivin et al,[76] 2000	Prospective cohort	Patients presenting to 3 outpatient clinics	100	Flulike illness of <72 h duration	PCR and culture from nasopharyngeal swab	Cough and fever (>38°C): Sens of 77.6% Spec of 55.0% PPV of 86.8% NPV of 39.3%
Stein et al,[72] 2005	Prospective cohort	Adult patients presenting to the emergency department	258	New illness within the past 3 wk associated with cough, fever, or upper respiratory tract symptoms		Clinician judgment: Sens of 29% (95% CI 18%–43%) Spec of 92% (95% CI 87%–95%) PLR of 3.8 (95% CI 1.9–7.5) NLR of 0.8 (95% CI 0.6–0.9) Decision rule (cough and fever): Sens of 40% (95% CI 27%–54%) Spec of 92% (95% CI 87%–95%) PLR of 5.1 (95% CI 2.7–9.6) NLR of 0.7 (95% CI 0.5–0.8)

| Dugas et al,[77] 2015 | Prospective cohort | Adult patients presenting to the emergency department | 270 | Fever or any respiratory-related symptom | PCR from nasopharyngeal swab | Clinical judgment: Sens of 36% (95% CI 22%–52%) Spec of 78% (95% CI 72%–83%) PLR of 1.63 (95% CI 1.01–2.62) NLR of 0.82 (95% CI 0.65–1.04) Influenzalike illness (fever $\geq$37.8°C with either cough or sore throat): Sens of 31% (95% CI 18%–47%) Spec of 88% (95% CI 83%–92%) PLR of 2.61 (95% CI 1.47–4.64) NLR of 0.78 (95% CI 0.64–0.96) |

Abbreviations: CI, confidence interval; NLR, negative likelihood ratio; NPV, negative predictive value; PCR, polymerase chain reaction; PLR, positive likelihood ratio; PPV, positive predictive value; Sens, sensitivity; Spec, specificity.

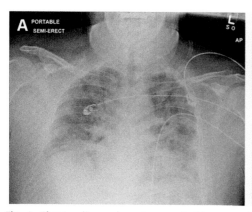
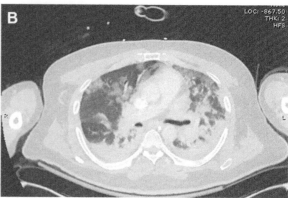

Fig. 4. Chest radiograph and computed tomography of the chest of a 42-year-old male patient admitted with pneumonia and 2009 H1N1 influenza infection leading to acute respiratory failure. Chest radiograph (*A*) reveals diffuse consolidation, and the computed tomography of the chest (*B*) reveals bilateral patchy ground-glass opacities and dense consolidation in the dorsal areas.

fever (61%), and runny nose (58%). On physical examination, the most common findings were wheezing (53%), rhonchi (46%), and crackles (40%).[81]

Just as in pneumonia caused by influenza or respiratory syncytial virus, there are no specific clinical manifestations of pneumonia caused by other respiratory viruses. In fact, symptoms and signs are not specific enough to differentiate viral from bacterial pneumonia.[82] The usual clinical manifestations of pneumonia, including fever higher than 37.8°C, heart rate faster than 100 beats per minute, crackles, and decreased breath sounds,[83] are to be expected in pneumonia caused by any of the respiratory viruses. In the end, the diagnosis of viral infection in patients with pneumonia relies on the recognition that respiratory viruses are a common etiology of pneumonia, and on the systematic performance of viral microbiology studies on these patients.

Radiological Manifestations

The chest radiograph of patients with viral pneumonia can show different patterns, including ground-glass opacities, consolidation, and nodular opacities. In general, patients present with faint opacities, commonly described as a ground-glass pattern. The second most commonly reported pattern is consolidation. Nodular opacities are less common but can occur. The opacities are often patchy in distribution.[80,84–87] Bilateral involvement is fairly common, and some series in influenza pneumonia show that bilateral involvement is slightly more common than unilateral involvement.[84] On the other hand, other series in respiratory syncytial virus or coronavirus pneumonia show that unilateral involvement is more common.[80,85] Pleural effusions are not usual but have

been reported.[87] On computed tomography of the chest, the most common pattern, ground-glass opacity, becomes even more noticeable, often in a patchy and bilateral distribution. Other patterns, such as consolidation, nodular opacities, and interlobular thickening, also can be present[86] (**Figs. 4 and 5**).

Similar to the clinical manifestations, the radiological findings are not specific and do not allow for the differentiation of viral from bacterial infection in patients with pneumonia, let alone the identification of a specific virus. The radiological findings, however, can help corroborate the diagnosis of viral pneumonia. For instance, in a patient in whom a viral pathogen has been identified by oropharyngeal swab, the demonstration of patchy ground-glass opacities in the lung are suggestive of a viral pneumonic infiltrate.

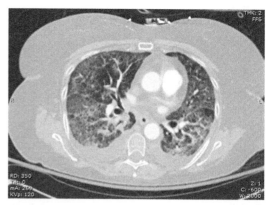

Fig. 5. Computed tomography of the chest revealing diffuse ground-glass opacities and small bilateral pleural effusion in a 62-year-old female patient with respiratory syncytial virus infection who developed pneumonia and acute respiratory distress syndrome.

PATHOGEN-DIRECTED THERAPY

Influenza

The 2 main classes of antiviral drugs for treatment of influenza include neuraminidase inhibitors and adamantanes.[7] Influenza viruses infect cells through the binding of its surface glycoprotein hemagglutinin to the sialic acid receptor. The attached virus is then released into the cells by another surface glycoprotein, neuraminidase, which is the target of neuraminidase inhibitors.[88] The adamantanes, which include amantadine and rimantadine, block the M2 protein, a membrane protein with ion channel activity.[89] They exhibit activity against influenza A but not against influenza B. The antiviral drugs currently approved by the US Food and Drug Administration are the neuraminidase inhibitors oral oseltamivir, inhaled zanamivir, and intravenous peramivir.[90] The adamantanes are not recommended for the treatment of influenza because of high resistance of influenza A against these drugs.[90]

There are a number of clinical trials that assessed the effect of oseltamivir for influenza. A comprehensive systematic review summarized the effect of oseltamivir for prophylaxis and treatment in adults and children. For the assessment of time to alleviation of symptoms in adults with influenza, 8 studies were pooled, totaling 2208 patients in the oseltamivir group and 1746 in the placebo group. Oseltamivir led to earlier relief of symptoms (16.8 hours; 95% CI 8.4–25.1 hours; $P < .001$). For the assessment of pneumonia prevention in adults with influenza, 8 studies were pooled, which included 2694 patients in the oseltamivir group and 1758 in the placebo group. Oseltamivir led to a reduction in pneumonia (risk difference of 1% [0.22%–1.49%]). For the assessment of hospitalization prevention in adults with influenza, 7 studies were pooled that included 2663 patients in the oseltamivir group and 1731 in the placebo group. There was no difference in need for hospitalization (risk ratio 0.92; 95% CI 0.57–1.5; $P = .73$). The pooling of 8 studies in adults, which included 2694 patients in the oseltamivir group and 1758 in the control group, showed that oseltamivir led to more nausea (risk ratio 1.57; 95% CI 1.14–2.15; $P = .005$) and more vomiting (risk ratio 2.43; 95% CI 1.75–3.38; $P<.001$]).[91] In aggregate, these meta-analyses indicate that influenza-infected patients treated with oseltamivir have a modest benefit in relief of symptoms and prevention of pneumonia. This comes at the expense of more nausea and vomiting. It should be noted, however, that the patients included in these trials did not appear ill. For instance, studies that enrolled patients with immunosuppressive conditions such as human immunodeficiency virus infection or malignancy were not included in the meta-analyses. The inclusion criteria for the pooled studies were the presence of influenzalike illness rather than pneumonia. Additionally, only 1 death was reported among all trials that included the adult population.

An earlier systematic review included observational studies that evaluated antiviral therapy versus no therapy or other antiviral therapy in patients with laboratory-confirmed or a clinical diagnosis of influenza. This review of observational studies had important distinctions from the review of randomized clinical trials. First, here the investigators pooled studies that included hospitalized patients, a high-risk population. The pooling of 3 studies (total of 681 patients) that adjusted for confounders showed that oseltamivir, as compared with no antiviral therapy, was associated with a reduction in mortality (OR 0.23; CI 0.13–0.43).[92] The quality of the evidence generated by this review was generally low because it relied on observational studies, which are at risk of confounding despite adjustment in the analyses. However, these observational studies and their meta-analyses fill in important knowledge gaps that were not and likely will not be addressed by clinical trials.

The Centers for Disease Control and Prevention recommends that treatment be initiated as soon as possible for those hospitalized; patients with severe, complicated, or progressive disease; and those at higher risk for influenza complications.[90] We agree with the Centers for Disease Control and Prevention recommendations and as such we submit that all influenza-infected patients with pneumonia, a complication from influenza, should receive antiviral therapy, which currently should be a neuraminidase inhibitor. In the absence of a sensitive point-of-care polymerase chain reaction, clinicians have to decide whether to initiate empiric treatment for influenza pneumonia. Strong consideration should be given to surveillance data and risk factors for influenza. It is important to note that not only an influenza diagnosis is often missed but also clinicians often fail to prescribe antiviral influenza treatment when a clinical diagnosis of influenza is made and there is indication for treatment.[93,94] The benefit from treatment is greatest when it is started early but a survival benefit has been demonstrated with treatment up to 5 days after symptom initiation[95] (**Fig. 6**).

Other Respiratory Viruses

For the treatment of pneumonia caused by respiratory viruses other than influenza, defining whether the patient is immunocompetent or

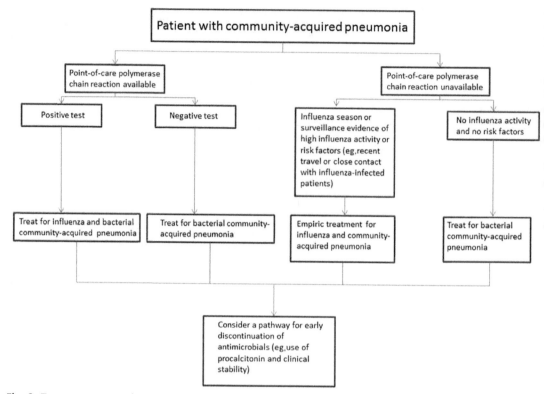

Fig. 6. Treatment approach in patients presenting with community-acquired pneumonia.

immunosuppressed is important. In immunocompetent patients, current antiviral treatment options are limited, generally reserved for severely ill patients, and based on anecdotal data. For instance, case reports and series have reported the use of cidofovir for the treatment of severe pneumonia caused by adenovirus in non-immunocompromised patients.[96,97] Even though patients had clinical improvement in these series, those studies were uncontrolled and thus do not allow a firm conclusion as to the efficacy of cidofovir. Antiviral treatment for pneumonia caused by viruses of the Herpesviridae family in immunocompetent hosts has been reported in severe cases.[98,99] In pregnant women with varicella zoster virus pneumonia, the mortality is high, and treatment with intravenous acyclovir is indicated.[100]

In immunosuppressed patients, aerosolized ribavirin, oral ribavirin, intravenous immunoglobulin, hyperimmunoglobulin, and palivizumab are treatment options that have been used in respiratory syncytial virus infection, particularly in patients with hematological malignancy or transplant recipients.[101] For cytomegalovirus pneumonia, treatment includes intravenous ganciclovir.[102] The addition of cytomegalovirus immunoglobulin to ganciclovir appears to lead to

improved survival according to a case series.[103] An alternative treatment for cytomegalovirus pneumonia is intravenous foscarnet.[104] For the treatment of varicella pneumonia, the indicated treatment is intravenous acyclovir.[105] Similarly, herpes simplex virus pneumonia is treated with intravenous acyclovir.[106] The evidence for the use of these therapies is weak and comes in the form of observational studies (**Fig. 7**).

DISCONTINUATION OF ANTIBIOTIC THERAPY

The identification of a viral pathogen in pneumonia should not in itself prompt a clinician to discontinue the initial empirical antibiotics because dual bacterial-viral infection is common. In fact, the recognition that dual bacterial-viral is common seems to be reflected in clinical practice. In an observational study, most patients with respiratory tract infection admitted to the hospital who turned out to have an identified viral pathogen did not have their antibiotics discontinued.[107] On the other hand, the use of a clinical pathway integrating the results of viral microbiology testing with clinical findings and procalcitonin testing could have a role in the safe discontinuation of antibiotics. It is now well established that use of procalcitonin to guide initiation and discontinuation of antibiotic in

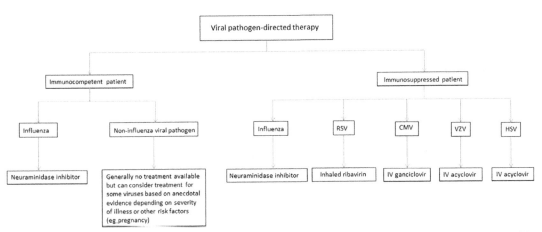

Fig. 7. Viral pathogen-directed therapy. CMV, cytomegalovirus; HSV, herpes simplex virus; IV, intravenous; RSV, respiratory syncytial virus; VZV, varicella zoster virus.

patients with acute respiratory tract infection leads to less use of antibiotics without worsening the outcomes.[108]

In a randomized clinical trial of 300 hospitalized patients with lower respiratory tract infection, the use of combined procalcitonin and viral polymerase chain reaction tests was compared with standard care. Both groups had similar antibiotic exposure. However, a lower proportion of patients with a positive viral polymerase chain reaction test and low procalcitonin received antibiotic on discharge as compared with standard care.[109] This study suggests that the result of a viral polymerase chain reaction test has the impact to further influence decision making even after procalcitonin and clinical evolution are factored in. It should be noted, however, that this was a feasibility study and patients with pneumonia were excluded. Additionally, viral polymerase chain reaction test result may not influence antibiotic decision in the absence of a protocol. This was shown in an observational, retrospective study in which only 10.5% of patients had antibiotic discontinued within 48 hours of a positive viral respiratory panel and a low procalcitonin result.[110]

Another randomized clinical trial assessed the effect of point-of-care respiratory viral panel in patients with acute respiratory illness or fever. The study enrolled 720 patients. There was no difference in the primary endpoint, which was the proportion of patients treated with antibiotics. However, the relevance of the primary outcome was impaired because many patients received antibiotics before the results of the point-of-care test. A significantly greater proportion of patients in the point-of-care group received only a single dose of antibiotics (10% vs 3%) or antibiotics for less than 48 hours (17% vs 9%).[111]

In summary, there is weak but mounting evidence that the use of nucleic acid amplification tests have the potential to aid in the decision to discontinue antibiotics in patients with respiratory infection (including pneumonia) but it is more likely to do so if integrated with clinical findings and procalcitonin. Additionally, continuing clinician education will be important to ensure implementation of strategies to minimize antibiotic exposure.

CORTICOSTEROID THERAPY

An exuberant inflammatory response can play a major role in the morbidity and mortality of patients with pneumonia. Corticosteroid has been used as a way of mitigating the exacerbated inflammatory response in these patients. A systematic review has synthesized the results of clinical trials assessing systemic corticosteroids. The clinical trials are mostly small with sample sizes ranging from 30 to 784 patients. Although no statistically significant improvement in mortality was observed in general, corticosteroids led to a reduction in mortality in patients with severe community-acquired pneumonia (risk ratio 0.39; CI 0.20–0.77).[112] Corticosteroids may be particularly beneficial in patients with community-acquired pneumonia and heightened inflammatory state, as demonstrated in a trial that enrolled patients with severe community-acquired pneumonia and a C-reactive protein greater than 150 mg/L.[113] In summary, despite the small sample size of most trials, the weight of evidence currently favors the use of systemic corticosteroids in patients with community-acquired pneumonia admitted to the hospital, particularly in patients with a high inflammatory state and severe pneumonia. Our approach currently is to reserve the use of corticosteroids for patients with community-acquired pneumonia with C-reactive protein greater than 150 mg/L and a lactic acid greater than 4 nmol/L or acidosis with pH <7.30.[114]

The 2009 H1N1 pandemic brought to light the use of systemic corticosteroid in influenza pneumonia. Some studies revealed that 40% to 50% of patients with severe influenza pneumonia received corticosteroid during the pandemic.[115,116] Unfortunately, although corticosteroid appears to be beneficial in patients with severe community-acquired pneumonia, the same does not hold true for patients with influenza pneumonia, a condition in which corticosteroids may actually be detrimental, as demonstrated in the systematic review. In this study, the investigators pooled 10 observational studies (total of 1497 patients) and found that corticosteroid therapy was associated with higher odds of death (OR 2.12; 95% CI 1.36–3.29). Of note, the studies included in the meta-analysis were predominantly conducted during the 2009 H1N1 influenza pandemic and in the ICU setting.[117]

A clinical trial designed to evaluate the effect of systemic corticosteroid in ICU patients with the 2009 H1N1 influenza pneumonia was unable to enroll the planned number of patients, highlighting the difficulties in conducting a clinical trial during a pandemic.[116] A limitation of the observational studies assessing corticosteroid therapy in influenza pneumonia is the possibility of confounding by indication; that is, the possibility that sicker patients are more often prescribed systemic corticosteroid. This has the potential to cause the false impression that corticosteroid therapy leads to worse outcomes in influenza pneumonia. Some studies adjusted for confounding factors, but residual confounding can still occur. In the absence of randomized clinical trials, and in view of the results of observational studies, it is our opinion that currently corticosteroid therapy should not be administered in influenza pneumonia. The effect of corticosteroid in patients with noninfluenza viral pneumonia is unclear.

FUTURE RESEARCH

The advent of nucleic acid amplification tests improved our understanding of the epidemiology of viral infections in pneumonia, and enables an etiologic diagnosis of viral infection in a large proportion of patients with pneumonia. However, one of the downsides of nucleic acid amplifications tests was a relatively long turnaround, limiting its clinical utility. This has been overcome by the development of "point-of-care" polymerase chain reaction tests that have a turnaround time of approximately 1 hour.[118] The assessment of these point-of-care tests in clinical pathways is a promising venue for clinical investigation. As these tests are being rapidly integrated into clinical practice, it is important to study their cost-effectiveness and whether they influence outcomes or decision making.

Ongoing research on antiviral treatment is promising. Just as for bacterial infection, combination therapy has been studied in influenza infection with different goals, such as preventing pathogen resistance,[119,120] mitigating the inflammatory response,[121] or achieving synergy.[122,123] There has been development of new compounds for the treatment of respiratory syncytial virus. These include a fusion inhibitor, which prevents the fusion of respiratory syncytial virus viral envelope with the host cell membrane, and a nucleoside analog, which prevents respiratory syncytial virus replication.[124,125]

SUMMARY

Viral respiratory infection is common in pneumonia and is present in approximately 25% of patients with community-acquired pneumonia. It is also common in immunosuppressed patients, but the latter are susceptible not only to the usual community-acquired respiratory viruses but also to viruses of the Herpesviridae family. Recent data show that respiratory viruses are also identified in hospital-acquired infections. The clinical diagnosis of viral infection is challenging. Clinical prediction rules have been developed for the diagnosis of influenza infection but they showed only modest accuracy. Similarly, radiological studies are nonspecific. In the end, the diagnosis of viral infection relies on the recognition that respiratory viruses are commonly present in pneumonia, and on the systematic performance of viral microbiology studies, particularly nucleic acid amplifications tests. The treatment of influenza pneumonia is currently with a neuraminidase inhibitor. The treatment options for pneumonia caused by other viruses in immunocompetent patients with pneumonia are limited, and the data are largely anecdotal. In immunosuppressed patients with infection by respiratory syncytial virus or a virus of the Herpesviridae family, there are antiviral treatments available. There is ongoing research involved with the development and testing of new treatment strategies both for influenza and noninfluenza viruses.

REFERENCES

1. Iuliano AD, Roguski KM, Chang HH, et al. Estimates of global seasonal influenza-associated respiratory mortality: a modelling study. Lancet 2017; 391(10127):1285–300.

2. Jain S, Self WH, Wunderink RG, et al. Community-acquired pneumonia requiring hospitalization among U.S. adults. N Engl J Med 2015;373(5):415–27.

3. Horimoto T, Kawaoka Y. Influenza: lessons from past pandemics, warnings from current incidents. Nat Rev Microbiol 2005;3(8):591–600.

4. Zimmer SM, Burke DS. Historical perspective—emergence of influenza A (H1N1) viruses. N Engl J Med 2009;361(3):279–85.

5. De Clercq E, Li G. Approved antiviral drugs over the past 50 years. Clin Microbiol Rev 2016;29(3):695–747.

6. Blanton L, Alabi N, Mustaquim D, et al. Update: influenza activity in the United States during the 2016-17 season and composition of the 2017-18 influenza vaccine. MMWR Morb Mortal Wkly Rep 2017;66(25):668–76.

7. Kamali A, Holodniy M. Influenza treatment and prophylaxis with neuraminidase inhibitors: a review. Infect Drug Resist 2013;6:187–98.

8. Bouvier NM, Palese P. The biology of influenza viruses. Vaccine 2008;26(Suppl 4):D49–53.

9. McLellan JS, Ray WC, Peeples ME. Structure and function of respiratory syncytial virus surface glycoproteins. Curr Top Microbiol Immunol 2013;372:83–104.

10. Jacobs SE, Lamson DM, St George K, et al. Human rhinoviruses. Clin Microbiol Rev 2013;26(1):135–62.

11. San Martin C. Latest insights on adenovirus structure and assembly. Viruses 2012;4(5):847–77.

12. Henrickson KJ. Parainfluenza viruses. Clin Microbiol Rev 2003;16(2):242–64.

13. de Haan CA, Kuo L, Masters PS, et al. Coronavirus particle assembly: primary structure requirements of the membrane protein. J Virol 1998;72(8):6838–50.

14. Wen X, Krause JC, Leser GP, et al. Structure of the human metapneumovirus fusion protein with neutralizing antibody identifies a pneumovirus antigenic site. Nat Struct Mol Biol 2012;19(4):461–3.

15. Gurda BL, Parent KN, Bladek H, et al. Human bocavirus capsid structure: insights into the structural repertoire of the Parvoviridae. J Virol 2010;84(12):5880–9.

16. Melero JA, Mas V. The Pneumovirinae fusion (F) protein: a common target for vaccines and antivirals. Virus Res 2015;209:128–35.

17. Thibaut HJ, De Palma AM, Neyts J. Combating enterovirus replication: state-of-the-art on antiviral research. Biochem Pharmacol 2012;83(2):185–92.

18. Olson NH, Kolatkar PR, Oliveira MA, et al. Structure of a human rhinovirus complexed with its receptor molecule. Proc Natl Acad Sci U S A 1993;90(2):507–11.

19. Burk M, El-Kersh K, Saad M, et al. Viral infection in community-acquired pneumonia: a systematic review and meta-analysis. Eur Respir Rev 2016;25(140):178–88.

20. Yin YD, Zhao F, Ren LL, et al. Evaluation of the Japanese respiratory society guidelines for the identification of mycoplasma pneumoniae pneumonia. Respirology 2012;17(7):1131–6.

21. Choi SH, Hong SB, Ko GB, et al. Viral infection in patients with severe pneumonia requiring intensive care unit admission. Am J Respir Crit Care Med 2012;186(4):325–32.

22. Karhu J, Ala-Kokko TI, Vuorinen T, et al. Lower respiratory tract virus findings in mechanically ventilated patients with severe community-acquired pneumonia. Clin Infect Dis 2014;59(1):62–70.

23. Couch RB, Englund JA, Whimbey E. Respiratory viral infections in immunocompetent and immunocompromised persons. Am J Med 1997;102(3A):2–9 [discussion: 25–6].

24. Meyers JD, Flournoy N, Thomas ED. Nonbacterial pneumonia after allogeneic marrow transplantation: a review of ten years' experience. Rev Infect Dis 1982;4(6):1119–32.

25. Kim DH, Messner H, Minden M, et al. Factors influencing varicella zoster virus infection after allogeneic peripheral blood stem cell transplantation: low-dose acyclovir prophylaxis and pre-transplant diagnosis of lymphoproliferative disorders. Transpl Infect Dis 2008;10(2):90–8.

26. Koc Y, Miller KB, Schenkein DP, et al. Varicella zoster virus infections following allogeneic bone marrow transplantation: frequency, risk factors, and clinical outcome. Biol Blood Marrow Transplant 2000;6(1):44–9.

27. Green ML. Viral pneumonia in patients with hematopoietic cell transplantation and hematologic malignancies. Clin Chest Med 2017;38(2):295–305.

28. Hong HL, Hong SB, Ko GB, et al. Viral infection is not uncommon in adult patients with severe hospital-acquired pneumonia. PLoS One 2014;9(4):e95865.

29. Dawood FS, Iuliano AD, Reed C, et al. Estimated global mortality associated with the first 12 months of 2009 pandemic influenza A H1N1 virus circulation: a modelling study. Lancet Infect Dis 2012;12(9):687–95.

30. Lee N, Hui D, Wu A, et al. A major outbreak of severe acute respiratory syndrome in Hong Kong. N Engl J Med 2003;348(20):1986–94.

31. Ksiazek TG, Erdman D, Goldsmith CS, et al. A novel coronavirus associated with severe acute respiratory syndrome. N Engl J Med 2003;348(20):1953–66.

32. Drosten C, Gunther S, Preiser W, et al. Identification of a novel coronavirus in patients with severe acute respiratory syndrome. N Engl J Med 2003;348(20):1967–76.

33. Zaki AM, van Boheemen S, Bestebroer TM, et al. Isolation of a novel coronavirus from a man with pneumonia in Saudi Arabia. N Engl J Med 2012; 367(19):1814–20.

34. de Groot RJ, Baker SC, Baric RS, et al. Middle East respiratory syndrome coronavirus (MERS-CoV): announcement of the coronavirus study group. J Virol 2013;87(14):7790–2.

35. Lim YX, Ng YL, Tam JP, et al. Human coronaviruses: a review of virus-host interactions. Diseases 2016; 4(3). https://doi.org/10.3390/diseases4030026.

36. Guery B, Poissy J, el Mansouf L, et al. Clinical features and viral diagnosis of two cases of infection with Middle East respiratory syndrome coronavirus: a report of nosocomial transmission. Lancet 2013; 381(9885):2265–72.

37. Assiri A, McGeer A, Perl TM, et al. Hospital outbreak of Middle East respiratory syndrome coronavirus. N Engl J Med 2013;369(5):407–16.

38. Bialek SR, Allen D, Alvarado-Ramy F, et al. First confirmed cases of Middle East respiratory syndrome coronavirus (MERS-CoV) infection in the United States, updated information on the epidemiology of MERS-CoV infection, and guidance for the public, clinicians, and public health authorities - May 2014. MMWR Morb Mortal Wkly Rep 2014; 63(19):431–6.

39. Chunara R, Goldstein E, Patterson-Lomba O, et al. Estimating influenza attack rates in the United States using a participatory cohort. Sci Rep 2015; 5:9540.

40. Dao CN, Kamimoto L, Nowell M, et al. Adult hospitalizations for laboratory-positive influenza during the 2005-2006 through 2007-2008 seasons in the United States. J Infect Dis 2010;202(6):881–8.

41. Casalino E, Antoniol S, Fidouh N, et al. Influenza virus infections among patients attending emergency department according to main reason to presenting to ED: a 3-year prospective observational study during seasonal epidemic periods. PLoS One 2017;12(8):e0182191.

42. Garg S, Jain S, Dawood FS, et al. Pneumonia among adults hospitalized with laboratory-confirmed seasonal influenza virus infection—United States, 2005-2008. BMC Infect Dis 2015;15:369.

43. Maruyama T, Fujisawa T, Suga S, et al. Outcomes and prognostic features of patients with influenza requiring hospitalization and receiving early antiviral therapy: a prospective multicenter cohort study. Chest 2016;149(2):526–34.

44. Blanton L, Mustaquim D, Alabi N, et al. Update: influenza activity—United States, October 2, 2016-February 4, 2017. MMWR Morb Mortal Wkly Rep 2017;66(6):159–66.

45. Falsey AR, Hennessey PA, Formica MA, et al. Respiratory syncytial virus infection in elderly and high-risk adults. N Engl J Med 2005;352(17):1749–59.

46. Zhou H, Thompson WW, Viboud CG, et al. Hospitalizations associated with influenza and respiratory syncytial virus in the United States, 1993-2008. Clin Infect Dis 2012;54(10):1427–36.

47. Gwaltney JM. Clinical significance and pathogenesis of viral respiratory infections. Am J Med 2002;112(Suppl 6A):13S–8S.

48. Monto AS. The seasonality of rhinovirus infections and its implications for clinical recognition. Clin Ther 2002;24(12):1987–97.

49. Gaunt ER, Hardie A, Claas EC, et al. Epidemiology and clinical presentations of the four human coronaviruses 229E, HKU1, NL63, and OC43 detected over 3 years using a novel multiplex real-time PCR method. J Clin Microbiol 2010;48(8):2940–7.

50. Gerna G, Percivalle E, Sarasini A, et al. Human respiratory coronavirus HKU1 versus other coronavirus infections in Italian hospitalised patients. J Clin Virol 2007;38(3):244–50.

51. Ruuskanen O, Mertsola J, Meurman O. Adenovirus infection in families. Arch Dis Child 1988;63(10): 1250–3.

52. Tan D, Zhu H, Fu Y, et al. Severe community-acquired pneumonia caused by human adenovirus in immunocompetent adults: a multicenter case series. PLoS One 2016;11(3):e0151199.

53. Cao B, Huang GH, Pu ZH, et al. Emergence of community-acquired adenovirus type 55 as a cause of community-onset pneumonia. Chest 2014;145(1):79–86.

54. Shields AF, Hackman RC, Fife KH, et al. Adenovirus infections in patients undergoing bone-marrow transplantation. N Engl J Med 1985; 312(9):529–33.

55. Berciaud S, Rayne F, Kassab S, et al. Adenovirus infections in Bordeaux University Hospital 2008-2010: clinical and virological features. J Clin Virol 2012;54(4):302–7.

56. Park JY, Kim BJ, Lee EJ, et al. Clinical features and courses of adenovirus pneumonia in healthy young adults during an outbreak among Korean military personnel. PLoS One 2017;12(1):e0170592.

57. Klinger JR, Sanchez MP, Curtin LA, et al. Multiple cases of life-threatening adenovirus pneumonia in a mental health care center. Am J Respir Crit Care Med 1998;157(2):645–9.

58. Cassir N, Hraiech S, Nougairede A, et al. Outbreak of adenovirus type 1 severe pneumonia in a French intensive care unit, September-October 2012. Euro Surveill 2014;19(39) [pii:20914].

59. Weinberg GA, Hall CB, Iwane MK, et al. Parainfluenza virus infection of young children: estimates of the population-based burden of hospitalization. J Pediatr 2009;154(5):694–9.

60. Liu WK, Liu Q, Chen DH, et al. Epidemiology and clinical presentation of the four human parainfluenza virus types. BMC Infect Dis 2013;13:28.

61. Marx A, Gary HE Jr, Marston BJ, et al. Parainfluenza virus infection among adults hospitalized for lower respiratory tract infection. Clin Infect Dis 1999;29(1):134–40.

62. Falsey AR, Erdman D, Anderson LJ, et al. Human metapneumovirus infections in young and elderly adults. J Infect Dis 2003;187(5):785–90.

63. Johnstone J, Majumdar SR, Fox JD, et al. Human metapneumovirus pneumonia in adults: results of a prospective study. Clin Infect Dis 2008;46(4):571–4.

64. Longtin J, Bastien M, Gilca R, et al. Human bocavirus infections in hospitalized children and adults. Emerg Infect Dis 2008;14(2):217–21.

65. Ghietto LM, Majul D, Ferreyra Soaje P, et al. Comorbidity and high viral load linked to clinical presentation of respiratory human bocavirus infection. Arch Virol 2015;160(1):117–27.

66. Jula A, Waris M, Kantola K, et al. Primary and secondary human bocavirus 1 infections in a family, Finland. Emerg Infect Dis 2013;19(8):1328–31.

67. Mori D, Ranawaka U, Yamada K, et al. Human bocavirus in patients with encephalitis, Sri Lanka, 2009-2010. Emerg Infect Dis 2013;19(11):1859–62.

68. Yu JM, Chen QQ, Hao YX, et al. Identification of human bocaviruses in the cerebrospinal fluid of children hospitalized with encephalitis in China. J Clin Virol 2013;57(4):374–7.

69. Windisch W, Schildgen V, Malecki M, et al. Detection of HBoV DNA in idiopathic lung fibrosis, cologne, Germany. J Clin Virol 2013;58(1):325–7.

70. Krakau M, Brockmann M, Titius B, et al. Acute human bocavirus infection in MDS patient, Cologne, Germany. J Clin Virol 2015;69:44–7.

71. Falcone V, Ridder GJ, Panning M, et al. Human bocavirus DNA in paranasal sinus mucosa. Emerg Infect Dis 2011;17(8):1564–5.

72. Stein J, Louie J, Flanders S, et al. Performance characteristics of clinical diagnosis, a clinical decision rule, and a rapid influenza test in the detection of influenza infection in a community sample of adults. Ann Emerg Med 2005;46(5):412–9.

73. Oliveira EC, Marik PE, Colice G. Influenza pneumonia: a descriptive study. Chest 2001;119(6):1717–23.

74. Michiels B, Thomas I, Van Royen P, et al. Clinical prediction rules combining signs, symptoms and epidemiological context to distinguish influenza from influenza-like illnesses in primary care: a cross sectional study. BMC Fam Pract 2011;12:4.

75. Ebell MH, Afonso A. A systematic review of clinical decision rules for the diagnosis of influenza. Ann Fam Med 2011;9(1):69–77.

76. Boivin G, Hardy I, Tellier G, et al. Predicting influenza infections during epidemics with use of a clinical case definition. Clin Infect Dis 2000;31(5):1166–9.

77. Dugas AF, Valsamakis A, Atreya MR, et al. Clinical diagnosis of influenza in the ED. Am J Emerg Med 2015;33(6):770–5.

78. McGee S. Simplifying likelihood ratios. J Gen Intern Med 2002;17(8):646–9.

79. Saha S, Chadha M, Al Mamun A, et al. Influenza seasonality and vaccination timing in tropical and subtropical areas of southern and southeastern Asia. Bull World Health Organ 2014;92(5):318–30.

80. Walsh EE, Peterson DR, Falsey AR. Is clinical recognition of respiratory syncytial virus infection in hospitalized elderly and high-risk adults possible? J Infect Dis 2007;195(7):1046–51.

81. Dowell SF, Anderson LJ, Gary HE Jr, et al. Respiratory syncytial virus is an important cause of community-acquired lower respiratory infection among hospitalized adults. J Infect Dis 1996;174(3):456–62.

82. Huijskens EG, Koopmans M, Palmen FM, et al. The value of signs and symptoms in differentiating between bacterial, viral and mixed aetiology in patients with community-acquired pneumonia. J Med Microbiol 2014;63(Pt 3):441–52.

83. Heckerling PS, Tape TG, Wigton RS, et al. Clinical prediction rule for pulmonary infiltrates. Ann Intern Med 1990;113(9):664–70.

84. Aviram G, Bar-Shai A, Sosna J, et al. H1N1 influenza: initial chest radiographic findings in helping predict patient outcome. Radiology 2010;255(1):252–9.

85. Woo PC, Lau SK, Tsoi HW, et al. Clinical and molecular epidemiological features of coronavirus HKU1-associated community-acquired pneumonia. J Infect Dis 2005;192(11):1898–907.

86. Chong S, Lee KS, Kim TS, et al. Adenovirus pneumonia in adults: radiographic and high-resolution CT findings in five patients. AJR Am J Roentgenol 2006;186(5):1288–93.

87. Wang K, Xi W, Yang D, et al. Rhinovirus is associated with severe adult community-acquired pneumonia in China. J Thorac Dis 2017;9(11):4502–11.

88. Moscona A. Neuraminidase inhibitors for influenza. N Engl J Med 2005;353(13):1363–73.

89. Wang C, Takeuchi K, Pinto LH, et al. Ion channel activity of influenza A virus M2 protein: characterization of the amantadine block. J Virol 1993;67(9):5585–94.

90. Available at: https://www.cdc.gov/flu/professionals/antivirals/summary-clinicians.htm. Accessed January 13, 2018.

91. Jefferson T, Jones M, Doshi P, et al. Oseltamivir for influenza in adults and children: systematic review of clinical study reports and summary of regulatory comments. BMJ 2014;348:g2545.

92. Hsu J, Santesso N, Mustafa R, et al. Antivirals for treatment of influenza: a systematic review and

meta-analysis of observational studies. Ann Intern Med 2012;156(7):512–24.

93. Biggerstaff M, Jhung MA, Reed C, et al. Impact of medical and behavioural factors on influenza-like illness, healthcare-seeking, and antiviral treatment during the 2009 H1N1 pandemic: USA, 2009-2010. Epidemiol Infect 2014;142(1):114–25.

94. Lindegren ML, Schaffner W. Treatment with neur-aminidase inhibitors for high-risk patients with influenza: why is adherence to antiviral treatment recommendations so low? J Infect Dis 2014; 210(4):510–3.

95. Louie JK, Yang S, Acosta M, et al. Treatment with neuraminidase inhibitors for critically ill patients with influenza A (H1N1)pdm09. Clin Infect Dis 2012;55(9):1198–204.

96. Kim SJ, Kim K, Park SB, et al. Outcomes of early administration of cidofovir in non-immunocompromised patients with severe adenovirus pneumonia. PLoS One 2015;10(4):e0122642.

97. Lee M, Kim S, Kwon OJ, et al. Treatment of adenoviral acute respiratory distress syndrome using cidofovir with extracorporeal membrane oxygenation. J Intensive Care Med 2017;32(3):231–8.

98. Grilli E, Galati V, Bordi L, et al. Cytomegalovirus pneumonia in immunocompetent host: case report and literature review. J Clin Virol 2012;55(4):356–9.

99. Hunt DP, Muse VV, Pitman MB. Case records of the Massachusetts General Hospital. Case 12-2013. An 18-year-old woman with pulmonary infiltrates and respiratory failure. N Engl J Med 2013; 368(16):1537–45.

100. Broussard RC, Payne DK, George RB. Treatment with acyclovir of varicella pneumonia in pregnancy. Chest 1991;99(4):1045–7.

101. Khanna N, Widmer AF, Decker M, et al. Respiratory syncytial virus infection in patients with hematological diseases: single-center study and review of the literature. Clin Infect Dis 2008; 46(3):402–12.

102. Tan BH. Cytomegalovirus treatment. Curr Treat Options Infect Dis 2014;6(3):256–70.

103. Reed EC, Bowden RA, Dandliker PS, et al. Treatment of cytomegalovirus pneumonia with ganciclovir and intravenous cytomegalovirus immunoglobulin in patients with bone marrow transplants. Ann Intern Med 1988;109(10):783–8.

104. Farthing C, Anderson MG, Ellis ME, et al. Treatment of cytomegalovirus pneumonitis with foscarnet (trisodium phosphonoformate) in patients with AIDS. J Med Virol 1987;22(2):157–62.

105. Mohsen AH, McKendrick M. Varicella pneumonia in adults. Eur Respir J 2003;21(5):886–91.

106. Ferrari A, Luppi M, Potenza L, et al. Herpes simplex virus pneumonia during standard induction chemotherapy for acute leukemia: case report and review of literature. Leukemia 2005;19(11):2019–21.

107. Yee C, Suarthana E, Dendukuri N, et al. Evaluating the impact of the multiplex respiratory virus panel polymerase chain reaction test on the clinical management of suspected respiratory viral infections in adult patients in a hospital setting. Am J Infect Control 2016;44(11):1396–8.

108. Schuetz P, Wirz Y, Sager R, et al. Procalcitonin to initiate or discontinue antibiotics in acute respiratory tract infections. Cochrane Database Syst Rev 2017;(10):CD007498.

109. Branche AR, Walsh EE, Vargas R, et al. Serum procalcitonin measurement and viral testing to guide antibiotic use for respiratory infections in hospitalized adults: a randomized controlled trial. J Infect Dis 2015;212(11):1692–700.

110. Timbrook T, Maxam M, Bosso J. Antibiotic discontinuation rates associated with positive respiratory viral panel and low procalcitonin results in proven or suspected respiratory infections. Infect Dis Ther 2015;4(3):297–306.

111. Brendish NJ, Malachira AK, Armstrong L, et al. Routine molecular point-of-care testing for respiratory viruses in adults presenting to hospital with acute respiratory illness (ResPOC): a pragmatic, open-label, randomised controlled trial. Lancet Respir Med 2017;5(5):401–11.

112. Siemieniuk RA, Meade MO, Alonso-Coello P, et al. Corticosteroid therapy for patients hospitalized with community-acquired pneumonia: a systematic review and meta-analysis. Ann Intern Med 2015; 163(7):519–28.

113. Torres A, Sibila O, Ferrer M, et al. Effect of corticosteroids on treatment failure among hospitalized patients with severe community-acquired pneumonia and high inflammatory response: a randomized clinical trial. JAMA 2015;313(7): 677–86.

114. Cavallazzi R, Ramirez JA. Using steroids in patients with community-acquired pneumonia at the university of Louisville Hospital: who, what, and when. Univ Louisville J Respir Infect 2017;1(4):4–6.

115. Brun-Buisson C, Richard JC, Mercat A, et al, REVA-SRLF A/H1N1v 2009 Registry Group. Early corticosteroids in severe influenza A/H1N1 pneumonia and acute respiratory distress syndrome. Am J Respir Crit Care Med 2011;183(9):1200–6.

116. Annane D, Antona M, Lehmann B, et al. Designing and conducting a randomized trial for pandemic critical illness: the 2009 H1N1 influenza pandemic. Intensive Care Med 2012;38(1):29–39.

117. Rodrigo C, Leonardi-Bee J, Nguyen-Van-Tam JS, et al. Effect of corticosteroid therapy on influenza-related mortality: a systematic review and meta-analysis. J Infect Dis 2015;212(2):183–94.

118. Somerville LK, Ratnamohan VM, Dwyer DE, et al. Molecular diagnosis of respiratory viruses. Pathology 2015;47(3):243–9.

119. Pires de Mello CP, Drusano GL, Adams JR, et al. Oseltamivir-zanamivir combination therapy suppresses drug-resistant H1N1 influenza A viruses in the hollow fiber infection model (HFIM) system. Eur J Pharm Sci 2018;111:443–9.

120. Duval X, van der Werf S, Blanchon T, et al. Efficacy of oseltamivir-zanamivir combination compared to each monotherapy for seasonal influenza: a randomized placebo-controlled trial. PLoS Med 2010;7(11):e1000362.

121. Hung IFN, To KKW, Chan JFW, et al. Efficacy of clarithromycin-naproxen-oseltamivir combination in the treatment of patients hospitalized for influenza A(H3N2) infection: an open-label randomized, controlled, phase IIb/III trial. Chest 2017;151(5): 1069–80.

122. Nguyen JT, Hoopes JD, Le MH, et al. Triple combination of amantadine, ribavirin, and oseltamivir is highly active and synergistic against drug resistant influenza virus strains in vitro. PLoS One 2010;5(2): e9332.

123. Smee DF, Hurst BL, Wong MH, et al. Effects of double combinations of amantadine, oseltamivir, and ribavirin on influenza A (H5N1) virus infections in cell culture and in mice. Antimicrob Agents Chemother 2009;53(5):2120–8.

124. DeVincenzo JP, Whitley RJ, Mackman RL, et al. Oral GS-5806 activity in a respiratory syncytial virus challenge study. N Engl J Med 2014;371(8): 711–22.

125. DeVincenzo JP, McClure MW, Symons JA, et al. Activity of oral ALS-008176 in a respiratory syncytial virus challenge study. N Engl J Med 2015; 373(21):2048–58.

126. Self WH, Williams DJ, Zhu Y, et al. Respiratory viral detection in children and adults: comparing asymptomatic controls and patients with community-acquired pneumonia. J Infect Dis 2016;213(4): 584–91.

127. Korteweg C, Gu J. Pathology, molecular biology, and pathogenesis of avian influenza A (H5N1) infection in humans. Am J Pathol 2008;172(5):1155–70.

128. van der Sluijs KF, van der Poll T, Lutter R, et al. Bench-to-bedside review: bacterial pneumonia with influenza pathogenesis and clinical implications. Crit Care 2010;14(2):219.

129. Grabowska K, Hogberg L, Penttinen P, et al. Occurrence of invasive pneumococcal disease and number of excess cases due to influenza. BMC Infect Dis 2006;6:58.

130. Jartti T, Lehtinen P, Vuorinen T, et al. Persistence of rhinovirus and enterovirus RNA after acute respiratory illness in children. J Med Virol 2004;72(4): 695–9.

Guidelines to Manage Community-Acquired Pneumonia

Richard G. Wunderink, MD

KEYWORDS

- Pneumonia • Community-acquired pneumonia • Macrolide • Viral pneumonia • Corticosteroids
- Procalcitonin

KEY POINTS

- Community-acquired pneumonia (CAP) accounts for 78% of deaths from infectious diseases in the United States, but outcomes continue to be highly variable even on a county level.
- The preponderance of evidence favors use of β-lactam/macrolide combination therapy over β-lactam monotherapy for hospitalized, non–intensive care unit patients.
- The decreasing incidence of pneumococcal pneumonia and greater viral detections in CAP due to public health efforts, especially pneumococcal conjugate vaccine, will impact future guideline management recommendations.
- The health care–associated pneumonia definition overestimates the small subgroup of CAP patients with pathogens resistant to the usual antibiotic regimens; new risk stratification is needed for individual pathogens, such as methicillin-resistant *Staphylococcus aureus*.

In the areas of pulmonary, infectious diseases, and critical care medicine, no guideline has greater validity and acceptance than that for management of community-acquired pneumonia (CAP).[1] These guidelines have been incorporated into quality metrics, pay-for-performance, and public reporting of physician and hospital care. Because pneumonia is the leading cause of adult admissions in the United States,[2] the leading cause of infectious deaths,[3] and in the differential of the most frequent symptom complexes in outpatient primary care,[4] this attention to CAP guidelines is neither surprising nor inappropriate. Of all infectious deaths in the United States, lower respiratory tract infection accounted for 78.8%, a log greater than human immunodeficiency virus/AIDS (7.0%) and 2 logs greater than tuberculosis (0.75%).[3] However, despite this high level of acceptance, areas in the guidelines remain controversial, and new challenges continue to emerge. Outcomes for lower respiratory tract infections also remain highly variable even on a county-by-county level, much higher than for other major infectious diseases.[3] This review addresses the current status and discusses areas of current debate.

RATIONALE FOR COMMUNITY-ACQUIRED PNEUMONIA GUIDELINES

The rationale for CAP guidelines has evolved over the last few decades. Significant variability in antibiotic prescription for CAP without differences in outcome was a primary driver of the initial efforts to derive guidelines. Almost every new antibiotic received a US Food and Drug Administration (FDA) indication for CAP, resulting in a plethora of individual antibiotics among which to choose. The cost/benefit relationship of these new more

Disclosure: Dr R.G. Wunderink has personally received consulting fees from Accelerate Diagnostics, Arsanis, Biotest, Curetis, GenMark, Glaxo/Smith/Klein, Inflarex, KBP Biosciences, Merck, Nabriva, Pfizer, Roche.
Department of Medicine, Pulmonary and Critical Care, Northwestern University Feinberg School of Medicine, 240 East Huron Street, McGaw M-336, Chicago, IL 60611, USA
E-mail address: r-wunderink@northwestern.edu

Clin Chest Med 39 (2018) 723–731
https://doi.org/10.1016/j.ccm.2018.07.006
0272-5231/18/© 2018 Elsevier Inc. All rights reserved.

expensive agents compared with each other and to generic antibiotics was unclear. Initial CAP guidelines attempted to address these issues through the opinion of experts in the field and were sponsored by professional societies. In the United States, the American Thoracic Society (ATS) and the Infectious Diseases Society of America (IDSA) led these efforts.[1,5,6]

Despite the basis of expert opinion only and a lack of randomized controlled trials specifically comparing guideline-recommended therapy to usual care, subsequent studies consistently demonstrated improved outcomes as a greater proportion of CAP patients were managed according to ATS/IDSA CAP guidelines.[7–9] The Centers for Medicare and Medicaid Services recognized the benefit of compliance with these guidelines by incorporating antibiotic choices consistent with ATS/IDSA guidelines as a major quality metric for public reporting.

The guidelines have expanded to address other issues, including appropriate diagnostic testing and the use of adjunctive therapies. New challenges for antibiotic management have also arisen, including the role of Legionella and community-acquired methicillin-resistant Staphylococcus aureus (MRSA),[10] and the emergence of CAP cases with other resistant pathogens typically associated with nosocomial infections and temporarily designated as health care–associated pneumonia (HCAP).[11]

CURRENT GUIDELINES

The current IDSA/ATS CAP guidelines were published in 2007,[1] and a new revision is anticipated soon. The current recommended antibiotic choices are listed in **Table 1** and do not differ substantially from previous versions.

Many other countries and regions have also developed CAP guidelines, including published guidelines from Great Britain,[12] Spain,[13] the Netherlands,[14] Sweden,[15] Japan,[16] and China.[17] Most guidelines roughly parallel those of the IDSA/ATS or northern Europe. Although differences are relatively minimal, these local and regional differences are actual internally consistent with a major emphasis in most guidelines for local adaptation of recommendations.

The major difference between the IDSA/ATS CAP guidelines[1] and those of northern European countries[12,14,15] is the need for macrolide combination with beta-lactams for hospitalized, non-ICU patients. Several justifications for macrolide combination exist. The primary is coverage of atypical bacterial pathogens (Mycoplasma, Chlamydophila, and Legionella). Because detection of these pathogens was difficult, empirical coverage was recommended. However, rates of Mycoplasma and Chlamydophila vary by seasons and can occur in occult epidemics.[18,19] Other potential benefits include an anti-inflammatory effect on host immune response,[20] as well as suppression of the pore-forming exotoxin pneumolysin,[21] a major virulence factor for Streptococcus pneumoniae.[22]

Despite these theoretic benefits of macrolides, the major driving force for the IDSA/ATS guideline recommendation for beta-lactam/macrolide combination therapy was a consistent survival benefit for combination therapy in large public and administrative databases.[18,23–28] Theoretic benefits of macrolides were only explored to explain the observed effect.

In contrast, proponents of beta-lactam monotherapy base their recommendation on the overwhelming dominance of pneumococcus (in addition of other Streptococci) as the cause of

Table 1		
Current recommended antibiotic therapy for community-acquired pneumonia		
Patient Category	**Recommended**	**Alternative**
Outpatient: previously healthy	Macrolide	Doxycycline
Outpatient: underlying disease/ previous treatment	Fluoroquinolone	Beta-lactam combined with macrolide or doxycycline
Non-ICU inpatient	Beta-lactam combined with macrolide or fluoroquinolone monotherapy	Beta-lactam combined with doxycycline
ICU patient	Beta-lactam combined with macrolide or beta-lactam combined with fluoroquinolone	Add linezolid or vancomycin for suspected MRSA Change to anti-pseudomonal beta-lactam and quinolone if suspect pseudomonas

CAP.[12,14,15] Atypical pathogen coverage is then reserved for patients with specific risk factors or failure of prior beta-lactam therapy. Routine macrolide combination therapy is not warranted, outside of intensive care unit (ICU) admissions, based on drug toxicity and the potential for development of resistance.

Three informative major studies have been published since the last guidelines. First, the large multicenter Centers for Disease Control and Prevention-sponsored Epidemiology of Pneumonia In the Community (EPIC) study found that the proportion of adults with detection of an atypical bacterial pathogen was 3.7%.[29] In contrast, pneumococcal detection occurred in only 5.1%, despite extensive diagnostic testing. Additional cases of pneumococcal pneumonia were subsequently found with research-only diagnostic tests[30] but still remain less than 15% of all detections. These dramatically lower detection rates for the pneumococcus compared with previous epidemiologic studies[31] likely represent the effect of near universal pediatric conjugate pneumococcal vaccination[32,33] and increased smoking cessation efforts.

A large multicenter cluster-randomized trial in the Netherlands appeared to support beta-lactam monotherapy as equivalent to both IDSA/ATS-recommended treatment regimens.[34] However, many aspects of the trial design call into question this conclusion. Because of a public health orientation, the chosen primary endpoint was 90-day mortality. This endpoint is compromised by a greater effect of underlying diseases, such as metastatic cancer, and intercurrent illnesses, especially cardiovascular events. The latter may be related to CAP, but the relationship to type of antibiotic treatment is very unclear. A more pertinent endpoint is need for alteration of the antibiotic regimen, which was 8.8% for beta-lactam monotherapy compared with 6.1% for combination and 3.7% for fluoroquinolone monotherapy. The study was also compromised by a large proportion of patients who crossed over treatment from that assigned. Differences in health care systems are relevant: the hospital length of stay (LOS) for the Netherlands is greater than 6 days in contrast to approximately 3 days in the United States.[34–36] This longer observation time allows recognition of failing therapy before discharge, thus avoiding readmission, which is now a major issue for public reporting of the quality of CAP management in the United States.

A head-to-head randomized controlled trial of macrolide/beta-lactam combination with monotherapy with the identical beta-lactam for non-ICU hospitalized CAP patients has finally been published.[37] Designed similar to antibiotic FDA-registration trials,[38] the primary endpoint was the more clinically relevant time to clinical stability, a measurement associated with safe discharge and low risk of readmission.[39] The difference in proportions achieving clinical stability by day 7 was 7.6% (95% confidence interval of the difference 0.8%–16%). In addition, serious adverse events of death and ICU transfer only occurred in monotherapy patients, and readmission rates were higher in the monotherapy group. Based on this study, if beta-lactam monotherapy was a new antibiotic, the probability of FDA approval would be very low.

A synthesis of these data is that a large proportion of CAP patients can be treated successfully with beta-lactam monotherapy but are more likely to fail without careful attention and potentially longer hospitalization. If the role of guidelines is to indicate the best treatment of most CAP patients, especially for primary care physicians and hospitalists, combination therapy clearly gives more consistent and lower risk. An analysis of risk benefit confirms that macrolides are not benign but that the mortality cost of not including macrolides with beta-lactams outweighs this risk.

CHALLENGES FOR CURRENT AND FUTURE COMMUNITY-ACQUIRED PNEUMONIA GUIDELINES

Evidence-based guidelines for an infectious disease are difficult, with continued evolution in antibiotic resistance, diagnostic tests, and new antibiotics invalidating older studies and their resultant recommendations. Many important clinical questions do not have sufficient high-quality studies to include in meta-analyses, and therefore, recommendations are often weak or there is no recommendation. Issues that current and future guidelines committees may face include the following.

Minimizing Fluoroquinolone Use

Lost in the debate regarding the need for macrolides are the excellent results with respiratory fluoroquinolones, which have CAP outcomes equivalent or better than beta-lactam/macrolide combination therapy. However, a major emphasis of current antibiotic stewardship efforts is to minimize use of quinolones when other legitimate alternatives exist.[40] This pressure to minimize quinolones is based on emerging data on toxicities and the fact that quinolones remain one of the few orally active agents for serious gram-negative infections.[41] These factors may alter the IDSA/ATS guideline recommendation of fluoroquinolones as equivalent to beta-lactam/macrolide combination therapy for non-ICU hospitalized CAP.

Only one antibiotic with an entirely new mechanism of action is on the FDA fast track for approval for CAP. Lefamulin, the first of the pleuromutilin class of antibiotics,[42] appears to have activity equivalent to moxifloxacin, arguably the best fluoroquinolone for CAP, while having a spectrum that includes MRSA. Drawbacks include limited gram-negative coverage, even for the occasional CAP pathogen. The entirely different mechanism of action makes salvage therapy for prior failures for either fluoroquinolones or beta-lactam/macrolide attractive. Other new antibiotics are next generations of currently available antibiotic classes (macrolides, quinolones). Although covering holes in the current regimens, including MRSA, beta-lactam resistance, and macrolide resistance, the cost/benefit equation for these agents is less favorable.

Increasing Evidence of Viral Cause in Adult Community-Acquired Pneumonia

The EPIC study found that viral detections were significantly more common in adult CAP than bacterial.[29] A large proportion (65%) of the EPIC patients without etiologic detections had procalcitonin (PCT) levels in the range ($\leq$0.25 ng/dL) seen with viral infection and safely managed without antibiotics.[43–46] The combination of more extensive use of respiratory viral panels and increased availability of PCT offers the opportunity to not only diagnose viral CAP but also, more importantly, avoid prolonged courses of antibiotics. Several meta-analyses demonstrate the safety of avoiding antibiotics in patients with persistently low PCT levels, and a guideline committee will have to address this approach.[46,47] Although demonstrated safe in a variety of CAP settings in European studies, concern remains regarding the need to use antibiotics for prevention of secondary bacterial pneumonia following viral infection. A critical aspect of these PCT protocols was a repeat assay if initially negative, because a small proportion of patients will have increased levels with time or in response to a dose of antibiotics. A compromise compatible with the US health care system emphasis on time to first antibiotic dose for suspected infections would be to give a single dose of antibiotics while awaiting a respiratory viral panel and repeat PCT level. Persistently low PCT, especially in the setting of a positive respiratory panel, can be used to stop antibiotics and shift to symptomatic care.

The only viral pneumonia with a legitimate treatment option currently is influenza. The development of other antivirals will significantly change the equation for respiratory viral testing. Treatment of respiratory syncytial virus is in late stage trials, and others are under development.

New Diagnostic Platforms

One of the other major findings of the EPIC study is that routine diagnostic testing for CAP cause is restricted and incomplete: 64% of adults had no pathogen detected.[29] Bacteremia rates have fallen dramatically, partially because of greater emphasis on rapid delivery of antibiotics. Even a single dose of antibiotic may be enough to make blood and respiratory tract cultures negative.

Molecular diagnostics offer an alternative to traditional culture-based methods. They are already the standard for respiratory viral diagnosis. Several platforms under development use various technologies. The greatest limitation is the inability to detect pathogens directly from blood, and therefore pathogens are susceptible to some of the same limitations as sputum cultures. Their highest yield and most likely benefit will be with lower respiratory specimens from intubated patients, especially those with suspected infection with more resistant pathogens, such as *Pseudomonas*, *Enterobacteriaceae*, and MRSA.

Most molecular tests will only detect the presence of a pathogen and offer no data on antibiotic susceptibility, similar to what is currently available with urinary antigen detection of *S pneumoniae* or *Legionella pneumophila*. The number of mutations giving rise to beta-lactam resistance in *S pneumoniae* is too extensive for any polymerase chain reaction–based technology to use for antibiotic susceptibility. Conversely, detection of the mecA gene in *S aureus* is highly predictive of beta-lactam resistance, as is a specific mutation for macrolide resistance in *Mycoplasma*.

No study yet has compared management based on these rapid diagnostic tests to standard limited testing and empirical antibiotic therapy. The ability to detect *S pneumoniae* or *Haemophilus influenzae* is unlikely to dramatically change antibiotic therapy if standard regimens are used, although a positive detection in a patient being treated with broad spectrum agents may have clinical value.

Management of Severe Community-Acquired Pneumonia

No prospective randomized controlled trial has been performed specifically on antibiotic treatment of severe CAP patients. The definition of severe CAP is variable but, specifically, mechanically ventilated and vasopressor-dependent CAP patients are routinely excluded from antibiotic trials.

Therefore, treatment regimens are based on case series or cohort studies, often retrospective.[48,49] Most guidelines recommend use of combination therapy with a beta-lactam and either a macrolide or a fluoroquinolone. Support for the former includes retrospective studies of bacteremic cases, although not all studies find a survival advantage for combination therapy.[50–53]

Consistently, retrospective studies demonstrate prolonged time to appropriate therapy is associated with an increased risk for adverse clinical consequences in CAP, including mechanical ventilation, acute respiratory distress syndrome, septic shock, and acute kidney injury.[54–58] Many studies also demonstrate a slight but clearly higher incidence of less common CAP pathogens in severe CAP,[29,59] mainly S aureus but also including those bacteria often associated with hospital-acquired infections. The tendency to use broad-spectrum treatment is somewhat understandable. However, the current level of evidence, although retrospective, suggests worse outcome with broad spectrum therapy. These contrasting findings result in an additional 2 different challenges to CAP guideline development: definition of patients who do benefit from broad-spectrum therapy and, alternatively, need for adjunctive therapy in severe CAP patients on appropriate antibiotics.

Alternative to Health Care–Associated Pneumonia Risk Factors for Resistant Community-Acquired Pneumonia Pathogens

The original HCAP definition was developed for cases of primary bacteremia and then was applied to pneumonia cases.[11] A small subgroup of patients with community-onset pneumonia will have pathogens resistant to the usual CAP antibiotic regimens. Unfortunately, the original HCAP definitions grossly overestimated that population, and

data demonstrate worse outcome with broad-spectrum antibiotics compared with usual CAP therapy.[60–64] New guidelines will have to address this small subgroup with alternative risk stratification.

An important strategy is to avoid combining pathogens with different risk factors and antibiotic treatment, such as MRSA, *Pseudomonas*, and *Acinetobacter*, into the single entity of HCAP. MRSA is difficult because of separate risks for true community-acquired strains (USA300 and 400)[10,65] and the more traditional hospital-acquired strains that extend into the community.[60,66] Treatment of these 2 MRSA categories may also vary, with a greater need for toxin-suppression therapy in the true community-acquired strain.[67] **Table 2** lists some risk factors for these drug-resistant pathogens[60,68]; application of these risk factors to define antibiotic treatment has not been prospectively validated.

Corticosteroids and Other Immunomodulatory Agents

Given the frequency of hospital and ICU admission and the associated mortality despite appropriate antibiotics, severe CAP is a likely target for immunomodulatory therapy. In fact, CAP predominates in most studies of immunomodulatory treatment of septic shock, and CAP subgroups often demonstrate the greatest benefit.[69–72] However, no agent is currently on the market, now that drotrecogin alfa activated has been withdrawn.[73]

Although routinely available and inexpensive, corticosteroid use in CAP remains very controversial. Meta-analysis suggests that steroid treatment can decrease hospitalization by a day,[74] but these studies were performed in settings wherein the usual LOS was 6 to 7 days and combination therapy with macrolides was rarely used.[35,36] The

Table 2
Risk factors for pathogens resistant to usual community-acquired pneumonia treatment

All drug-resistant pathogens	1. Prior broad-spectrum antibiotic therapy 2. Recent hospitalization 3. Immunocompromising drugs or conditions 4. Prior colonization/infection with drug-resistant pathogen 5. Nursing home patients unable to perform activities of daily living, gastrostomy, tracheostomy		
CA-MRSA	Hospital Strains MRSA	Pseudomonas	*Enterobacteriaceae*
Hemoptysis Influenza season Neutropenia from infection	Hemodialysis Congestive heart failure	Structural lung disease Severe chronic obstructive pulmonary disease Bronchiectasis	Alcoholism Cigarette smoking Gastric acid suppression

greatest theoretic benefit was demonstrated in a randomized controlled trial of CAP patients with very high inflammatory biomarkers, but this population is very infrequent.[75]

SUMMARY

Current guidelines for CAP have had a demonstrated benefit on outcomes and are widely accepted. Differences among guidelines likely reflect the local health care systems and, as such, are appropriately different. Despite this, new data, diagnostic testing, and evolving resistance will require regular updates to guidelines but will challenge consensus.

REFERENCES

1. Mandell LA, Wunderink RG, Anzueto A, et al. Infectious Diseases Society of America/American Thoracic Society consensus guidelines on the management of community-acquired pneumonia in adults. Clin Infect Dis 2007;44(Suppl 2):S27–72.
2. Pfuntner A, Wier LM, Stocks C. Most frequent conditions in U.S. Hospitals, 2011: statistical brief #162. Healthcare cost and utilization project (HCUP) statistical briefs. Rockville (MD): Agency for Healthcare Research and Quality; 2013. Available at: http://www.ncbi.nlm.nih.gov/pubmed/24228292.
3. El Bcheraoui C, Mokdad AH, Dwyer-Lindgren L, et al. Trends and patterns of differences in infectious disease mortality among US Counties, 1980-2014. JAMA 2018;319(12):1248–60.
4. Schappert SM, Burt CW. Ambulatory care visits to physician offices, hospital outpatient departments, and emergency departments: United States, 2001-02. Vital Health Stat 13 2006;(159):1–66.
5. Niederman MS, Bass JB Jr, Campbell GD, et al. Guidelines for the initial management of adults with community-acquired pneumonia: diagnosis, assessment of severity, and initial antimicrobial therapy. American Thoracic Society. Medical Section of the American Lung Association. Am Rev Respir Dis 1993;148(5):1418–26.
6. Niederman MS, Mandell LA, Anzueto A, et al. Guidelines for the management of adults with community-acquired pneumonia. Diagnosis, assessment of severity, antimicrobial therapy, and prevention. Am J Respir Crit Care Med 2001;163(7):1730–54.
7. Dean NC, Bateman KA, Donnelly SM, et al. Improved clinical outcomes with utilization of a community-acquired pneumonia guideline. Chest 2006;130(3):794–9.
8. Dean NC, Silver MP, Bateman KA, et al. Decreased mortality after implementation of a treatment guideline for community-acquired pneumonia. Am J Med 2001;110(6):451–7.
9. Gattarello S, Borgatta B, Sole-Violan J, et al. Decrease in mortality in severe community-acquired pneumococcal pneumonia: impact of improving antibiotic strategies (2000-2013). Chest 2014;146(1):22–31.
10. Lobo LJ, Reed KD, Wunderink RG. Expanded clinical presentation of community-acquired methicillin-resistant Staphylococcus aureus pneumonia. Chest 2010;138(1):130–6.
11. Guidelines for the management of adults with hospital-acquired, ventilator-associated, and healthcare-associated pneumonia. Am J Respir Crit Care Med 2005;171(4):388–416.
12. Eccles S, Pincus C, Higgins B, et al, Guideline Development Group. Diagnosis and management of community and hospital acquired pneumonia in adults: summary of NICE guidance. BMJ 2014; 349:g6722.
13. Alfageme I, Aspa J, Bello S, et al. Guidelines for the diagnosis and management of community-acquired pneumonia. Spanish Society of Pulmonology and Thoracic Surgery (SEPAR). Arch Bronconeumol 2005;41(5):272–89 [in Spanish].
14. Wiersinga WJ, Bonten MJ, Boersma WG, et al. SWAB/NVALT (Dutch Working Party on Antibiotic Policy and Dutch Association of Chest Physicians) guidelines on the management of community-acquired pneumonia in adults. Neth J Med 2012; 70(2):90–101.
15. Hedlund J, Stralin K, Ortqvist A, et al. Swedish guidelines for the management of community-acquired pneumonia in immunocompetent adults. Scand J Infect Dis 2005;37(11–12):791–805.
16. Miyashita N, Matsushima T, Oka M, et al, Japanese Respiratory Society. The JRS guidelines for the management of community-acquired pneumonia in adults: an update and new recommendations. Intern Med 2006;45(7):419–28.
17. Cao B, Huang Y, She DY, et al. Diagnosis and treatment of community-acquired pneumonia in adults: 2016 clinical practice guidelines by the Chinese Thoracic Society, Chinese Medical Association. Clin Respir J 2018;12(4):1320–60.
18. Houck PM, MacLehose RF, Niederman MS, et al. Empiric antibiotic therapy and mortality among medicare pneumonia inpatients in 10 western states : 1993, 1995, and 1997. Chest 2001;119(5):1420–6.
19. Diaz MH, Benitez AJ, Cross KE, et al. Molecular detection and characterization of mycoplasma pneumoniae among patients hospitalized with community-acquired pneumonia in the United States. Open Forum Infect Dis 2015;2(3):ofv106.
20. Amsden GW. Anti-inflammatory effects of macrolides—an underappreciated benefit in the treatment of community-acquired respiratory tract infections and chronic inflammatory pulmonary conditions? J Antimicrob Chemother 2005;55(1):10–21.

21. Anderson R, Steel HC, Cockeran R, et al. Clarithro-mycin alone and in combination with ceftriaxone inhibits the production of pneumolysin by both macrolide-susceptible and macrolide-resistant strains of Streptococcus pneumoniae. J Antimicrob Chemother 2007;59(2):224–9.

22. Dessing MC, Hirst RA, de Vos AF, et al. Role of Toll-like receptors 2 and 4 in pulmonary inflammation and injury induced by pneumolysin in mice. PLoS One 2009;4(11):e7993.

23. Meehan TP, Fine MJ, Krumholz HM, et al. Quality of care, process, and outcomes in elderly patients with pneumonia. JAMA 1997;278(23):2080–4.

24. Brown RB, Iannini P, Gross P, et al. Impact of initial antibiotic choice on clinical outcomes in community-acquired pneumonia: analysis of a hospital claims-made database. Chest 2003;123(5):1503–11.

25. Garcia Vazquez E, Mensa J, Martinez JA, et al. Lower mortality among patients with community-acquired pneumonia treated with a macrolide plus a beta-lactam agent versus a beta-lactam agent alone. Eur J Clin Microbiol Infect Dis 2005;24(3):190–5.

26. Gleason PP, Meehan TP, Fine JM, et al. Associations between initial antimicrobial therapy and medical outcomes for hospitalized elderly patients with pneumonia. Arch Intern Med 1999;159(21):2562–72.

27. Rodrigo C, McKeever TM, Woodhead M, et al. Single versus combination antibiotic therapy in adults hospitalised with community acquired pneumonia. Thorax 2013;68(5):493–5.

28. Tessmer A, Welte T, Martus P, et al. Impact of intravenous b-lactam/macrolide versus b-lactam monotherapy on mortality in hospitalized patients with community-acquired pneumonia. J Antimicrob Chemother 2009;63(5):1025–33.

29. Jain S, Self WH, Wunderink RG, et al. Community-acquired pneumonia requiring hospitalization among U.S. adults. N Engl J Med 2015;373(5):415–27.

30. Wunderink RG, Self WH, Anderson EJ, et al. Pneumococcal community-acquired pneumonia detected by serotype-specific urinary antigen detection assays. Clin Infect Dis 2018;66(10):1504–10.

31. Marston BJ, Plouffe JF, File TM Jr, et al. Incidence of community-acquired pneumonia requiring hospitalization. Results of a population-based active surveillance Study in Ohio. The Community-Based Pneumonia Incidence Study Group. Arch Intern Med 1997;157(15):1709–18.

32. Griffin MR, Zhu Y, Moore MR, et al. U.S. hospitalizations for pneumonia after a decade of pneumococcal vaccination. N Engl J Med 2013;369(2):155–63.

33. Whitney CG, Farley MM, Hadler J, et al. Decline in invasive pneumococcal disease after the introduction of protein-polysaccharide conjugate vaccine. N Engl J Med 2003;348(18):1737–46.

34. Postma DF, van Werkhoven CH, van Elden LJ, et al. Antibiotic treatment strategies for community-acquired pneumonia in adults. N Engl J Med 2015;372(14):1312–23.

35. Meijvis SC, Hardeman H, Remmelts HH, et al. Dexamethasone and length of hospital stay in patients with community-acquired pneumonia: a randomised, double-blind, placebo-controlled trial. Lancet 2011;377(9782):2023–30.

36. Snijders D, Daniels JM, de Graaff CS, et al. Efficacy of corticosteroids in community-acquired pneumonia: a randomized double-blinded clinical trial. Am J Respir Crit Care Med 2010;181(9):975–82.

37. Garin N, Genne D, Carballo S, et al. beta-Lactam monotherapy vs beta-lactam-macrolide combination treatment in moderately severe community-acquired pneumonia: a randomized noninferiority trial. JAMA Intern Med 2014;174(12):1894–901.

38. Spellberg B, Fleming TR, Gilbert DN. Executive summary: workshop on issues in the design and conduct of clinical trials of antibacterial drugs in the treatment of community-acquired pneumonia. Clin Infect Dis 2008;47(Suppl 3):S105–7.

39. Halm EA, Fine MJ, Marrie TJ, et al. Time to clinical stability in patients hospitalized with community-acquired pneumonia: implications for practice guidelines. JAMA 1998;279:1452–7.

40. Weiss K, Tillotson GS. Fluoroquinolones for respiratory infection: too valuable to overuse (and too valuable to misuse!). Chest 2002;122(3):1102–3 [author reply: 1103].

41. Spellberg B. Community-acquired pneumonia. N Engl J Med 2014;370(19):1861–2.

42. Mendes RE, Farrell DJ, Flamm RK, et al. In vitro activity of lefamulin tested against streptococcus pneumoniae with defined serotypes, including multidrug-resistant isolates causing lower respiratory tract infections in the United States. Antimicrob Agents Chemother 2016;60(7):4407–11.

43. Self WH, Wunderink RG, Jain S, et al, Etiology of Pneumonia in the Community (EPIC) Study Investigators. Procalcitonin as a marker of etiology in adults hospitalized with community-acquired pneumonia. Clin Infect Dis 2018;66(10):1640–1.

44. Christ-Crain M, Jaccard-Stolz D, Bingisser R, et al. Effect of procalcitonin-guided treatment on antibiotic use and outcome in lower respiratory tract infections: cluster-randomised, single-blinded intervention trial. Lancet 2004;363(9409):600–7.

45. Christ-Crain M, Stolz D, Bingisser R, et al. Procalcitonin guidance of antibiotic therapy in community-acquired pneumonia: a randomized trial. Am J Respir Crit Care Med 2006;174(1):84–93.

46. Schuetz P, Briel M, Christ-Crain M, et al. Procalcitonin to guide initiation and duration of antibiotic treatment in acute respiratory infections: an individual

patient data meta-analysis. Clin Infect Dis 2012; 55(5):651–62.

47. Soni NJ, Samson DJ, Galaydick JL, et al. Procalcitonin-guided antibiotic therapy: a systematic review and meta-analysis. J Hosp Med 2013;8(9): 530–40.

48. Frei CR, Attridge RT, Mortensen EM, et al. Guideline-concordant antibiotic use and survival among patients with community-acquired pneumonia admitted to the intensive care unit. Clin Ther 2010; 32(2):293–9.

49. Rodriguez A, Mendia A, Sirvent JM, et al. Combination antibiotic therapy improves survival in patients with community-acquired pneumonia and shock. Crit Care Med 2007;35(6):1493–8.

50. Baddour LM, Yu VL, Klugman KP, et al. Combination antibiotic therapy lowers mortality among severely ill patients with pneumococcal bacteremia. Am J Respir Crit Care Med 2004;170(4):440–4.

51. Harbarth S, Garbino J, Pugin J, et al. Lack of effect of combination antibiotic therapy on mortality in patients with pneumococcal sepsis. Eur J Clin Microbiol Infect Dis 2005;24(10):688–90.

52. Martinez JA, Horcajada JP, Almela M, et al. Addition of a macrolide to a beta-lactam-based empirical antibiotic regimen is associated with lower in-hospital mortality for patients with bacteremic pneumococcal pneumonia. Clin Infect Dis 2003;36(4): 389–95.

53. Waterer GW, Somes GW, Wunderink RG. Monotherapy may be suboptimal for severe bacteremic pneumococcal pneumonia. Arch Intern Med 2001; 161(15):1837–42.

54. Rodriguez A, Lisboa T, Blot S, et al. Mortality in ICU patients with bacterial community-acquired pneumonia: when antibiotics are not enough. Intensive Care Med 2009;35(3):430–8.

55. Kojicic M, Li G, Hanson AC, et al. Risk factors for the development of acute lung injury in patients with infectious pneumonia. Crit Care 2012; 16(2):R46.

56. Garcia-Vidal C, Fernandez-Sabe N, Carratala J, et al. Early mortality in patients with community-acquired pneumonia: causes and risk factors. Eur Respir J 2008;32(3):733–9.

57. Leroy O, Santre C, Beuscart C, et al. A five-year study of severe community-acquired pneumonia with emphasis on prognosis in patients admitted to an intensive care unit. Intensive Care Med 1995; 21(1):24–31.

58. Gattarello S, Lagunes L, Vidaur L, et al. Improvement of antibiotic therapy and ICU survival in severe non-pneumococcal community-acquired pneumonia: a matched case-control study. Crit Care 2015;19:335.

59. van der Eerden MM, Vlaspolder F, de Graaff CS, et al. Comparison between pathogen directed antibiotic treatment and empirical broad spectrum antibiotic treatment in patients with community acquired pneumonia: a prospective randomised study. Thorax 2005;60(8):672–8.

60. Shindo Y, Ito R, Kobayashi D, et al. Risk factors for drug-resistant pathogens in community-acquired and healthcare-associated pneumonia. Am J Respir Crit Care Med 2013;188(8):985–95.

61. Attridge RT, Frei CR, Restrepo MI, et al. Guideline-concordant therapy and outcomes in healthcare-associated pneumonia. Eur Respir J 2011;38(4): 878–87.

62. Chalmers JD, Rother C, Salih W, et al. Healthcare-associated pneumonia does not accurately identify potentially resistant pathogens: a systematic review and meta-analysis. Clin Infect Dis 2014; 58(3):330–9.

63. Garcia-Vidal C, Viasus D, Roset A, et al. Low incidence of multidrug-resistant organisms in patients with healthcare-associated pneumonia requiring hospitalization. Clin Microbiol Infect 2011;17(11): 1659–65.

64. Webb BJ, Dangerfield BS, Pasha JS, et al. Guideline-concordant antibiotic therapy and clinical outcomes in healthcare-associated pneumonia. Respir Med 2012;106(11):1606–12.

65. Gillet Y, Vanhems P, Lina G, et al. Factors predicting mortality in necrotizing community-acquired pneumonia caused by Staphylococcus aureus containing Panton-Valentine leukocidin. Clin Infect Dis 2007; 45(3):315–21.

66. Kollef MH, Shorr A, Tabak YP, et al. Epidemiology and outcomes of health-care-associated pneumonia: results from a large US database of culture-positive pneumonia. Chest 2005;128(6): 3854–62.

67. Sicot N, Khanafer N, Meyssonnier V, et al. Methicillin resistance is not a predictor of severity in community-acquired Staphylococcus aureus necrotizing pneumonia–results of a prospective observational study. Clin Microbiol Infect 2013;19(3):E142–8.

68. Wunderink RG, Waterer GW. Clinical practice. Community-acquired pneumonia. N Engl J Med 2014;370(6):543–51.

69. Abraham E, Anzueto A, Gutierrez G, et al. Double-blind randomised controlled trial of monoclonal antibody to human tumour necrosis factor in treatment of septic shock. NORASEPT II Study Group. Lancet 1998;351(9107):929–33.

70. Laterre PF, Garber G, Levy H, et al. Severe community-acquired pneumonia as a cause of severe sepsis: data from the PROWESS study. Crit Care Med 2005;33(5):952–61.

71. Wunderink RG, Laterre PF, Francois B, et al. Recombinant tissue factor pathway inhibitor in severe community-acquired pneumonia: a randomized trial. Am J Respir Crit Care Med 2011;183(11):1561–8.

72. Wunderink RG, Leeper KV Jr, Schein R, et al. Filgrastim in patients with pneumonia and severe sepsis or septic shock. Chest 2001;119:523–9.

73. Ranieri VM, Thompson BT, Barie PS, et al. Drotrecogin alfa (activated) in adults with septic shock. N Engl J Med 2012;366(22):2055–64.

74. Siemieniuk RA, Meade MO, Alonso-Coello P, et al. Corticosteroid therapy for patients hospitalized with community-acquired pneumonia: a systematic review and meta-analysis. Ann Intern Med 2015; 163(7):519–28.

75. Torres A, Sibila O, Ferrer M, et al. Effect of corticosteroids on treatment failure among hospitalized patients with severe community-acquired pneumonia and high inflammatory response: a randomized clinical trial. JAMA 2015;313(7):677–86.

Vaccines to Prevent Pneumococcal Community-Acquired Pneumonia

Cornelis H. van Werkhoven, MD, PhD[a],*,
Susanne M. Huijts, MD, PhD[b]

KEYWORDS

- Streptococcus pneumoniae • Community-acquired pneumonia • Invasive pneumococcal disease
- Pneumococcal vaccines • Pneumococcal conjugate vaccine
- Pneumococcal polysaccharide vaccine

KEY POINTS

- In the elderly, pneumococcal polysaccharide vaccines are efficacious in preventing invasive pneumococcal disease, but efficacy against pneumococcal pneumonia has not been established.
- The 13-valent pneumococcal conjugate vaccine has been demonstrated to be effective in prevention of vaccine type community-acquired pneumonia and vaccine-type invasive pneumococcal disease in immunocompetent elderly populations.
- The benefit of pneumococcal vaccination among adults mainly depends on the incidence of vaccine-preventable pneumococcal disease and vaccine efficacy.
- Vaccine-preventable pneumococcal disease incidence is decreasing owing to childhood immunization with pneumococcal conjugate vaccines.

INTRODUCTION

Lower respiratory infections, including pneumonia, are among the top 10-causes of death according to the World Health Organization, causing 3.2 million deaths worldwide in 2015.[1] The most frequent pathogen causing pneumonia is *Streptococcus pneumoniae*.[2] The elderly and young children are especially at risk for developing pneumococcal pneumonia and prevention by vaccination has been the subject of attention for many decades.

In this article, we review the epidemiology of pneumococcal community-acquired pneumonia (CAP), history of pneumococcal vaccination, immunogenicity, indirect effects of child immunization, efficacy of both pneumococcal polysaccharide (PPVs) and pneumococcal conjugate (PCVs) vaccines in adults and the benefit of adult pneumococcal vaccination.

EPIDEMIOLOGY OF PNEUMOCOCCAL COMMUNITY-ACQUIRED PNEUMONIA

Although there are more than 90 known serotypes of the pneumococcus, only a part of these serotypes cause infection. Infections can vary from mild mucosal infections like otitis media to severe invasive infections like CAP, meningitis, and other invasive infections. *S pneumoniae* is the most common causative agent of CAP. In a metaanalysis that included studies conducted in hospitalized

Disclosure Statement: C.H. van Werkhoven reports speaker fees and financial support for thesis printing from Pfizer, and speaker fees from Merck/MSD. S.M. Huijts reports financial support from Pfizer for thesis printing. Both authors were involved in research funded by Pfizer through their institution.

[a] Julius Center for Health Sciences and Primary Care, University Medical Center Utrecht, PO-Box 85500, Utrecht 3508 GA, The Netherlands; [b] Department of Respiratory Medicine, University Medical Center Utrecht, PO-Box 85500, Utrecht 3508 GA, The Netherlands
* Corresponding author.
E-mail address: c.h.vanwerkhoven@umcutrecht.nl

Clin Chest Med 39 (2018) 733–752
https://doi.org/10.1016/j.ccm.2018.07.007

patients with bacterial CAP, *S pneumoniae* was found in 7.5% to 26.0% of cases, depending on the diagnostic test.[3] In radiologically confirmed CAP in the primary care setting, the proportion of confirmed pneumococcal etiology varies from less than 10% to more than 30%, depending on country, microbiological testing performed, and health care setting.[4–6] In more than 50% of CAP cases, the causative agent remains undetected, potentially representing in part undetected pneumococcal infection.

Infection progresses through colonization of the upper respiratory tract, where *S pneumoniae* is part of the bacterial flora. Asymptomatic carriage of pneumococci usually lasts weeks to months and does not necessarily lead to infection; there is an inverse relationship between duration of carriage and infection rate of *S pneumoniae* serotypes.[7,8] The prevalence of carriage is age dependent: prevalence rates in developed countries are highest in young children (ranging from 24% to 70%) and decrease in older children and adults (8%–22%).[9–11] Since the introduction of PCVs in children, rates of vaccine-type pneumococcal carriage have decreased in individuals in both vaccine targeted and nontargeted age groups, but overall rates of pneumococcal carriage have not changed notably.[12,13]

Pneumococcal infections and especially pneumonia are a frequent cause of morbidity and mortality globally. Reported incidences of CAP in developed countries range from 1 to 11 per 1000 per year in the adult population and, with a global number of 3.2 million deaths owing to lower respiratory tract infections, it is the most important cause of mortality from infection.[14,15] In children, CAP is the number one cause of mortality worldwide.[1,16–18] The highest incidence rates of CAP requiring hospital admission are found in children up to 2 years of age (6–8 per 1000 per year) and in elderly individuals (35–40 per 1000 per year in those aged over 85 years of age).[19–22] Hospitalization rates of 20% to 40% have been reported in adult patients with CAP.[23–26]

Invasive pneumococcal disease (IPD) is defined as an infection in which *S pneumoniae* is isolated from normally sterile body fluids. The most common infections associated with IPD are pneumonia and meningitis. Bacteremia is present in 25% of pneumococcal CAP cases.[3] The incidence rates of IPD are greatest in young children, elderly patients, patients with chronic comorbid conditions such as chronic liver disease and chronic obstructive pulmonary disease, and immunocompromised patients, and these groups are also at increased risk of adverse outcomes.[27] Mortality in patients with IPD lies between 3% in young children and 18% in the elderly, but has decreased in the elderly group since the introduction of PCVs in national immunization programs.[28]

There is a clear seasonal pattern of CAP and IPD that coincides with influenza epidemics, although the magnitude of the influenza epidemic is only moderately correlated with the winter peak of IPD incidence.[29,30] The proportion of pneumococcal etiology in CAP may also vary between seasons.[31]

HISTORY

The first human experiment of pneumococcal vaccination, based on administration of a mixture of polysaccharides, was conducted in 1911 and the first hexavalent-vaccine was registered in 1946. However, these vaccines were soon withdrawn because of the discovery of penicillin, with the general expectation that this new treatment would eliminate the threat of pneumonia.[32] In the late 1970s, a 14-valent PPV was registered in the United States, containing purified polysaccharides of 14 pneumococcal serotypes 1, 2, 3, 4, 6A, 7F, 8, 9N, 12F, 14, 18C, 19F, 23F, and 25F. In 1983, this vaccine was replaced by a 23-valent PPV (PPV23). Serotype 25F was dropped and 10 additional serotypes were included (**Table 1**). In the following years, many countries implemented general PPV23 vaccination for people over 65 years of age and for those in certain risk groups.[33]

Until 2011, this vaccine remained the only pneumococcal vaccine for immunization of adults. The vaccine induces T-cell–independent B-cell responses, yielding antibodies in adults but not in young children. Because immunologic memory is not induced, vaccination needs to be repeated every 5 years.

Since the turn of the century, new pneumococcal vaccines have been made available, with polysaccharide capsular antigens conjugated to a protein (PCVs). The latter induces T-cell–dependent immune responses, yielding adequate antibody responses in adults and young children, and also resulting in immunologic memory. The first PCV, PCV7 was introduced in the United States in 2000 for use in infants, containing 7 serotypes (see **Table 1**). Introduction in Europe followed in 2001. In 2009, PCV10 was registered in Europe, followed by PCV13 in the same year (see **Table 1**). PCV13 was licensed in the United States in 2010. The PCVs were first only registered for use in children, because the vaccination trials for registration were carried out in this age group.

Since October 2011, PCV13 has been licensed for prevention of IPD in adults aged greater than 50 years of age in Europe. In June 2012, the US

Table 1
Overview of various pneumococcal vaccines

Vaccine	Year	1	2	3	4	5	6A	6B	7F	8	9N	9V	10A	11A	12F	14	15B	17F	18C	19A	19F	20	22F	23F	33	Description
PPV23	1983	x	x	x	x	x	—	x	x	x	x	x	x	x	x	x	x	x	x	x	x	x	x	x	x	Inducing T-cell–independent B-cell responses: no immunologic memory, no antibody response in children. Suitable for individuals of >2 y of age. Recommended in most countries for risk groups (see **Table 2**)
PCV7	2000	—	—	—	x	—	—	x	—	—	—	x	—	—	—	x	—	—	x	—	x	—	—	x	—	Polysaccharide capsular antigens conjugated to a protein inducing T-cell–dependent immune response: immunologic memory, adequate antibody response also in young children. Only licensed for use in children. Introduced in most developed countries in the infant immunization program from 2000 onward
PCV10	2009	x	—	—	x	x	—	x	x	—	—	x	—	—	—	x	—	—	x	—	x	—	—	x	—	See general remarks under PCV7. Part of infant immunization program in a few countries (see **Table 2**)
PCV13	2010	x	—	x	x	x	x	x	x	—	—	x	—	—	—	x	—	—	x	x	x	—	—	x	—	See general remarks under PCV7. Until today part of infant immunization program in most developed countries (see **Table 2**). 2011: also licensed for use in adults. 2014: ACIP recommendation to use as pneumococcal vaccine for adults >65 y of age

Abbreviations: ACIP, Advisory Committee on Immunization Practices; PCV, pneumococcal conjugate vaccine (number indicating valency); PPV23, 23-valent pneumococcal polysaccharide vaccine.

Food and Drug Administration approved PCV13 for all adults older than 50 years of age for the prevention of pneumonia and IPD.[34]

After the results of the CAPiTA study became available,[35] the Advisory Committee on Immunization Practices decided in September 2014 to include PCV13 vaccination in their recommendations: adults 65 years and older who have never received a pneumococcal vaccine should first receive a dose of PCV13 followed 6 to 12 months later by a dose of PPV23.[36] Other countries have now also implemented the use of PCV13 in adult immunization schedules (**Table 2**).

IMMUNOGENICITY

Immunogenicity is measured by the serotype specific IgG antibody levels and/or by functional antibody responses (opsonophagocytic activity). To evaluate the immune responses of the various vaccines, these measures are compared in prevaccination and postvaccination samples.[37]

In adults, a single dose of PCV7 yields higher or at least equal immune responses as a single dose of PPV23, both in immunocompetent and in immunocompromised adults.[38–42] Furthermore, 2 randomized, multicenter, immunogenicity studies conducted in the United States and Europe among older adults demonstrated that PCV13 induced an immune response as good as or better than that induced by PPV23 and independent of age and comorbidity.[43–45]

Although PCVs induce immunologic memory, it is unclear if the immune response lasts longer. One year after vaccination with PCV13 or PPV23 among 831 adults (60–64 years of age), the immune response decreased for both vaccines, varying per serotype (some showing a higher opsonophagocytic activity titer for PCV13 vaccination, but not consistently).[44] Among 181 patients with moderate to severe chronic obstructive pulmonary disease vaccinated with PCV7 or PPV23, the majority of the opsonophagocytic activity titers were higher at 1 and 2 years after vaccination for subjects vaccinated with PCV7.[46]

Because memory B cells are activated by the use of PCV, it was hypothesized that the use of PCVs might prime the immune system for a better immune response to PPV. There are a few studies that support this hypothesis. One study demonstrated higher antibody levels in subjects who received PPV23 1 year after PCV13[47] and similar results were found when the interval was extended to 4 years.[48] The first study also demonstrated that PCV13 followed after one year by PPV23 yielded higher immune responses after the second

vaccination compared to PPV23 followed by PCV13.[48] Therefore, the Advisory Committee on Immunization Practices in the United States recommends a dose of PCV13 first, followed by PPV23 with an interval of preferably 1 year and at least 8 weeks.[49]

INDIRECT EFFECTS FROM CHILD IMMUNIZATION WITH PNEUMOCOCCAL CONJUGATE VACCINES

PCV7 was introduced in the United States infant immunization program in 2000 and was replaced by PCV13 in 2010.[50,51] Both introductions were accompanied by a catch-up program in children younger than 5 years of age. Shortly after the introduction of PCV7, substantial decreases in the incidence of IPD were observed in children.[52] Indirect effects in adults also resulted in a reduced incidence of vaccine serotype (VT) IPD in adults, partly replaced by non-VT IPD.[52] Similar effects have been reported after the introduction of PCV13 (**Fig. 1**).[28,53–58]

In a few countries, PCV10 is used instead of PCV13 (see **Table 2**). PCV10 uses a different conjugation protein and the polysaccharide dosages are lower. Indirect effects have been described for PCV10, but data seem to be too limited to compare effect sizes with PCV7 and PCV13.[59–62] Nasopharyngeal pneumococcal colonization in children is considered to be the most important reservoir of pneumococcal infection in adults and indirect effects (also termed herd protection) for adults are, therefore, assumed to result from changes in the serotype distribution of pneumococci carried in children.[63] In a systematic review of randomized, controlled trials comparing one of the PCVs with controls, the effects of immunization on pneumococcal carriage in children aged 6 to 12 months were less for the single included study of an 11-valent PCV (the precursor of PCV10) compared with studies of PCV7.[64] In contrast, there was no difference in VT pneumococcal colonization in a trial comparing PCV10 with PCV7, although the effects may have been masked by universal child immunization with PCV7 during this trial[65] and PCV10 compared with no vaccine caused both direct and indirect (ie, in unvaccinated siblings) reductions in VT *S pneumoniae* carriage 2 studies.[66–68] A natural experiment conducted in Sweden, where 21 counties used either PCV10 or PCV13, revealed similar direct and indirect effects between PCV10 and PCV13.[69] Possible local differences, for example, in contact patterns between the elderly and children, hamper comparisons of the observed indirect effects. Yet, if PCV10

Table 2
Pneumococcal vaccination policies

Country	Children	Elderly[a]	Immunocompromised	Other	Guideline Sources
USA	PCV13	PCV13 followed by PPV23	PCV13 followed by PPV23	Adult smokers, alcoholics, selected comorbidities: PPV23	CDC 2017: https://www.cdc.gov/vaccines/vpd/pneumo/hcp/who-when-to-vaccinate.html
Australia	PCV13	PPV23	PCV13 followed by PPV23	Aboriginal and Torres Strait Islander people >50 y: PPV23 Aboriginal and Torres Strait Islander people 18–49 y with selected comorbidities/alcoholics/smokers: PPV23	http://www.immunise.health.gov.au/internet/immunise/publishing.nsf/Content/nips
UK	PCV13	PPV23	PCV13 followed by PPV23[b]	Asplenia, selected comorbidities, cochlear implant, CSF leakage: PPV23	h:tps://www.nhs.uk/conditions/vaccinations/pneumococcal-vaccination/?tabname=nhs-vaccination-schedule
Canada	PCV13	PPV23	PCV13 followed by 2 doses PPV23[c]	Selected comorbidities, long term care facilities, smokers, alcoholics, homeless: PPV23	https://www.canada.ca/en/public-health/services/publications/healthy-living/canadian-immunization-guide-part-4-active-vaccines/page-16-pneumococcal-vaccine.html
Netherlands	PVC10	None	PCV13 followed by PPV23	None	https://lci.rivm.nl/richtlijnen/pneumokokkenziekte-invasief#immunisatie
Belgium	PCV10[d]	PCV13 followed by PPV23	PCV13 followed by PPV23	Adults 50–85 y with selected comorbidities: PCV13 followed by PPV23	https://www.health.belgium.be/sites/default/files/uploads/fields/fpshealth_theme_file/19100960/Vaccinatie%20tegen%20pneumokokken%20-%20volwassenen%20%282014%29%20%28HGR%209210%29.pdf https://www.zorg-en-gezondheid.be/sites/default/files/atoms/files/vaccinatie%20fiche%20pneumokokken%20kinderen%202015.pdf https://kce.fgov.be/nl/welk-vaccin-om-ouderen-tegen-pneumokokken-te-beschermen

(continued on next page)

Table 2
(continued)

Country	Children	Elderly[a]	Immunocompromised	Other	Guideline Sources
Germany	PCV13	>60 y: PPV23	PCV13 followed by PPV23	Selected comorbidities: PPV23 Cochlear implant/CSF leakage: PCV13 followed by PPV23	https://www.rki.de/EN/Content/infections/Vaccination/recommandations/34_2017_engl.pdf?blob=publicationFile
Sweden	PCV13	PPV23	PPV23	Selected comorbidities, cochlear implant, CSF leakage: PPV23	https://www.folkhalsomyndigheten.se/the-public-health-agency-of-sweden/communicable-disease-control/vaccinations/vaccination-programmes/
Finland	PCV10	PCV13 and/or PPV23[e]	PCV13 followed by PPV23[f]	PCV13 and/or PPV23[e]	https://thl.fi/en/web/vaccination/national-vaccination-programme/vaccination-programme-for-children-and-adolescents https://thl.fi/fi/web/rokottaminen/rokotteet/pneumokokkirokote/taulukko-2
Denmark	PCV13	PPV23 or PCV13 followed by PPV23[g]	PCV13 followed by PPV23	Selected comorbidities, smoking, occupational risk: PCV13 followed by PPV23[g]	ECDC: https://ecdc.europa.eu/en/immunisation-vaccines/EU-vaccination-schedules https://www.ssi.dk/English/News/EPI-NEWS/2014/No%2040%20-%202014.aspx
Italy	PCV13	Mixed PPV23/PCV13 schedule	PCV13 + PPV23 (order not clearly described)	Selected comorbidities, alcoholism: PCV13 + PPV23 (order not clearly described)	ECDC: https://ecdc.europa.eu/en/immunisation-vaccines/EU-vaccination-schedules https://www.tandfonline.com/doi/full/10.1080/21645515.2017.1343773 http://www.epicentro.iss.it/temi/vaccinazioni/GruppiRischio.asp http://www.salute.gov.it/imgs/C_17_pubblicazioni_2571_allegato.pdf
France	PCV13	None	PCV13 followed by PPV23	Selected comorbidities, cancer: PCV13 followed by PPV23	https://www.mesvaccins.net/web/news/10638-les-nouveautes-du-calendrier-vaccinal-2017-meningocoques-et-pneumocoques-papillomavirus-bcg-varicelle-et-penuries

Country					Reference
Spain	PCV13	PCV13 followed by PPV23	PCV13 followed by PPV23	Selected comorbidities, alcoholism, smoking: PCV13 followed by PPV23	http://vacunasaep.org/familias/vacunas-una-a-una/vacuna-neumococo http://www.msal.gob.ar/images/stories/bes/graficos/0000000947cnt-Lineamientos_neumo_adultos_WEB.pdf
Japan	PCV13	PPV23	Not found	>60 y and with comorbidities or immunocompromised: PPV23	http://www.niid.go.jp/niid/images/vaccine/schedule/2016/EN20161001.jpg WHO: http://apps.who.int/immunization_monitoring/globalsummary/schedules?sc%5B%5D=JPN&sc%5Bd%5D=&sc%5Bv%5D%5B%5D=PNEUMO_CONJ&sc%5Bv%5D%5B%5D=PNEUMO_PS&sc%5BOK%5D=OK
Russia	PCV13 or PCV10[h]	PCV13 followed by PPV23	Not found	Not found	http://www.yaprivit.ru/o-vaccinah/vaccines/privivka-ot-pnevmokokkovoj-infekcii/
China	PCV13	None[i]	Not found	Not found	https://www.tandfonline.com/doi/pdf/10.1080/21645515.2017.1409316?needAccess=true
South Africa	PCV13	PCV13 followed by PPV23	PCV13 followed by PPV23	Severe underlying comorbid conditions: PCV13 followed by PPV23	http://www.nicd.ac.za/assets/files/NICD_Vaccine_Booklet_D132_FINAL.pdf https://www.ncbi.nlm.nih.gov/pmc/articles/PMC5506119/

Abbreviations: CSF, cerebrospinal fluid; PCV, pneumococcal conjugate vaccine (number indicating valency); PPV23, 23-valent pneumococcal polysaccharide vaccine.

a For those ≥65 years of age unless otherwise indicated.
b Only accounts for severe immunocompromised subjects: multiple myeloma, leukemia, bone marrow transplantation or genetic disorders affecting the immune system.
c Second dose concerns revaccination with PPV23 after 5 years of age.
d Between 2011 and 2015 use of PCV13.
e Recommended but not free of charge. Choice of vaccine depends on preference of patient and/or earlier vaccination.
f Only accounts for stem cell transplant patients.
g Recommended, but no reimbursement from Danish government.
h Both are mentioned in the national vaccination program.
i No recommendation in national immunization program, only available at own expenses.

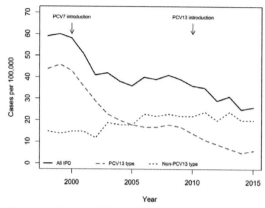

Fig. 1. Incidence of all-serotype, PCV13 serotype, and non-PCV13 serotype IPD in adults ≥65 years in the US. IPD, invasive pneumococcal disease; PCV, pneumococcal conjugate vaccine (number indicating valency). (*Data from* Centers for Disease Control and Prevention. Active Bacterial Core surveillance, Trends by Serotype Group, 1998–2015. 2016. Available at: https://www.cdc.gov/abcs/reports-findings/survreports/spneutypes.html.)

immunization of children (as compared with PCV7 or PCV13) would have fewer indirect effects in adults, this would have important consequences for policy making. Moreover, the 3 additional serotypes contained in PCV13 are among the most frequently observed replacing serotypes after PCV7 introduction.[70]

Although indirect effects are well-documented for IPD, the indirect effects on non-IPD pneumococcal CAP are less well-established. Because IPD represents only about 25% of all pneumococcal infections in adults, the evaluation of indirect effects based on IPD may not accurately reflect those for non-IPD pneumococcal CAP.[3] Assumptions regarding indirect effects for non-IPD pneumococcal CAP are essential in cost-effectiveness analyses.[71] The limited available data on indirect effects for non-IPD pneumococcal CAP suggest that the relative indirect effects are similar to those seen in IPD, although the assumption that absolute effects are also similar cannot be corroborated with data.[72]

EFFICACY OF PNEUMOCOCCAL POLYSACCHARIDE VACCINES

Although many countries have implemented routine PPV23 immunization for the elderly (see **Table 2**), the efficacy to prevent pneumococcal pneumonia remains debated. There is broad consensus that PPV23 is efficacious in preventing IPD in all populations except those less than 2 years of age and pneumococcal pneumonia in

young adults. However, for pneumococcal pneumonia in at-risk populations (the elderly and those with chronic comorbidities), the conclusions are less straightforward.[73–78] The trials performed so far are clinically heterogeneous, most have an inadequate sample size to draw firm conclusions, and many use suboptimal microbiological tests for confirmation of pneumococcal etiology. We have summarized the evidence in **Table 3**, with a focus on the elderly or patients with chronic comorbidities, because most countries use these criteria to determine the target population. Here we discuss the most important trials.

In the open population of elderly, a large, open-label trial has been performed in 26,925 community-dwelling adults over 65 years of age in Finland.[79] They received PPV23 together with influenza vaccine or influenza vaccine alone based on year of birth. No difference was found for the number of all-cause or pneumococcal pneumonias with a trend in favor of the group receiving the influenza vaccine only. This study was criticized for using serology to determine pneumococcal etiology, which has a low specificity and for this reason has been ignored in policy making.[80] However, even if this test has a very poor specificity (which leads to bias toward no effect), a trend toward a negative effect of the size observed in this study would be unlikely if the vaccine has a meaningful protective effect. Another trial in the elderly in the general population that was adequately powered only showed an effect on pneumococcal pneumonia in a subgroup at increased risk of pneumonia.[81] However, because as many as 7 subgroup analyses were performed, there is a high risk of false-positive findings. Other trials had too low sample sizes or too few outcomes to draw any conclusion on clinical outcomes.[82,83]

Two large trials in nursing home residents have been performed. In France, nursing and elderly home residents were randomized to PPV14 or no vaccine in an open-label trial; 40 patients contracted suspected pneumococcal pneumonia over a 2 year follow-up period.[84] A decrease in both suspected pneumococcal pneumonia and microbiologically confirmed pneumococcal pneumonia of about 75% was observed, although only the first was statistically significant. In Japan, 1006 nursing home residents were randomized to PPV23 or placebo.[85] They found a vaccine efficacy (VE) of 44.8% for all-cause pneumonia and 63.8% for pneumococcal pneumonia. In both studies, high incidences of pneumonia were observed in the control groups: about 5% in 2 years in the first and 91 per 1000 person-years in the second study. In both studies, there was no impact on all-cause

Table 3
Trials of PPV and PCV in elderly and at-risk adults

Author, Year	Country, Study Period	Size	Domain	Intervention (Vaccine)	Randomization and Blinding	Results	Limitations
PPV: General population							
Austrian,[82] 1980 (B)	USA Study period unknown	13,600	Adults with health insurance plan	PPV12 vs placebo	Randomized; placebo used but blinding not described	IPD VE: 89% (−107% to 99%)[b] All-cause pneumonia VE: 2% (−17% to 17%)[b]	Primary study not accessible
Koivula et al,[81] 1997	Finland 1982–1985	2837	Subject >65 y old	PPV14 + influenza vs influenza	Randomized by computer; single blinded	All subjects: Pneumococcal pneumonia: VE 15% (95% CI, −43% to 50%) All-cause pneumonia: VE −17% (95% CI, −65% to 17%).	Pneumolysin antibodies used to define etiology, no cultures
Honkanen et al,[79] 1999	Finland 1992–1995	26,925	Community-dwelling adults ≥65 y old	PPV23 + influenza vs influenza	Randomized based on year of birth (even or odd); open label	All-cause pneumonia: VE −20% (95% CI, −50% to 10%) Pneumococcal pneumonia: VE −20% (95% CI, −90% to 20%) IPD: VE 60% (95% CI, −40% to 90%)[a]	Used nonspecific serologic test for pneumococcal pneumonia
Kawakami et al,[83] 2010	Japan 2005-2007	778	Those ≥65 y old receiving influenza vaccination	PPV23 + influenza vs influenza	Randomized, open label: subject choosing sealed envelope with card indicating PPV or only influenza	All-cause pneumonia: VE 24.8% (95% CI, −18.5% to 52.8%) Admission owing to all-cause pneumonia: VE 27.3% (95% CI, −16.3% to 55.8%)	No determination of CAP etiology (pneumococcal CAP)

(continued on next page)

Table 3
(continued)

PPV: Long-term care setting

Author, Year	Country, Study Period	Size	Domain	Intervention (Vaccine)	Randomization and Blinding	Results	Limitations
Austrian,[82] 1980 (A)	USA Study period unknown	1300	Patients with mental illness in long-term care	PPV12 vs placebo	Randomized; double blind.	All-cause pneumonia VE: −30% (95% CI, −68% to 0%)[b]	Primary study not accessible
Gaillat et al,[84] 1985	France 1981–1982	1827	Elderly people in hospital or nursing home	PPV14 vs no vaccine	Randomization stratified by type of institution and proportion at risk; blinding not described, no placebo	Pneumonia: VE 79% (95% CI, 55% to 90%)	Hospitalized or nursing home residents, so officially not fulfilling criteria for CAP Six non-VT cases excluded from analysis (2 [PPV14] vs 4 [no vaccine])
Maruyama et al,[85] 2010	Japan 2006–2009	1006	Nursing home residents	PPV23 vs placebo	Randomized by random syringe numbers; double blind	All cause pneumonia: VE 44.8% (95% CI, 22.4%–60.8%) Pneumococcal pneumonia: VE 63.8% (95% CI, 32.1%–80.7%)	Nursing home residents, so officially not fulfilling criteria for CAP Very high incidence of pneumonia (72.8/1000 person-years); representative for other populations?

PPV: Comorbidity groups

Study	Country, Year	N	Population	Comparison	Methods	Results	Limitations
Simberkoff et al,[86] 1986	USA 1981–1985	2295	Veterans at high risk for pneumococcal infection owing to comorbidity	PPV14 vs placebo	Fixed block randomization scheme; placebo used but blinding not described	Proven pneumococcal infection: 2 (PPV14) vs 1 (placebo) Probable pneumococcal pneumonia: VE −27% (95% CI, −144% to 34%)[a] Probable pneumococcal bronchitis: VE −84% (95% CI, −262% to 6%)	Method of follow-up not clearly described Numbers too small to evaluate impact on IPD
Klastersky et al,[87] 1986	Belgium Study period not described	50	Patients with bronchogenic carcinoma	PPV17 vs placebo	Placebo-controlled, randomization method, or blinding not described	VE pneumococcal infections 39.4% (95% CI, −141% to 84.8%)[a]	Very small sample size Very specific study population Three subjects loss to follow-up not included in analyses
Leech et al,[88] 1987	Canada 1981–1983	189	Patients with COPD with FEV$_1$ <1.5L	PPV14 + influenza vs placebo + influenza	Stratification by age and FEV$_1$, randomization procedure not described; double blind	Admission owing to pneumonia: VE −280% (95% CI, −809% to −58%)[a]	Small sample size Relatively high proportion lost to follow-up Data collection interview based; possible recall bias No standard determination of etiology

(continued on next page)

Table 3
(continued)

Author, Year	Country, Study Period	Size	Domain	Intervention (Vaccine)	Randomization and Blinding	Results	Limitations
Davis et al,[89] 1987	USA	103	Patients with COPD	PPV14 vs placebo	Randomized, double blinded	Pneumonia: 3 (PPV14) vs 7 (placebo) subjects with 4 vs 7 episodes	Small number of events
Ortqvist et al,[90] 1998	Sweden 1991–1994	691	Patients who had been treated in hospital for CAP	PPV23 vs placebo	Random number allocation to syringe by manufacturer; double blinded	Pneumonia: VE, -20% (95% CI, -72% to 11%) Pneumococcal pneumonia: VE. -28% (95% CI, -150% to 34%)	Study concerns 'secondary prophylaxis' after CAP High incidence and recurrence rate: population representative?
French et al,[91] 2000	Uganda 1995–1998	1323	Adult (15+) HIV patients, WHO clinical stage 1, 2, 3	PPV23 vs placebo	Randomization 1:1; blocks of 20, stratified for clinic; double blind	IPD: VE, -47% (95% CI, -227% to 34%) VT-IPD: VE, -110% (95% CI, -416%–14%) All pneumococcal disease: VE, -40% (95% CI, -178% to 29%) All-cause pneumonia: VE, -89% (95% CI, -221% to -12%)	Young participants (mean age, 31 y)
Alfageme et al,[92] 2006	Spain 1999–2004	600	Patients with spirometric diagnosis of COPD	PPV23 vs no vaccine	Randomized in fixed blocks; no blinding.	CAP of pneumococcal or unknown etiology VE: 24% (95% CI, -24% to 54%) First episode of pneumococcal pneumonia: 0 (PPV23) vs 5 (placebo)	Small number of events

	Country	Years	N	Population	Intervention	Design	Outcomes	Comments
Furumoto et al,[93] 2008	Japan	2001–2004	191	Stable chronic lung disease with history of acute exacerbation	PPV23 + influenza vaccine vs influenza vaccine	Randomized; 1:1 blocks per center; open label	Pneumonia VE: 0% (−99% to 50%)[a] Infective acute exacerbation: 33% (7% to 52%)[a] Pneumococcal acute exacerbation VE: 82% (11% to 96%)[a] Non-infectious acute exacerbation: −38% (−245% to 45%)[a]	Small sample size Patients with incomplete follow-up excluded (7 in PPV23 vs 17 in placebo group)
Izumi et al,[94] 2017	Japan		900	Patients with rheumatoid arthritis	PPV23 vs placebo	Randomized, double blinded	Pneumococcal pneumonia: 2 (PPV23) vs 1 (placebo) episodes Nonpneumococcal pneumonia: VE −1% (95% CI, −101% to 50%) All-cause pneumonia: VE −6% (95% CI, −106% to 45%)	Trial did not reach required sample size of 1600 because it was ended prematurely owing to introduction of routine vaccination in elderly
PCV								
French et al,[91] 2000	Malawi	2003–2007	496	Adults who had recovered from documented IPD	2 doses of PCV7 vs placebo	Randomization in random sized blocks double blind	VT-IPD (including 6A): VE 74% (95% CI, 30%–90%)	88% HIV positive Secondary prophylaxis
Bonten et al,[35] 2015	Netherlands	2008–2013	84,496	Immunocompetent adults >65 y of age	PCV13 vs placebo	Randomized in fixed blocks; double blind	VT-CAP: VE, 45.6% (95.2% CI, 21.8%–62.5%)[c] noninvasive VT-CAP: VE, 45.0% (95.2% CI, 14.2%–65.3%)[c] VT-IPD: VE, 75.0% (CI 95% CI, 41.4%–90.8%)[c]	Pneumococcal Vaccine naïve subjects owing to no general PPV23 vaccination for elderly Limited to immunocompetent subjects

Abbreviations: CAP, community-acquired pneumonia; CI, confidence interval; COPD, chronic obstructive pulmonary disease; HIV, human immunodeficiency virus; IPD, invasive pneumococcal disease; PCV, pneumococcal conjugate vaccine (number indicating valency); PPV, pneumococcal polysaccharide vaccine (number indicating valency); VE, vaccine efficacy; VT, vaccine type; WHO, World Health Organization.

[a] Calculated from reported crude data or relative risk.

[b] Derived from metaanalysis.[74]

[c] Per-protocol analysis.

mortality. An older trial with PPV12 in patients with mental illness in long-term care showed a marginally significant opposite effect on all-cause pneumonia.[82]

Other trials that were performed in different at-risk populations were generally underpowered for clinical endpoints, resulting in wide confidence intervals (CIs), and none of them demonstrated a clear protective effect.[86–94]

Observational studies are prone to confounding by indication or healthy user bias. Recently, the test-negative case control design was proposed to solve this issue, which builds on the assumption that confounding effects are similar for the vaccine-preventable and non–vaccine-preventable outcomes,[95] although the validity of this approach has been challenged as well.[96]

Because it is not reasonable to assume that PPVs only protect nursing home residents against nonbacteremic pneumococcal pneumonia, there is a remaining challenge to solve why it was protective in 2 trials in nursing homes, whereas it does not seem to be effective in the general elderly population with or without comorbidities.

EFFICACY OF PNEUMOCOCCAL CONJUGATE VACCINES

The efficacy of PCVs in preventing pneumococcal disease in young children has been well established, with estimated VEs of 80% (95% CI, 58%–90%) and 27% (95% CI, 15%–36%) for vaccine type IPD and radiographically confirmed pneumonia, respectively.[97]

The efficacy of PCVs in adults have only been evaluated in 2 randomized clinical trials: one among patients infected with the human immunodeficiency virus (HIV)[98] and one in an immunocompetent elderly population.[35]

The first trial was conducted in Malawi, where 496 adults (88.5% with HIV) who had recovered from IPD were randomly assigned to receive 2 doses of PCV7 (n = 248) or placebo (n = 248). After a median follow-up of 1.2 years, the unadjusted VE to prevent a new episode of VT-IPD (PCV7 serotypes + serotype 6A) was 74% (95% CI, 30%–90%). VE adjusted for age, sex, viral load, clinical stage, and CD4 count was 69% (95% CI, 16%–89%). There were no significant beneficial effects on all-cause IPD (adjusted VE, 20%; 95% CI, -44% to 55%) or mortality (adjusted VE, -24%; 95% CI, -75% to 12%). This was the first trial to demonstrate efficacy of PCV in adults. However, the study participants were mainly HIV positive and pneumococcal vaccination was evaluated as secondary prophylaxis, which is not representative for pneumococcal vaccination in

the general population. However, the trial demonstrated that the vaccine was even effective in the immunocompromised individuals with a CD4$^+$ T-cell count of less than 200 cells/mm^3 at baseline.

The second trial, the CAPiTA study, a randomized placebo-controlled trial conducted in the Netherlands, included 84,496 immunocompetent adults 65 years of age and older. The mean follow-up time was almost 4 years. The trial demonstrated a VE of PCV13 of 75% for VT-IPD and 45% for VT-CAP (per-protocol analysis). This trial was the first to demonstrate the efficacy of PCV in immunocompetent adults and in the prevention of noninvasive VT-CAP. However, the trial was conducted among subjects who had never received a pneumococcal vaccination before. The degree of observed VE may vary in other populations, depending on the epidemiology of pneumococcal serotypes and susceptibility to pneumococcal infections.

The results of these trials are in line with previous effects demonstrated in children, especially concerning the efficacy against VT-IPD (80% in children, 74% in HIV-positive patients, and 75% in the immunocompetent elderly population). The CAPiTA trial was the first trial to demonstrate VE against VT-CAP, including protection against noninvasive VT-CAP.

BENEFITS OF ADULT PNEUMOCOCCAL VACCINATION IN THE POSTPNEUMOCOCCAL CONJUGATE VACCINE ERA

Assuming that the immunization of the elderly with PPV23 or PCV13 will not induce indirect effects,[99] the benefit of PPV23 and PCV13 depends mainly on 2 parameters: VE against IPD and non-IPD pneumococcal CAP and the absolute number of VT-CAP and VT-IPD events that can be prevented. Since the introduction of PCVs in childhood immunization programs, decreased incidences of VT-IPD have consistently been reported in all age groups, with decreases of more than 80% among the elderly in the UK.[53,56,100] These indirect effects generally take 5 to 7 years to be maximized, presumably depending on whether a catchup program among children was implemented.[70,100]

Naturally, the amount of herd protection will be influenced by the coverage of childhood immunization programs. Universal vaccination of elderly with PCV13 may be justified when there is sufficient disease burden caused by VT *S pneumoniae*, which may be the case in an early stage of child immunization with PCV13, if lower valency vaccines are used in children, or if PCV13 coverage in children is low. However, if PCV13 for child immunization has a high uptake, the cost–benefit ratio for vaccination of adults is expected to change considerably in the 5 to 7 years after the introduction of PCV13. The discontinuation of such a program among adults based on an updated cost-effectiveness analyses may arouse ethical discussions, as was seen after recommendations to decrease screening intensity for breast cancer.[101] Therefore, it might be appropriate to define the criteria for future policy adaptations before implementing an adult immunization program if a reduction in vaccine-preventable disease incidence is expected. In their 2014 recommendation, the Advisory Committee on Immunization Practices committed to reevaluate the recommendation to routinely vaccinate adults over 65 years of age in 2018, however, without indicating the criteria to revert the recommendation.[36]

If the VE of PPV23 and PCV13 in the elderly are comparable, naturally, PPV23 will offer greater absolute risk reduction because of the higher valency. However, as discussed elsewhere in this article, although the VE for IPD has been established for both vaccines and seems relatively comparable, the VE for non-IPD pneumococcal CAP has only been clearly demonstrated for PCV13. In 2003, the Dutch Health Council decided that there was not enough evidence to justify the routine vaccination of the elderly with PPV23 and uptake of pneumococcal vaccines is, therefore, still low in the Netherlands.[102] Recently, after reviewing the new evidence, the recommendation was made to offer PPV23 once every 5 years to people aged 60 to 75 years,[103] despite the fact that the evidence for PPV23 is still conflicting. It is hoped that the health authorities will take this unique opportunity to set up a well-designed experiment to determine the VE of PPV23 in elderly in the general population.

In the meantime, it would be worthwhile to extend the valency of existing vaccines or to develop a new PCV for adults containing the non-VTs that cause most replacement disease in adults but not in children, provided that the incidence of CAP and IPD caused by these serotypes is high enough to reach cost effectiveness. With this approach, the elderly would be protected against the serotypes included in the pediatric vaccine through indirect effects and to additional serotypes through direct immunization. Other approaches, such as whole cell pneumococcal vaccines and pneumococcal protein vaccines, seem promising, although it will take several years to further develop these vaccines and demonstrate their safety and efficacy in randomized, controlled trials.[104]

SUMMARY

PCVs have greatly reduced the pneumococcal diseases burden in children. Owing to indirect effects, incidences of vaccine-preventable pneumococcal disease has substantially declined in the adult population, which was partly replaced by non–vaccine-preventable pneumococcal disease. As a result, the potential benefit of pneumococcal vaccination for adults, particularly of PCVs but also of PPV23, is decreased. The efficacy of PPV23 in preventing IPD has been demonstrated, but efficacy against pneumonia has not firmly been established. PCV13 is effective in prevention of VT-CAP and VT-IPD. Well-designed trials to determine the VE of old and new vaccines are desirable.

REFERENCES

1. World Health Organization (WHO). The top 10 causes of death. 2017. Available at: http://www.who.int/mediacentre/factsheets/fs310/en/. Accessed March 6, 2018.
2. Prina E, Ranzani OT, Torres A. Community-acquired pneumonia. Lancet 2015;386(9998):1097–108.
3. Said MA, Johnson HL, Nonyane BAS, et al. Estimating the burden of pneumococcal pneumonia among adults: a systematic review and meta-analysis of diagnostic techniques. PLoS One 2013;8(4):e60273.
4. Postma DF, van Werkhoven CH, Huijts SM, et al. New trends in the prevention and management of community-acquired pneumonia. Neth J Med 2012;70(8):337–48.
5. Rozenbaum MH, Pechlivanoglou P, van der Werf TS, et al. The role of Streptococcus pneumoniae in community-acquired pneumonia among adults in Europe: a meta-analysis. Eur J Clin Microbiol Infect Dis 2013;32(3):305–16.
6. Musher DM, Abers MS, Bartlett JG. Evolving understanding of the causes of pneumonia in adults, with special attention to the role of pneumococcus. Clin Infect Dis 2017;65(10):1736–44.
7. Ekdahl K, Ahlinder I, Hansson HB, et al. Duration of nasopharyngeal carriage of penicillin-resistant Streptococcus pneumoniae: experiences from the South Swedish Pneumococcal Intervention Project. Clin Infect Dis 1997;25(5):1113–7.
8. Sleeman KL, Griffiths D, Shackley F, et al. Capsular serotype–specific attack rates and duration of carriage of streptococcus pneumoniae in a population of children. J Infect Dis 2006;194(5):682–8.
9. Le Polain De Waroux O, Flasche S, Prieto-Merino D, et al. Age-dependent prevalence of nasopharyngeal carriage of streptococcus pneumoniae before conjugate vaccine introduction: a prediction model

based on a meta-analysis. PLoS One 2014;9(1): e86136.

10. van Gils EJM, Veenhoven RH, Rodenburg GD, et al. Effect of 7-valent pneumococcal conjugate vaccine on nasopharyngeal carriage with Haemophilus influenzae and Moraxella catarrhalis in a randomized controlled trial. Vaccine 2011;29(44):7595–8.

11. Goldblatt D, Hussain M, Andrews N, et al. Antibody responses to nasopharyngeal carriage of Streptococcus pneumoniae in adults: a longitudinal household study. J Infect Dis 2005;192(3):387–93.

12. Nicholls TR, Leach AJ, Morris PS. The short-term impact of each primary dose of pneumococcal conjugate vaccine on nasopharyngeal carriage: systematic review and meta-analyses of randomised controlled trials. Vaccine 2015;34(6):703–13.

13. Davis SM, Deloria-Knoll M, Kassa HT, et al. Impact of pneumococcal conjugate vaccines on nasopharyngeal carriage and invasive disease among unvaccinated people: review of evidence on indirect effects. Vaccine 2013;32(1):133–45.

14. World Health Organization (WHO). Global health estimates 2015: deaths by cause, age, sex, by country and by region, 2000-2015. Geneva (Switzerland); 2016. Available at: http://www.who.int/healthinfo/global_burden_disease/estimates/en/index1.html. Accessed March 12, 2018.

15. Welte T, Torres A, Nathwani D. Clinical and economic burden of community-acquired pneumonia among adults in Europe. Thorax 2012;67(1):71–9.

16. Bjerre LM, Verheij TJ, Kochen MM. Antibiotics for community acquired pneumonia in adult outpatients. Cochrane Database Syst Rev 2009;(4):1–41.

17. Mandell LA, Wunderink RG, Anzueto A, et al. Infectious Diseases Society of America/American Thoracic Society consensus guidelines on the management of community-acquired pneumonia in adults. Clin Infect Dis 2007;44(Suppl 2):S27–72.

18. World Health Organization (WHO). Causes of child mortality, 2016. Available at: http://www.who.int/gho/child_health/mortality/causes/en/. Accessed August 29, 2018.

19. Jain S, Williams DJ, Arnold SR, et al. Community-acquired pneumonia requiring hospitalization among U.S. children. N Engl J Med 2015;372(9):835–45.

20. Rozenbaum MH, Mangen M-JJ, Huijts SM, et al. Incidence, direct costs and duration of hospitalization of patients hospitalized with community acquired pneumonia: a nationwide retrospective claims database analysis. Vaccine 2015;33(28):3193–9.

21. Ewig S, Birkner N, Strauss R, et al. New perspectives on community-acquired pneumonia in 388 406 patients. Results from a nationwide mandatory performance measurement programme in healthcare quality. Thorax 2009;64(12):1062–9.

22. Ramirez JA, Wiemken TL, Peyrani P, et al. Adults hospitalized with pneumonia in the United States: incidence, epidemiology, and mortality. Clin Infect Dis 2017;65(11):1806–12.

23. Woodhead MA, Macfarlane JT, Mccracken JS, et al. Prospective study of the aetiology and outcome of pneumonia in the community. Lancet 1987;329(8534):671–4.

24. Niederman MS, Mecombs JS, Unger AN, et al. The cost of treating community-acquired pneumonia. Clin Ther 1998;20(4):820–37.

25. Capelastegui A, Espana PP, Bilbao A, et al. Study of community-acquired pneumonia: incidence, patterns of care, and outcomes in primary and hospital care. J Infect 2010;61(5):364–71.

26. Colice GL, Morley MA, Asche C, et al. Treatment costs of community-acquired pneumonia in an employed population. Chest 2004;125(8):2140–5.

27. Chalmers JD, Campling J, Dicker A, et al. A systematic review of the burden of vaccine preventable pneumococcal disease in UK adults. BMC Pulm Med 2016;16(1):77.

28. Harboe ZB, Dalby T, Weinberger DM, et al. Impact of 13-valent pneumococcal conjugate vaccination in invasive pneumococcal disease incidence and mortality. Clin Infect Dis 2014;59(8):1066–73.

29. Domenech de Cellès M, Arduin H, Varon E, et al. Characterizing and comparing the seasonality of influenza-like illnesses and invasive pneumococcal diseases using seasonal waveforms. Am J Epidemiol 2017;187(5):1029–39.

30. Weinberger DM, Harboe ZB, Viboud C, et al. Pneumococcal disease seasonality: incidence, severity and the role of influenza activity. Eur Respir J 2014;43(3):833–41.

31. Cilloniz C, Ewig S, Gabarrus A, et al. Seasonality of pathogens causing community-acquired pneumonia. Respirology 2017;22(4):778–85.

32. Siber GR, Klugman KP, Mäkelä PH, editors. Pneumococcal vaccines: the impact of conjugate vaccine. 1st edition. Washington, DC: ASM Press; 2008.

33. Centers for Disease Control and Prevention (CDC). Update: pneumococcal polysaccharide vaccine usage–United States. MMWR Morb Mortal Wkly Rep 1984;33(20):273–6, 281.

34. Centers for Disease Control and Prevention (CDC). Licensure of 13-valent pneumococcal conjugate vaccine for adults aged 50 years and older. MMWR Morb Mortal Wkly Rep 2012;61(21):394–5.

35. Bonten MJM, Huijts SM, Bolkenbaas M, et al. Polysaccharide conjugate vaccine against pneumococcal pneumonia in adults. N Engl J Med 2015;372(12):1114–25.

36. Tomczyk S, Bennett NM, Stoecker C, et al. Use of 13-valent pneumococcal conjugate vaccine and 23-valent pneumococcal polysaccharide vaccine among adults aged ≥65 years: recommendations of the Advisory Committee on Immunization Practices (ACIP). MMWR Morb Mortal Wkly Rep 2014; 63(37):822–5.

37. World Health Organization (WHO). Guidelines on clinical evaluation of vaccines: regulatory expectations, 9. Annex. Geneva: World Health Organization; 2017.

38. Dransfield MT, Nahm MH, Han MK, et al. Superior immune response to protein-conjugate versus free pneumococcal polysaccharide vaccine in chronic obstructive pulmonary disease. Am J Respir Crit Care Med 2009;180(1535–4970):499–505.

39. Goldblatt D, Southern J, Andrews N, et al. The immunogenicity of 7-valent pneumococcal conjugate vaccine versus 23-valent polysaccharide vaccine in adults aged 50-80 years. Clin Infect Dis 2009;49(1537–6591):1318–25.

40. de Roux A, Schmöle-Thoma B, Schmöele-Thoma B, et al. Comparison of pneumococcal conjugate polysaccharide and free polysaccharide vaccines in elderly adults: conjugate vaccine elicits improved antibacterial immune responses and immunological memory. Clin Infect Dis 2008; 46(7):1015–23.

41. Kumar D, Rotstein C, Miyata G, et al. Randomized, double-blind, controlled trial of pneumococcal vaccination in renal transplant recipients. J Infect Dis 2003;187(10):1639–45.

42. Kapetanovic MC, Roseman C, Jonsson G, et al. Heptavalent pneumococcal conjugate vaccine elicits similar antibody response as standard 23-valent polysaccharide vaccine in adult patients with RA treated with immunomodulating drugs. Clin Rheumatol 2011;30(1434–9949):1555–61.

43. Jackson LA, Gurtman A, Rice K, et al. Immunogenicity and safety of a 13-valent pneumococcal conjugate vaccine in adults 70 years of age and older previously vaccinated with 23-valent pneumococcal polysaccharide vaccine. Vaccine 2013; 31(35):3585–93.

44. Jackson LA, Gurtman A, van Cleeff M, et al. Immunogenicity and safety of a 13-valent pneumococcal conjugate vaccine compared to a 23-valent pneumococcal polysaccharide vaccine in pneumococcal vaccine-naive adults. Vaccine 2013; 31(35):3577–84.

45. van Deursen AMM, van Houten MA, Webber C, et al. Immunogenicity of the 13-valent pneumococcal conjugate vaccine in older adults with and without comorbidities in the community-acquired pneumonia immunization trial in adults (CAPiTA). Clin Infect Dis 2017;65(5):787–95.

46. Dransfield MT, Harnden S, Burton RL, et al. Long-term comparative immunogenicity of protein conjugate and free polysaccharide pneumococcal vaccines in chronic obstructive pulmonary disease. Clin Infect Dis 2012;55(5):e35–44.

47. Greenberg RN, Gurtman A, Frenck RW, et al. Sequential administration of 13-valent pneumococcal conjugate vaccine and 23-valent pneumococcal polysaccharide vaccine in pneumococcal vaccine-naïve adults 60-64 years of age. Vaccine 2014;32(20):2364–74.

48. Jackson LA, Gurtman A, van Cleeff M, et al. Influence of initial vaccination with 13-valent pneumococcal conjugate vaccine or 23-valent pneumococcal polysaccharide vaccine on anti-pneumococcal responses following subsequent pneumococcal vaccination in adults 50 years and older. Vaccine 2013;31(35):3594–602.

49. Kobayashi M, Bennett NM, Gierke R, et al. Intervals between PCV13 and PPSV23 vaccines: recommendations of the advisory committee on immunization practices (ACIP). MMWR Morb Mortal Wkly Rep 2015;64(34):944–7.

50. Advisory Committee on Immunization Practices (ACIP).. Preventing pneumococcal disease among infants and young children. recommendations of the advisory committee on immunization practices (ACIP). MMWR Recomm Rep 2000;49(RR-9):1–35.

51. Centers for Disease Control and Prevention (CDC). Licensure of a 13-valent pneumococcal conjugate vaccine (PCV13) and recommendations for use among children - advisory Committee on Immunization Practices (ACIP). MMWR Morb Mortal Wkly Rep 2010;59(9):258–61.

52. Centers for Disease Control and Prevention (CDC). Direct and indirect effects of routine vaccination of children with 7-valent pneumococcal conjugate vaccine on incidence of invasive pneumococcal disease–United States, 1998-2003. MMWR Morb Mortal Wkly Rep 2005;54(36):893–7.

53. Moore MR, Link-Gelles R, Schaffner W, et al. Effect of use of 13-valent pneumococcal conjugate vaccine in children on invasive pneumococcal disease in children and adults in the USA: analysis of multisite, population-based surveillance. Lancet Infect Dis 2015;15(3):301–9.

54. Miller E, Andrews NJ, Waight PA, et al. Effectiveness of the new serotypes in the 13-valent pneumococcal conjugate vaccine. Vaccine 2011;29(49):9127–31.

55. Steens A, Bergsaker MAR, Aaberge IS, et al. Prompt effect of replacing the 7-valent pneumococcal conjugate vaccine with the 13-valent vaccine on the epidemiology of invasive pneumococcal disease in Norway. Vaccine 2013;31(52):6232–8.

56. Regev-Yochay G, Paran Y, Bishara J, et al. Early impact of PCV7/PCV13 sequential introduction to the national pediatric immunization plan, on adult invasive pneumococcal disease: a nationwide surveillance study. Vaccine 2015;33(9):1135–42.

57. Griffin MR, Zhu Y, Moore MR, et al. U.S. hospitalizations for pneumonia after a decade of pneumococcal vaccination. N Engl J Med 2013;369(2): 155–63.

58. Centers for Disease Control and Prevention (CDC). Active bacterial core surveillance, Trends by Serotype Group, 1998–2015. 2016. Available at: https://www.cdc.gov/abcs/reports-findings/survreports/spneu-types.html. Accessed February 6, 2018.

59. National Institute for Public Health and the Environment. The National Immunisation Programme in the Netherlands, Surveillance and developments in 2013-2014. 2014. p. 71–7. Available at: http://www.rivm.nl/Documenten_en_publicaties/Wetenschappelijk/Rapporten/2014/november/The_National_Immunisation_Programme_in_the_Netherlands_Surveillance_and_developments_in_2013_2014. Accessed March 24, 2015.

60. Instituto de Salud Pública de Chile. Vigilancia de Enfermedad Invasora Streptococcus pneumoniae. Chile, 2007 – 2013. Santiago: Boletin Instituto de Salud Pública de Chile; 2014. Available at: http://www.ispch.cl/sites/default/files/Boletin_Neumo_21-03-2014.pdf. Accessed March 3, 2014.

61. National Institute for Health and Welfare Finland. Incidence of invasive pneumococcal disease in Finland. 2014. Available at: https://thl.fi/fi/web/thlfi-en/research-and-expertwork/projects-and-programmes/monitoring-the-population-effectiveness-of-pneumococcal-conjugate-vaccination-in-the-finnish-national-vaccination-programme/incidence-of-invasive-pneumococcal-disease-in-finland.

62. dos Santos SR, Passadore LF, Takagi EH, et al. Serotype distribution of Streptococcus pneumoniae isolated from patients with invasive pneumococcal disease in Brazil before and after ten-pneumococcal conjugate vaccine implementation. Vaccine 2013;31(51):6150–4.

63. Huang SS, Hinrichsen VL, Stevenson AE, et al. Continued impact of pneumococcal conjugate vaccine on carriage in young children. Pediatrics 2009;124(1):e1–11.

64. Fleming-Dutra KE, Conklin L, Loo JD, et al. Systematic review of the effect of pneumococcal conjugate vaccine dosing schedules on vaccine-type nasopharyngeal carriage. Pediatr Infect Dis J 2014;33(Suppl 2):S152–60.

65. van den Bergh MR, Spijkerman J, Swinnen KM, et al. Effects of the 10-valent pneumococcal non-typeable Haemophilus influenzae protein D-conjugate vaccine on nasopharyngeal bacterial colonization in young children: a randomized controlled trial. Clin Infect Dis 2013;56(3):e30–9.

66. Jokinen J, Kilpi TM, Kaijalainen T, et al. Indirect effectiveness of ten-valent pneumococcal haemophilus influenzae protein d conjugate vaccine (PHiD-CV10) against nasopharyngeal carriage: finip indirect carriage study. Milan (Italy): ESPID; 2013. Available at: http://w3.kenes-group.com/apps/espid2013/abstracts/pdf/208.pdf.

67. Vesikari T, Forstén A, Seppä I, et al. Impact of the 10-valent pneumococcal non-typeable Haemophilus influenzae protein D conjugate vaccine (PHiD-CV) on bacterial nasopharyngeal carriage in Finnish children: a cluster-randomized controlled trial. Berlin: ECCMID; 2013. Available at: https://www.escmid.org/escmid_library/online_lecture_library/material/?mid=6529.

68. Hammitt LL, Akech DO, Morpeth SC, et al. Population effect of 10-valent pneumococcal conjugate vaccine on nasopharyngeal carriage of Streptococcus pneumoniae and non-typeable Haemophilus influenzae in Kilifi, Kenya: findings from cross-sectional carriage studies. Lancet Glob Health 2014;2(7):e397–405.

69. Naucler P, Galanis I, Morfeldt E, et al. Comparison of the impact of pneumococcal conjugate vaccine 10 or pneumococcal conjugate vaccine 13 on invasive pneumococcal disease in equivalent populations. Clin Infect Dis 2017;65(11): 1780–9.

70. Feikin DR, Kagucia EW, Loo JD, et al. Serotype-specific changes in invasive pneumococcal disease after pneumococcal conjugate vaccine introduction: a pooled analysis of multiple surveillance sites. PLoS Med 2013;10(9):e1001517.

71. Smith KJ, Wateska AR, Nowalk MP, et al. Cost-effectiveness of adult vaccination strategies using pneumococcal conjugate vaccine compared with pneumococcal polysaccharide vaccine. JAMA 2012;307(8):804–12.

72. van Werkhoven CH. Herd effects of child vaccination with pneumococcal conjugate vaccine against pneumococcal non-invasive community-acquired pneumonia: what is the evidence? Hum Vaccin Immunother 2016;13(5):1177–81.

73. Huss A, Scott P, Stuck AE, et al. Efficacy of pneumococcal vaccination in adults: a meta-analysis. CMAJ 2009;180(1488–2329):48–58.

74. Moberley S, Holden J, Tatham DP, et al. Vaccines for preventing pneumococcal infection in adults. Cochrane Database Syst Rev 2013;(1):CD000422.

75. Diao W-Q, Shen N, Yu P-X, et al. Efficacy of 23-valent pneumococcal polysaccharide vaccine in preventing community-acquired pneumonia among immunocompetent adults: a systematic review and meta-analysis of randomized trials. Vaccine 2016;34(13):1496–503.

76. Kraicer-Melamed H, O'Donnell S, Quach C. The effectiveness of pneumococcal polysaccharide vaccine 23 (PPV23) in the general population of 50 years of age and older: a systematic review and meta-analysis. Vaccine 2016;34(13):1540–50.

77. Schiffner-Rohe J, Witt A, Hemmerling J, et al. Efficacy of PPV23 in preventing pneumococcal pneumonia in adults at increased risk - a systematic review and meta-analysis. PLoS One 2016;11(1):e0146338.

78. Falkenhorst G, Remschmidt C, Harder T, et al. Effectiveness of the 23-valent pneumococcal polysaccharide vaccine (ppv23) against pneumococcal disease in the elderly: systematic review and meta-analysis. PLoS One 2017;12(1): e0169368.

79. Honkanen PO, Keistinen T, Miettinen L, et al. Incremental effectiveness of pneumococcal vaccine on simultaneously administered influenza vaccine in preventing pneumonia and pneumococcal pneumonia among persons aged 65 years or older. Vaccine 1999;17(20–21):2493–500.

80. Falkenhorst G, Remschmidt C, Harder T, et al. Background paper to the updated pneumococcal vaccination recommendation for older adults in Germany. Bundesgesundheitsblatt Gesundheitsforschung Gesundheitsschutz 2016;59(12): 1623–57.

81. Koivula I, Stén M, Leinonen M, et al. Clinical efficacy of pneumococcal vaccine in the elderly: a randomized, single-blind population-based trial. Am J Med 1997;103(4):281–90.

82. Austrian R. Surveillance of pneumococcal infection for field trials of polyvalent pneumococcal vaccines. [report no. DAB-VDP-12-84]. Bethesda (MD): National Institute of Allergy and Infectious Diseases; 1980. p. 184–94.

83. Kawakami K, Ohkusa Y, Kuroki R, et al. Effectiveness of pneumococcal polysaccharide vaccine against pneumonia and cost analysis for the elderly who receive seasonal influenza vaccine in Japan. Vaccine 2010;28(43):7063–9.

84. Gaillat J, Zmirou D, Mallaret MR, et al. [Clinical trial of an antipneumococcal vaccine in elderly subjects living in institutions]. Rev Epidemiol Sante Publique 1985;33(6):437–44.

85. Maruyama T, Taguchi O, Niederman MS, et al. Efficacy of 23-valent pneumococcal vaccine in preventing pneumonia and improving survival in nursing home residents: double blind, randomised and placebo controlled trial. BMJ 2010;340:c1004.

86. Simberkoff MS, Cross AP, Al-Ibrahim M, et al. Efficacy of pneumococcal vaccine in high-risk patients. results of a veterans administration cooperative study. N Engl J Med 1986;315(21):1318–27.

87. Klastersky J, Mommen P, Cantraine F, et al. Placebo controlled pneumococcal immunization in patients with bronchogenic carcinoma. Eur J Cancer Clin Oncol 1986;22(7):807–13.

88. Leech JA, Gervais A, Ruben FL. Efficacy of pneumococcal vaccine in severe chronic obstructive pulmonary disease. CMAJ 1987;136(4):361–5.

89. Davis AL, Aranda CP, Schiffman G, et al. Pneumococcal infection and immunologic response to pneumococcal vaccine in chronic obstructive pulmonary disease. A Pilot Study. Chest 1987;92(2): 204–12.

90. Ortqvist A, Hedlund J, Burman LA, et al. Randomised trial of 23-valent pneumococcal capsular polysaccharide vaccine in prevention of pneumonia in middle-aged and elderly people. Swedish Pneumococcal Vaccination Study Group. Lancet 1998;351(9100):399–403.

91. French N, Nakiyingi J, Carpenter LM, et al. 23-Valent pneumococcal polysaccharide vaccine in HIV-1-infected Ugandan adults: double-blind, randomised and placebo controlled trial. Lancet 2000;355(9221):2106–11.

92. Alfageme I, Vazquez R, Reyes N, et al. Clinical efficacy of anti-pneumococcal vaccination in patients with COPD. Thorax 2006;61(3):189–95.

93. Furumoto A, Ohkusa Y, Chen M, et al. Additive effect of pneumococcal vaccine and influenza vaccine on acute exacerbation in patients with chronic lung disease. Vaccine 2008;26(33):4284–9.

94. Izumi Y, Akazawa M, Akeda Y, et al. The 23-valent pneumococcal polysaccharide vaccine in patients with rheumatoid arthritis: a double-blinded, randomized, placebo-controlled trial. Arthritis Res Ther 2017;19(1):15.

95. Suzuki M, Dhoubhadel BG, Ishifuji T, et al. Serotype-specific effectiveness of 23-valent pneumococcal polysaccharide vaccine against pneumococcal pneumonia in adults aged 65 years or older: a multicentre, prospective, test-negative design study. Lancet Infect Dis 2017; 17(3):313–21.

96. Lewnard JA, Tedijanto C, Cowling BJ, et al. Measurement of vaccine direct effects under the test-negative design. Am J Epidemiol 2018. [Epub ahead of print].

97. Lucero MG, Dulalia VE, Nillos LT, et al. Pneumococcal conjugate vaccines for preventing vaccine-type invasive pneumococcal disease and X-ray defined pneumonia in children less than two years of age. Cochrane Database Syst Rev 2009;(4):CD004977.

98. French N, Gordon SB, Mwalukomo T, et al. A trial of a 7-valent pneumococcal conjugate vaccine in HIV-infected adults. N Engl J Med 2010;362(9): 812–22.

99. van Deursen AMM, van Houten MA, Webber C, et al. The impact of the 13-valent pneumococcal conjugate vaccine on pneumococcal carriage in the community acquired pneumonia immunization trial in adults (CAPiTA) study. Clin Infect Dis 2018; 67(1):42–9.

100. Waight PA, Andrews NJ, Ladhani SN, et al. Effect of the 13-valent pneumococcal conjugate vaccine on

invasive pneumococcal disease in England and Wales 4 years after its introduction: an observational cohort study. Lancet Infect Dis 2015;15(6): 629.

101. Plutynski A. Ethical issues in cancer screening and prevention. J Med Philos 2012;37(3): 310–23.

102. Health council of the Netherlands. Pneumococcal vaccine in elderly adults and risk groups. The Hague (the Netherlands): Health Council of the Netherlands; 2003. Available at: https://www. gezondheidsraad.nl/en/task-and-procedure/areas-of-activity/prevention/pneumococcal-vaccine-in-elderly-adults-and-risk.

103. Health council of the Netherlands. Pneumococcal vaccination for older persons, executive summary. The Hague (the Netherlands). 2018. Available at: https://www.gezondheidsraad.nl/sites/default/files/ grpublication/executive_summary_pneumococcal _vaccination_for_older_persons.pdf. Accessed March 12, 2018.

104. Principi N, Esposito S. Development of pneumococcal vaccines over the last 10 years. Expert Opin Biol Ther 2018;18(1):7–17.

Adjunctive Therapies for Community-Acquired Pneumonia

Adrian Ceccato, MD[a], Miquel Ferrer, MD, PhD[a],
Enric Barbeta, MD[a], Antoni Torres, MD, PhD[a,b,*]

KEYWORDS

- Adjunctive treatments • Pneumonia • Corticosteroids

KEY POINTS

- Community-acquired pneumonia has high mortality, despite early and adequate antibiotic treatment.
- Several adjunctive treatments have been tested in community-acquired pneumonia.
- Corticosteroids have been shown to reduce the rate of treatment failure (including progression to acute respiratory distress syndrome), duration of stay, and time to clinical stability.
- Metaanalyses suggest that corticosteroids seem to decrease mortality in patients with severe community-acquired pneumonia.
- IgM-enriched immunoglobulin treatment in very severe community-acquired pneumonia is a promising adjunctive treatment.

Community-acquired pneumonia (CAP) is one of the leading causes of death worldwide.[1] With an estimated annual hospitalization rate of 649 patients per 100,000 inhabitants,[2] CAP has a mortality rate between 6% and 15%,[2,3] which may increase to more than 40% in cases of severe pneumonia, septic shock, or mechanical ventilation requirement.[4]

Mortality owing to pneumonia remains high, despite advances in health care,[5,6] even for patients receiving early and adequate antibiotic treatment.[7] Inappropriate initial treatment has been shown to be a risk factor in many studies[4,8,9]; however, the recommended empirical treatments[10] are effective against most pneumonia-causing germs.

The presence of underlying conditions, such as age or comorbidity, in addition to the initial response to infection, may increase the severity of the pneumonia and, as a result, the associated mortality.[11,12] An initial dysregulated host response can lead to severe sepsis and multiorgan dysfunction.[13,14] In addition, the initial antibiotic treatment may trigger an inflammatory response owing to a cascade of cytokines in patients with a high bacterial load.[15]

Pneumonia induces significant inflammation at both pulmonary and systemic levels.[16,17(p1),18–20] The first reaction of the host to infection generates a proinflammatory cascade causing tissue damage, followed by a compensatory antiinflammatory response.[18] Several host factors (underlying

This work was supported by Ciberes CB06/06/0028.

[a] Pneumology Department, Respiratory Institute (ICR), Hospital Clinic of Barcelona, Institut d'Investigacions Biomèdiques August Pi i Sunyer (IDIBAPS), University of Barcelona (UB), SGR 911 - Ciber de Enfermedades Respiratorias (CIBERES), ICREA Academia, Villarroel 170, Barcelona 08036, Spain; [b] Department of Pneumology, Hospital Clinic of Barcelona, Villarroel 140, Barcelona 08036, Spain

* Corresponding author. Department of Pneumology, Hospital Clinic of Barcelona, Villarroel 170, Barcelona 08036, Spain.

E-mail address: ATORRES@CLINIC.CAT

Clin Chest Med 39 (2018) 753–764
https://doi.org/10.1016/j.ccm.2018.07.008
0272-5231/18/© 2018 Elsevier Inc. All rights reserved.

chestmed.theclinics.com

diseases or immune status) and pathogen factors (load and virulence) are responsible of this initial response.[21]

Elevated inflammatory markers (interleukin [IL]-6) and antiinflammatory markers (IL-10) at hospital admission are directly associated with increased mortality.[18] This inadequate response presents clinically in the form of organ failure; septic shock is the maximum expression at the systemic level, and respiratory distress at the pulmonary level.[22]

Sepsis also alters coagulation.[23–26] Excess fibrin leads to the activation of the tissue factor, the protein C system, and antithrombin, generating an imbalance that can lead to disseminated intravascular coagulation.

Protease-activated receptors form the link between coagulation and inflammation.[23] Protease-activated receptors exert cytoprotective effects when stimulated with activated protein C or low doses of thrombin, but disrupt the barrier function of endothelial cells when activated with high doses of thrombin. The oxidative stress generated by the innate inflammatory response is a major cause of tissue damage[27–29] in critically ill patients.

Another interesting feature is the possibility of relative adrenal insufficiency in patients with severe pneumonia and sepsis.[30–33] The large-scale inflammation generated by the infection triggers the response of the hypothalamic–pituitary–adrenal axis. IL-1 induces a 2-phase response with an initial increase followed by a progressive reduction in adrenocorticotropic hormone concentrations; nitric oxide, free cortisol (stimulated by mechanisms unrelated to the axis), and certain drugs such as opioid analgesics and azole antifungals also lead to a decrease in adrenocorticotropic hormone levels or synthesis. Several enzymatic steps in steroidogenesis may also be inhibited by drugs. Another interesting point is the presence of tissue resistance to glucocorticoids, with a greater degree of evidence in the cases that present with acute respiratory distress syndrome.

The innate inflammatory response is followed by the adaptive response, mediated by lymphocytes, B cells and T cells. Recent studies have shown that in patients with pneumonia, those with less than 724 lymphocytes/mm^3 in serum at admission are at increased risk of mortality.[34] The mechanism underlying this finding is still unknown.[35]

Lymphocytes become plasma cells, which in turn produce antibodies. Low levels of immunoglobulins are also an important risk factor for mortality in pneumonia. Around 20% of patients admitted to the general ward and 40% admitted to the intensive care unit have low IgG levels; this proportion was 50% in patients who died.[36,37] Similar results have been observed in patients with sepsis, severe sepsis, and septic shock, but because these studies used different cut-off points their results cannot be compared.[38]

For all these reasons, CAP outcomes might be improved if these factors are modified (Fig. 1). In this article, we address the various adjuvant treatments that have been studied in the treatment of pneumonia.

MACROLIDES

Although their main mechanism of action is antibacterial, macrolides also show immunomodulatory activity. Thus, they have been used in

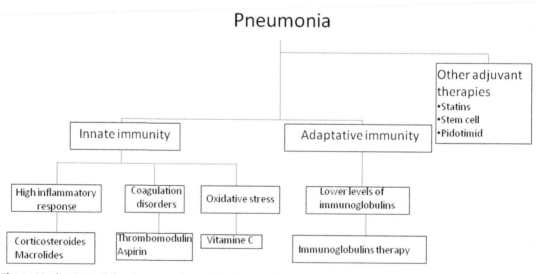

Fig. 1. Mechanisms of the disease and possible therapeutic targets.

multiple chronic respiratory diseases such as chronic obstructive pulmonary disease, bronchiectasis, and cystic fibrosis.[39-41]

Several studies have shown a benefit when using macrolides in the treatment of pneumonia and sepsis, even in patients presenting severe forms that require invasive ventilation or severe sepsis, or who have macrolide-resistant isolates.[42-45] Mortensen and colleagues,[42] in a retrospective study of more than 70,000 pneumonia patients, showed that the 30-day mortality (odds ratio [OR], 0.76; 95% confidence interval [CI], 0.73–0.80) and the 90-day mortality (OR, 0.73; 95% CI, 0.70–0.76) were significantly lower in patients who had received azithromycin. In turn, better outcomes have been observed in patients with bacteremic pneumococcal pneumonia who received macrolides.[46]

Macrolides decrease levels of proinflammatory cytokines such as IL-6 and increase levels of antiinflammatory cytokines such as IL-10. They also affect the structural cells of the respiratory tract, such as endothelial and epithelial cells, mainly regarding the expression of adhesion molecules, thus modifying the migration of inflammatory cells.[47,48]

Nevertheless, the results of randomized, controlled trials are controversial. Garin and colleagues[49] did not find noninferiority when comparing the combination of beta-lactams plus macrolides versus beta-lactam monotherapy in terms of time to clinical stability (in the monotherapy group 41.2% had not reached clinical stability at day 7 compared with 33.6% in the combination arm; $P = .07$). The absolute difference was 7.6%, with a 90% CI of 13.0% and a 2-sided 95% CI of −0.8% to 16.0%. This finding may be due to the inclusion of patients with severe pneumonia caused by *Legionella pneumophila* or by other atypical pathogens in the monotherapy group. No differences were found in mortality between groups. In a cluster randomized controlled trial, Postma and colleagues[50] found noninferiority for the strategy of beta-lactam monotherapy compared with the combination of beta-lactams with macrolides or fluoroquinolones alone in patients with nonsevere pneumonia. The absolute difference in the adjusted risk of death between beta-lactams and the beta-lactam–macrolide strategy was 1.9% (90% CI, −0.6 to 4.4) in favor of the beta-lactam monotherapy strategy, and −0.6% with fluoroquinolones (90% CI, −2 to 8–1.9).

For these reasons, new studies should evaluate the effect of macrolides in pneumonia, as well as the effect of their combination with other adjuvant treatments.

CORTICOSTEROIDS

Several studies have evaluated the use of corticosteroids as adjuvant treatment in pneumonia over the last 2 decades.[51-59] These studies have varied widely in terms of their outcomes, the drugs used, and the duration of treatment; however, with the exception of the study by Snijders and colleagues,[53] all have yielded positive results and they have been included in multiple metaanalyses and systematic reviews. The results of the main studies are summarized in **Table 1**.

Among the main outcomes, the studies do not show benefits in terms of mortality, although they were not designed or powered for this purpose. The data of the metaanalyses are controversial,[60-66] because those that included studies of lower quality show positive results. The benefit of corticosteroid use seems to be greater in patients with severe pneumonia; a Cochrane systematic review showed that it is necessary to treat 18 patients to prevent 1 death.[64] An interesting point to consider is the inclusion criterion used in the study by Torres and colleagues,[56] who admitted only severe pneumonia patients with a high inflammatory response defined by a C-reactive protein level of greater than 15 mg/dL. In that study, the outcome was defined as treatment failure (composite outcome) divided into early (first 72 hours) or late (between days 4 and 7); late treatment failure was significantly less in patients who received corticosteroids as compared with those who received placebo.

Several studies and metaanalyses have shown a reduction in the risk of progression to respiratory distress (risk ratio [RR], 0.24; 95% CI, 0.10–0.56),[60,61,66] a shorter time to clinical stability (weighted mean difference, −1.22; 95% CI, −2.08 to −0.35 days) and a shorter duration of hospital stay (weighted mean difference, −1.0; 95% CI, −1.79 to −0.21 days).[60] The results of these metaanalyses are summarized in **Fig. 2**.

Corticosteroids have an important role in patients in septic shock. Their use has been tested in multiple studies in patients with sepsis and septic shock, and the results are controversial.[67-70] A retrospective study by Tagami and colleagues[71] of 6900 patients with pneumonia requiring mechanical ventilation found significant differences in 28-day mortality, with a protective effect for corticosteroids only in patients who presented with septic shock and catecholamine requirement. Even though, in patients with septic shock, this condition reverts faster with the use of corticosteroids, no improvement in mortality has been found in patients with sepsis and septic shock. The guidelines propose the use of hydrocortisone

Table 1
RCTs of corticosteroids in CAP

References	Study Design and Population	Main Results	Adverse Events
Confalonieri et al,[52] 2005	Multicenter RCT Hydrocortisone vs placebo Patients with severe CAP	Improvement in Pao_2/Fio_2 ($P = .002$), chest radiograph score ($P<.0001$), reduction in C-reactive protein levels ($P = .01$), delayed septic shock ($P = .001$), reduction in duration of hospital stay ($P = .03$) and mortality ($P = .009$)	One digestive hemorrhage in each group.
Snijders et al,[53] 2010	Single-center RCT in the Netherlands Prednisolone vs placebo Hospitalized patients with CAP	Clinical cure at days 7 was 80.8% in the prednisolone group and 85.3% in the placebo group ($P = .38$) Clinical cure at days 30 was 66.3% in the prednisolone group and 77.1% in the placebo group ($P = .08$). Late failure (>72 h after admission) was more common in the prednisolone group than in the placebo group (19.2% vs 6.4%; $P = .04$ respectively)	Hyperglycemia in five (2.3%) patients in the prednisolone group and 2 (0.9%) patients in the placebo group ($P = .27$)
Fernandez-Serrano et al,[55] 2011	Single-center RCT in Spain Methylprednisolone vs placebo in Severe CAP	Improvement in Pao_2/Fio_2 ($P = .001$) and faster time to resolution (median 5 d in MPN group [IQR 2–6 d] vs 7 d in placebo group [IQR 3–10 d] $P<.05$)	One patient with hyperglycemia and one digestive hemorrhage in the MPN group
Meijvis et al,[51] 2011	Two-center RCT in Netherlands Dexamethasone vs placebo Patients with CAP	Decrease in duration of stay in dexamethasone group compared with the placebo group (6.5 d vs 7.5 d; $P = .048$, respectively)	Hyperglycemia in 67 (44%) of dexamethasone group compared with 35 (23%) of controls ($P<.0001$).
Torres et al,[56] 2015	Multicenter RCT in Spain Methylprednisolone vs placebo Patients with severe CAP and high inflammatory response	Corticosteroid treatment reduced the risk of treatment failure (OR, 0.34; 95% CI, 0.14–0.87; $P = .02$) In-hospital mortality did not differ between the 2 groups (10% in the methylprednisolone group vs 15% in the placebo group; $P = .37$)	Hyperglycemia occurred in 11 (18%) in the methylprednisolone group and in seven patients (12%) in the placebo group ($P = .34$). One patient in the methylprednisolone group had delirium and one patient in the placebo group had gastrointestinal bleeding

(continued on next page)

Table 1
(continued)

References	Study Design and Population	Main Results	Adverse Events
Blum et al,[57] 2015	Multicenter RCT in Switzerland Prednisone vs placebo Patients with CAP	Reduction of time to clinical stability in the prednisone group compared with the placebo group (3 d vs 4.4 d; P<.0001)	Hyperglycemia occurred in 76 (19%) in the Prednisone group and in 43 patients (11%) in the placebo group (P = .001). Gastrointestinal bleeding occurred in three (1%) in the Prednisone group and in four patients (1%) in the placebo group.

Abbreviations: CAP, community-acquired pneumonia; CI, confidence interval; IQR, interquartile range; MPN, methylpred-nisolone; OR, odds ratio; RCT, randomized, controlled trial.

only in patients who present with shock despite adequate fluid resuscitation and vasopressor support.[72]

Several metaanalyses have evaluated the use of corticosteroids in patients with pneumonia owing to influenza and have reported increases in mortality. A recent Cochrane review found an increase in mortality in patients who received corticosteroids (OR, 3.06; 95% CI, 1.58–5.92).[73] These results were confirmed by other investigators, even in

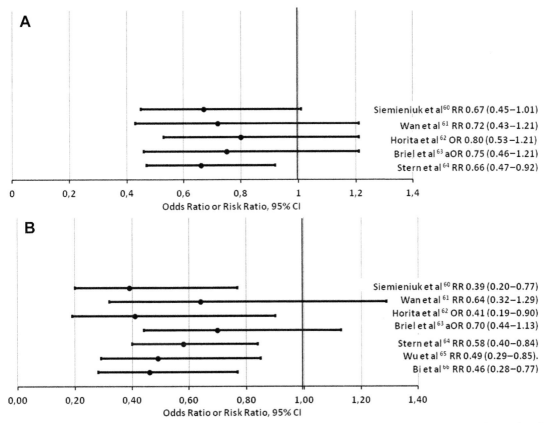

Fig. 2. Odds ratios (ORs) and risk ratios (RRs) for corticosteroids in community-acquired pneumonia (CAP; *A*) and severe CAP (*B*): results of metaanalyses published since 2015. aOR, adjusted odds ratio; CI, confidence interval.

patients who received low and moderate doses.[74,75] However, Delaney and colleagues[76] observed that this increased mortality risk disappeared after an analysis using marginal structural models to adjust the time-dependent differences between groups (OR, 0.96; 95% CI, 0.28–3.28; $P = .95$). It should be noted that few randomized clinical trials have been conducted in this specific population and so all these metaanalyses have included studies with low quality of evidence.

A recent post hoc study by Wirz and colleagues[77] observed a lower response to corticosteroids in patients with pneumococcal pneumonia, possibly because pneumolysin blocks the cytoplasmic receptor of the corticosteroids.

Corticosteroids have also shown a significant number of adverse effects; although not serious, these effects must be taken into account before corticosteroid treatment is initiated. Hyperglycemia, gastrointestinal bleeding, and neuropsychiatric disorders are the most important. Although hyperglycemia in diabetic patients may hinder clinical management, these patients have shown similar outcomes compared with nondiabetic patients.[78]

Interestingly, a recently guide published by Society of Critical Care Medicine and European Society of Intensive Care Medicine for management of critical illness-related corticosteroid insufficiency in critically ill patients recommended the use of corticosteroids for 5 to 7 days at a daily dose of less than 400 mg intravenous hydrocortisone or equivalent in hospitalized patients with CAP. This recommendation is conditional, with a moderate quality of evidence.[32]

The combination of corticosteroids and macrolides is an interesting strategy. A post hoc study found this combination to be safe,[79] and the study by Wirz and colleagues[77] observed fewer rehospitalizations in patients who received corticoids and macrolides jointly. Different corticosteroids and doses were evaluated in clinical studies. Methylprednisolone or prednisone 0.5 mg/kg/BID during 5 or 7 days, seems safe, and with lower mineralocorticoid effect than hydrocortisone. It is no clear the rebound effect observed by Snijders and colleagures,[53] with higher rate of late treatment failure in the corticosteroid group; probably the treatment should not be shorter than the time until clinical stability. Longer treatment than 5–7 days or higher doses may increase adverse events with the same anti-inflammatory effect.

VITAMIN C

A recent study evaluated the use of corticosteroids in combination with vitamin C and thiamine in patients with sepsis.[80] This combination was proposed in view of the fact that vitamin C attenuates proinflammatory mediators and prevents sepsis-induced coagulopathy.[81] Low concentrations of ascorbic acid in patients with sepsis are inversely correlated with the incidence of multiple organ failure and directly correlated with survival.[82] A phase I randomized controlled trial (RCT) showed that intravenous ascorbic acid infusion in patients with severe sepsis was safe and well-tolerated and may positively impact the extent of multiple organ failure and biomarkers of inflammation and endothelial injury.[83] The mechanism of vitamin C involves rebalancing the production and use of nitric oxide; changes in arteriolar reactivity in sepsis are mediated by the stimulation of nitric oxide synthase and vitamin C inhibits this mechanism.[84]

In a case-control study by Marik and colleagues[80] in patients with septic shock, the combination of vitamin C, hydrocortisone, and thiamine was a protective factor for mortality with an adjusted OR of 0.13 (95% CI, 0.04–0.48; $P = .002$). The duration of vasopressor treatment also decreased.

MODULATION OF COAGULATION

As described elsewhere in this article, the coagulation disorders triggered by the inflammatory cascade in sepsis represent an important target that needs to be modified. Several studies with different drugs have been performed.

Recombinant activated protein C or drotrecogin alpha (activated) was shown to be a promising drug after its first evaluation in 2001 in the PROWESS study, a phase III study that was prematurely terminated for efficacy.[85] The trial included 1960 patients with severe sepsis and showed a decrease in the relative risk of death of 19.4% (95% CI, 6.6–30.5). It also showed a tendency toward a greater risk of bleeding in patients in the treatment group. Despite these promising results, after subgroup analysis the US Food and Drug Administration approved its use only in patients with a very high risk of death. The positive results could not be replicated in 2 subsequent RCTs.[86,87] In a subsequent metaanalysis, drotrecogin alpha (activated) was associated with a significant decrease in in-hospital mortality and an increase in bleeding rates in patients with severe sepsis.[88]

Tifacogin, a recombinant inhibitor of the human tissue factor pathway, has also been tested in patients with CAP. This study showed no benefits in terms of mortality.[89]

A new soluble human recombinant agent thrombomodulin has been approved by Japanese Ministry of Health, Labour and Welfare in 2008 and is being used in clinical practice in Japan for the treatment of disseminated intravascular coagulopathy. In a retrospective study of patients with severe sepsis and disseminated intravascular coagulopathy, adjusted by a propensity score, the use of human recombinant agent thrombomodulin showed benefits in in-hospital mortality at 30, 60, and 90 days.[90–92] Results from RCTs are required for its approval by regulatory agencies in Europe and the United States.

Aspirin is an antiplatelet agent that is used in the primary and secondary prevention of cardiovascular diseases. A physiologic study reported that the intravenous infusion of acetylsalicylic acid resulted in a modest improvement in intrapulmonary shunt, probably by enhancing hypoxic pulmonary vasoconstriction, without significant changes in arterial oxygenation.[93] Subsequent observational studies have shown that the mortality owing to CAP is lower in patients using aspirin and that the combination of aspirin and macrolides improves survival in patients who present with septic shock owing to pneumonia.[94,95]

STATINS

Statins have shown antiinflammatory, immunomodulatory, and antioxidant effects in experimental and observational studies. A double-blind, placebo-controlled, phase II RCT was carried out to assess the effect of statins in patients with severe sepsis admitted to the intensive care unit, in which the drug chosen was atorvastatin.[96] The study showed that there were no differences in levels of IL-6 between the control group and placebo, nor were there any significant differences in mortality. However, in patients who received statins before admission, mortality was lower.

An RCT evaluating simvastatin in patients with CAP was interrupted owing to low recruitment; the results showed no benefits in the use of statins in terms of time to clinical stability or inflammatory cytokine levels.[97]

COLONY-STIMULATING FACTORS

The use of granulocytic colony-stimulating factors has shown some benefits in experimental models of pneumonia. As a result, it was studied in a phase III placebo-controlled RCT that included 700 patients with pneumonia and severe sepsis (community and hospital acquired). However, no benefits in mortality were found.[98]

IMMUNOGLOBULINS

Since the 1980s, several studies have assessed the use of immunoglobulins in patients with sepsis, severe sepsis, and septic shock. These studies have focused on IgG- and IgM-enriched polyclonal immunoglobulins and have found that polyvalent immunoglobulins improve bacterial opsonization, prevent nonspecific activation of complement, protect against antibiotic-induced endotoxin release, and neutralize endotoxin and superantigens.

Two metaanalyses have shown a benefit of immunoglobulin use in patients with severe sepsis and septic shock. A Cochrane metaanalysis published by Alejandria and colleagues[99] found a relative risk for mortality of 0.77 (95% CI, 0.68–0.87), with a greater benefit in studies that included enriched IgG (RR, 0.66; 95% CI, 0.51–0.85). Kreymann and colleagues[100] observed similar results in a metaanalysis with a relative risk of death of 0.79 (95% CI, 0.69–0.90) and a strong tendency in favor of an immunoglobulin preparation enriched with IgA and IgM (RR, 0.66; 95% CI, 0.51–0.84; $P<.0009$) compared with preparations containing only IgG (RR, 0.85; 95% CI, 0.73–0.99). Interestingly, a retrospective case-control study in patients with septic shock caused by gram-negative XDR bacteria showed improved survival in those patients who received IgG enriched with IgM and IgA.[101]

A phase II study evaluated the use of intravenous immunoglobulins with a novel product developed to generate a preparation that contains approximately 23% IgM, 23% IgA, and 54% IgG, in patients with CAP who required invasive mechanical ventilation. The outcome measure in the study was ventilation-free days.[102] Although the results have not yet been published, the laboratory promoting the trial reported a benefit in the use of immunoglobulins only in patients with low baseline levels of IgM or in those with a high inflammatory response. In view of these results, there are plans to conduct a phase III study in these specific subpopulations.

Although many of the agents discussed in this article are still being evaluated in clinical trials, we have designed a preliminary treatment algorithm (presented in **Fig. 3**).

FUTURE TRIALS

Mesenchymal stem cells show immunomodulatory properties and regulate the function of a large number of immune cells, including B lymphocytes, T lymphocytes, macrophages, and natural killer cells.[103–105] The molecular and cellular mechanisms involved in the immunoregulatory activity of mesenchymal stem cells depend on cell-to-cell interactions and soluble factors and the generation of cells with regulatory activity such as regulatory T lymphocytes or antiinflammatory macrophages, which play a central role in maintaining a

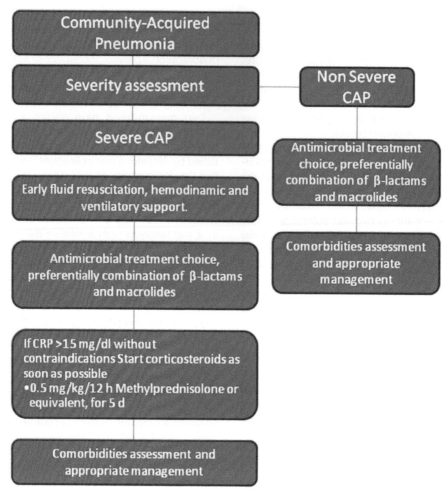

Fig. 3. Algorithm of treatment in patients with severe community-acquired pneumonia (CAP). CRP, C-reactive protein.

satisfactory balance in the immune system in health and disease. It has also been reported that mesenchymal stem cells show antimicrobial activities against different pathogens.[106] A phase Ib/IIa clinical trial is currently underway to evaluate the safety and viability of mesenchymal stem cell therapy in patients who develop severe sepsis owing to CAP (EudraCT: 2015–002994–39).

Pidotimod, a synthetic dipeptide (3-pyriglutamyl-1-thiazolidine-4-carboxylic acid), is an immunomodulator that affects both innate and adaptive immunity. It elicits higher expression of TLR2 and HLA-DR, induction of dendritic cell maturation and release of proinflammatory molecules, stimulation of T-lymphocyte proliferation and differentiation toward a T-helper 1 phenotype, as well as an increase in phagocytosis. This new drug was tested in a study with 16 patients who presented alterations in the inflammatory response; however, this finding did not translate into changes in the clinical response.[107]

SUMMARY

The use of adjuvant therapies is still in development. Combinations of antibiotics with macrolides seem to be the best option when there is no risk of resistance. The use of corticosteroids is the treatment of choice in patients with severe pneumonia and high inflammatory response who do not present contraindications for these drugs. The other drugs mentioned herein await confirmation of their benefit and should for the moment be used only on exceptional occasions.

REFERENCES

1. Prina E, Ranzani OT, Torres A. Community-acquired pneumonia. Lancet 2015;386(9998):1097–108.
2. Ramirez JA, Wiemken TL, Peyrani P, et al. Adults hospitalized with pneumonia in the United States: incidence, epidemiology, and mortality. Clin Infect Dis 2017;65(11):1806–12.

3. Ranzani OT, Prina E, Menéndez R, et al. New sepsis definition (Sepsis-3) and community-acquired pneumonia mortality: a validation and clinical decision-making study. Am J Respir Crit Care Med 2017;196(10):1287–97.

4. Liapikou A, Ferrer M, Polverino E, et al. Severe community-acquired pneumonia: validation of the Infectious Diseases Society of America/American Thoracic Society guidelines to predict an intensive care unit admission. Clin Infect Dis 2009;48(4): 377–85.

5. Jones DS, Podolsky SH, Greene JA. The burden of disease and the changing task of medicine. N Engl J Med 2012;366(25):2333–8.

6. Simonetti AF, Garcia-Vidal C, Viasus D, et al. Declining mortality among hospitalized patients with community-acquired pneumonia. Clin Microbiol Infect 2010;22(6):567–617.

7. Shindo Y, Ito R, Kobayashi D, et al. Risk factors for 30-day mortality in patients with pneumonia who receive appropriate initial antibiotics: an observational cohort study. Lancet Infect Dis 2015;15(9): 1055–65.

8. Bodí M, Rodríguez A, Solé-Violán J, et al. Antibiotic prescription for community-acquired pneumonia in the intensive care unit: impact of adherence to Infectious Diseases Society of America guidelines on survival. Clin Infect Dis 2005;41(12):1709–16.

9. Torres A, Cillóniz C, Ferrer M, et al. Bacteraemia and antibiotic-resistant pathogens in community acquired pneumonia: risk and prognosis. Eur Respir J 2015;45(5):1353–63.

10. Mandell LA, Wunderink RG, Anzueto A, et al. Infectious Diseases Society of America/American Thoracic Society consensus guidelines on the management of community-acquired pneumonia in adults. Clin Infect Dis 2007;44(Suppl 2): S27–72.

11. Cilloniz C, Ceccato A, San Jose A, et al. Clinical management of community acquired pneumonia in the elderly patient. Expert Rev Respir Med 2016. https://doi.org/10.1080/17476348.2016.1240037.

12. Cillóniz C, Polverino E, Ewig S, et al. Impact of age and comorbidity on cause and outcome in community-acquired pneumonia. Chest 2013; 144(3):999–1007.

13. Menéndez R, Cavalcanti M, Reyes S, et al. Markers of treatment failure in hospitalised community acquired pneumonia. Thorax 2008;63(5):447–52.

14. Menéndez R, Montull B, Reyes S, et al. Pneumonia presenting with organ dysfunctions: causative microorganisms, host factors and outcome. J Infect 2016;73(5):419–26.

15. Wunderink RG. Corticosteroids for severe community-acquired pneumonia: not for everyone. JAMA 2015;313(7):673–4.

16. Menéndez R, Torres A, Zalacaín R, et al. Risk factors of treatment failure in community acquired pneumonia: implications for disease outcome. Thorax 2004;59(11):960–5.

17. Fernandez-Botran R, Uriarte SM, Arnold FW, et al. Contrasting inflammatory responses in severe and non-severe community-acquired pneumonia. Inflammation 2014;37(4):1158–66.

18. Kellum JA, Kong L, Fink MP, et al. Understanding the inflammatory cytokine response in pneumonia and sepsis: results of the Genetic and inflammatory markers of sepsis (GenIMS) study. Arch Intern Med 2007;167(15):1655–63.

19. Torres A, Ramirez P, Montull B, et al. Biomarkers and community-acquired pneumonia: tailoring management with biological data. Semin Respir Crit Care Med 2012;33(3):266–71.

20. Paats MS, Bergen IM, Hanselaar WEJJ, et al. Local and systemic cytokine profiles in nonsevere and severe community-acquired pneumonia. Eur Respir J 2013;41(6):1378–85.

21. Angus DC, van der Poll T. Severe sepsis and septic shock. N Engl J Med 2013;369(9):840–51.

22. Singer M, Deutschman CS, Seymour CW, et al. The third international consensus definitions for sepsis and septic shock (Sepsis-3). JAMA 2016;315(8): 801–10.

23. Levi M, van der Poll T. Inflammation and coagulation. Crit Care Med 2010;38(2 Suppl):S26–34.

24. Dhainaut JF, Marin N, Mignon A, et al. Hepatic response to sepsis: interaction between coagulation and inflammatory processes. Crit Care Med 2001;29(7 Suppl):S42–7.

25. Petäjä J. Inflammation and coagulation. An overview. Thromb Res 2011;127(Suppl 2):S34–7.

26. Levi M. The coagulant response in sepsis and inflammation. Hamostaseologie 2010;30(1):10–2, 14–16.

27. Alonso de Vega JM, Díaz J, Serrano E, et al. Oxidative stress in critically ill patients with systemic inflammatory response syndrome. Crit Care Med 2002;30(8):1782–6.

28. Schieber M, Chandel NS. ROS function in redox signaling and oxidative stress. Curr Biol 2014; 24(10):R453–62.

29. Mittal M, Siddiqui MR, Tran K, et al. Reactive oxygen species in inflammation and tissue injury. Antioxid Redox Signal 2014;20(7):1126–67.

30. Marik PE, Zaloga GP. Adrenal insufficiency during septic shock. Crit Care Med 2003;31(1):141–5.

31. Annane D, Pastores SM, Rochwerg B, et al. Guidelines for the diagnosis and management of Critical Illness-Related Corticosteroid Insufficiency (CIRCI) in critically Ill patients (Part I): Society of Critical Care Medicine (SCCM) and European Society of Intensive Care Medicine (ESICM) 2017. Crit Care Med 2017;45(12):2078–88.

32. Pastores SM, Annane D, Rochwerg B. Esicm and the CGTF of S and. Guidelines for the diagnosis and management of Critical Illness-Related Corticosteroid Insufficiency (CIRCI) in critically Ill patients (Part II): Society of Critical Care Medicine (SCCM) and European Society of Intensive Care Medicine (ESICM) 2017. Crit Care Med 2018; 46(1):146.

33. Salluh JIF, Verdeal JC, Mello GW, et al. Cortisol levels in patients with severe community-acquired pneumonia. Intensive Care Med 2006; 32(4):595–8.

34. Bermejo-Martin JF, Cilloniz C, Mendez R, et al. Lymphopenic Community Acquired Pneumonia (L-CAP), an immunological phenotype associated with higher risk of mortality. EBioMedicine 2017; 24:231–6.

35. Bermejo-Martin JF, Almansa R, Martin-Fernandez M, et al. Immunological profiling to assess disease severity and prognosis in community-acquired pneumonia. Lancet Respir Med 2017;5(12):e35–6.

36. de la Torre MC, Torán P, Serra-Prat M, et al. Serum levels of immunoglobulins and severity of community-acquired pneumonia. BMJ Open Respir Res 2016;3(1):e000152.

37. de la Torre MC, Palomera E, Serra-Prat M, et al. IgG2 as an independent risk factor for mortality in patients with community-acquired pneumonia. J Crit Care 2016;35:115–9.

38. Martin-Loeches I, Muriel-Bombín A, Ferrer R, et al. The protective association of endogenous immunoglobulins against sepsis mortality is restricted to patients with moderate organ failure. Ann Intensive Care 2017;7(1):44.

39. Albert RK, Connett J, Bailey WC, et al. Azithromycin for prevention of exacerbations of COPD. N Engl J Med 2011;365(8):689–98.

40. Altenburg J, de Graaff CS, Stienstra Y, et al. Effect of azithromycin maintenance treatment on infectious exacerbations among patients with non-cystic fibrosis bronchiectasis: the BAT randomized controlled trial. JAMA 2013;309(12): 1251–9.

41. Saiman L, Marshall BC, Mayer-Hamblett N, et al. Azithromycin in patients with cystic fibrosis chronically infected with Pseudomonas aeruginosa: a randomized controlled trial. JAMA 2003;290(13): 1749–56.

42. Mortensen EM, Halm EA, Pugh MJ, et al. Association of azithromycin with mortality and cardiovascular events among older patients hospitalized with pneumonia. JAMA 2014;311(21):2199–208.

43. Restrepo MI, Mortensen EM, Waterer GW, et al. Impact of macrolide therapy on mortality for patients with severe sepsis due to pneumonia. Eur Respir J 2009;33(1):153–9.

44. Asadi L, Sligl WI, Eurich DT, et al. Macrolide-based regimens and mortality in hospitalized patients with community-acquired pneumonia: a systematic review and meta-analysis. Clin Infect Dis 2012; 55(3):371–80.

45. Martin-Loeches I, Lisboa T, Rodriguez A, et al. Combination antibiotic therapy with macrolides improves survival in intubated patients with community-acquired pneumonia. Intensive Care Med 2010;36(4):612–20.

46. Baddour LM, Yu VL, Klugman KP, et al. Combination antibiotic therapy lowers mortality among severely ill patients with pneumococcal bacteremia. Am J Respir Crit Care Med 2004;170(4): 440–4.

47. Giamarellos-Bourboulis EJ. Macrolides beyond the conventional antimicrobials: a class of potent immunomodulators. Int J Antimicrob Agents 2008; 31(1):12–20.

48. Kovaleva A, Remmelts HHF, Rijkers GT, et al. Immunomodulatory effects of macrolides during community-acquired pneumonia: a literature review. J Antimicrob Chemother 2012;67(3):530–40.

49. Garin N, Genné D, Carballo S, et al. β-Lactam monotherapy vs β-lactam-macrolide combination treatment in moderately severe community-acquired pneumonia: a randomized noninferiority trial. JAMA Intern Med 2014;174(12):1894–901.

50. Postma DF, van Werkhoven CH, van Elden LJR, et al. Antibiotic treatment strategies for community-acquired pneumonia in adults. N Engl J Med 2015;372(14):1312–23.

51. Meijvis SCA, Hardeman H, Remmelts HHF, et al. Dexamethasone and length of hospital stay in patients with community-acquired pneumonia: a randomised, double-blind, placebo-controlled trial. Lancet 2011;377(9782):2023–30.

52. Confalonieri M, Urbino R, Potena A, et al. Hydrocortisone infusion for severe community-acquired pneumonia: a preliminary randomized study. Am J Respir Crit Care Med 2005;171(3):242–8.

53. Snijders D, Daniels JMA, de Graaff CS, et al. Efficacy of corticosteroids in community-acquired pneumonia: a randomized double-blinded clinical trial. Am J Respir Crit Care Med 2010;181(9): 975–82.

54. Garcia-Vidal C, Calbo E, Pascual V, et al. Effects of systemic steroids in patients with severe community-acquired pneumonia. Eur Respir J 2007;30(5):951–6.

55. Fernández-Serrano S, Dorca J, Garcia-Vidal C, et al. Effect of corticosteroids on the clinical course of community-acquired pneumonia: a randomized controlled trial. Crit Care 2011;15(2):R96.

56. Torres A, Sibila O, Ferrer M, et al. Effect of corticosteroids on treatment failure among hospitalized patients with severe community-acquired pneumonia

and high inflammatory response: a randomized clinical trial. JAMA 2015;313(7):677–86.

57. Blum CA, Nigro N, Briel M, et al. Adjunct prednisone therapy for patients with community-acquired pneumonia: a multicentre, double-blind, randomised, placebo-controlled trial. Lancet 2015;385(9977):1511–8.

58. Sabry NA, Omar EE-D. Corticosteroids and ICU course of community acquired pneumonia in Egyptian settings. Pharmacol Pharm 2011; 2(2):73.

59. Nafae RM, Ragab MI, Amany FM, et al. Adjuvant role of corticosteroids in the treatment of community-acquired pneumonia. Egypt J Chest Dis Tuberc 2013;62(3):439–45.

60. Siemieniuk RAC, Meade MO, Alonso-Coello P, et al. Corticosteroid therapy for patients hospitalized with community-acquired pneumonia: a systematic review and meta-analysis. Ann Intern Med 2015; 163(7):519–28.

61. Wan Y-D, Sun T-W, Liu Z-Q, et al. Efficacy and safety of corticosteroids for community-acquired pneumonia: a systematic review and meta-analysis. Chest 2016;149(1):209–19.

62. Horita N, Otsuka T, Haranaga S, et al. Adjunctive systemic corticosteroids for hospitalized community-acquired pneumonia: systematic review and meta-analysis 2015 update. Sci Rep 2015;5: 14061.

63. Briel M, Spoorenberg SMC, Snijders D, et al. Corticosteroids in patients hospitalized with community-acquired pneumonia: systematic review and individual patient data metaanalysis. Clin Infect Dis 2018;66(3):346–54.

64. Stern A, Skalsky K, Avni T, et al. Corticosteroids for pneumonia. Cochrane Database Syst Rev 2017;12: CD007720.

65. Wu W-F, Fang Q, He G-J. Efficacy of corticosteroid treatment for severe community-acquired pneumonia: a meta-analysis. Am J Emerg Med 2017. https://doi.org/10.1016/j.ajem.2017.07.050.

66. Bi J, Yang J, Wang Y, et al. Efficacy and safety of adjunctive corticosteroids therapy for severe community-acquired pneumonia in adults: an updated systematic review and meta-analysis. PLoS One 2016;11(11):e0165942.

67. Keh D, Trips E, Marx G, et al. Effect of hydrocortisone on development of shock among patients with severe sepsis: the HYPRESS randomized clinical trial. JAMA 2016;316(17):1775–85.

68. Annane D, Bellissant E, Bollaert P-E, et al. Corticosteroids in the treatment of severe sepsis and septic shock in adults: a systematic review. JAMA 2009;301(22):2362–75.

69. Venkatesh B, Finfer S, Cohen J, et al. Adjunctive glucocorticoid therapy in patients with septic shock. N Engl J Med 2018;378(9):797–808.

70. Sprung CL, Annane D, Keh D, et al. Hydrocortisone therapy for patients with septic shock. N Engl J Med 2008;358(2):111–24.

71. Tagami T, Matsui H, Horiguchi H, et al. Low-dose corticosteroid use and mortality in severe community-acquired pneumonia patients. Eur Respir J 2015;45(2):463–72.

72. Rhodes A, Evans LE, Alhazzani W, et al. Surviving sepsis campaign: international guidelines for management of sepsis and septic shock: 2016. Intensive Care Med 2017;43(3):304–77.

73. Rodrigo C, Leonardi-Bee J, Nguyen-Van-Tam J, et al. Corticosteroids as adjunctive therapy in the treatment of influenza. Cochrane Database Syst Rev 2016;3:CD010406.

74. Zhang Y, Sun W, Svendsen ER, et al. Do corticosteroids reduce the mortality of influenza A (H1N1) infection? A meta-analysis. Crit Care 2015;19:46.

75. Yang J-W, Fan L-C, Miao X-Y, et al. Corticosteroids for the treatment of human infection with influenza virus: a systematic review and meta-analysis. Clin Microbiol Infect 2015;21(10):956–63.

76. Delaney JW, Pinto R, Long J, et al. The influence of corticosteroid treatment on the outcome of influenza A(H1N1pdm09)-related critical illness. Crit Care 2016;20:75.

77. Wirz SA, Blum CA, Schuetz P, et al. Pathogen- and antibiotic-specific effects of prednisone in community-acquired pneumonia. Eur Respir J 2016;48(4):1150–9.

78. Popovic M, Blum CA, Nigro N, et al. Benefit of adjunct corticosteroids for community-acquired pneumonia in diabetic patients. Diabetologia 2016;59(12):2552–60.

79. Ceccato A, Cilloniz C, Ranzani OT, et al. Treatment with macrolides and glucocorticosteroids in severe community-acquired pneumonia: a post-hoc exploratory analysis of a randomized controlled trial. PLoS One 2017;12(6):e0178022.

80. Marik PE, Khangoora V, Rivera R, et al. Hydrocortisone, Vitamin C, and thiamine for the treatment of severe sepsis and septic shock: a retrospective before-after study. Chest 2017;151(6):1229–38.

81. Wilson JX. Evaluation of vitamin C for adjuvant sepsis therapy. Antioxid Redox Signal 2013; 19(17):2129–40.

82. Borrelli E, Roux-Lombard P, Grau GE, et al. Plasma concentrations of cytokines, their soluble receptors, and antioxidant vitamins can predict the development of multiple organ failure in patients at risk. Crit Care Med 1996;24(3):392–7.

83. Fowler AA, Syed AA, Knowlson S, et al. Phase I safety trial of intravenous ascorbic acid in patients with severe sepsis. J Transl Med 2014;12:32.

84. Marik PE. "Vitamin S" (Steroids) and Vitamin C for the treatment of severe sepsis and septic shock! Crit Care Med 2016;44(6):1228–9.

85. Bernard GR, Vincent JL, Laterre PF, et al. Efficacy and safety of recombinant human activated protein C for severe sepsis. N Engl J Med 2001;344(10):699–709.

86. Annane D, Timsit J-F, Megarbane B, et al. Recombinant human activated protein C for adults with septic shock: a randomized controlled trial. Am J Respir Crit Care Med 2013;187(10):1091–7.

87. Ranieri VM, Thompson BT, Barie PS, et al. Drotrecogin alfa (activated) in adults with septic shock. N Engl J Med 2012;366(22):2055–64.

88. Martí-Carvajal AJ, Solà I, Gluud C, et al. Human recombinant protein C for severe sepsis and septic shock in adult and paediatric patients. Cochrane Database Syst Rev 2012;12:CD004388.

89. Wunderink RG, Laterre P-F, Francois B, et al. Recombinant tissue factor pathway inhibitor in severe community-acquired pneumonia: a randomized trial. Am J Respir Crit Care Med 2011;183(11):1561–8.

90. Yamakawa K, Ogura H, Fujimi S, et al. Recombinant human soluble thrombomodulin in sepsis-induced disseminated intravascular coagulation: a multicenter propensity score analysis. Intensive Care Med 2013;39(4):644–52.

91. Hayakawa M, Yamakawa K, Saito S, et al. Recombinant human soluble thrombomodulin and mortality in sepsis-induced disseminated intravascular coagulation. A multicentre retrospective study. Thromb Haemost 2016;115(6):1157–66.

92. Yoshimura J, Yamakawa K, Ogura H, et al. Benefit profile of recombinant human soluble thrombomodulin in sepsis-induced disseminated intravascular coagulation: a multicenter propensity score analysis. Crit Care 2015;19:78.

93. Ferrer M, Torres A, Baer R, et al. Effect of acetylsalicylic acid on pulmonary gas exchange in patients with severe pneumonia: a pilot study. Chest 1997;111(4):1094–100.

94. Falcone M, Russo A, Farcomeni A, et al. Septic shock from community-onset pneumonia: is there a role for aspirin plus macrolides combination? Intensive Care Med 2016;42(2):301–2.

95. Falcone M, Russo A, Cangemi R, et al. Lower mortality rate in elderly patients with community-onset pneumonia on treatment with aspirin. J Am Heart Assoc 2015;4(1):e001595.

96. Kruger P, Bailey M, Bellomo R, et al. A multicenter randomized trial of atorvastatin therapy in intensive care patients with severe sepsis. Am J Respir Crit Care Med 2013;187(7):743–50.

97. Viasus D, Garcia-Vidal C, Simonetti AF, et al. The effect of simvastatin on inflammatory cytokines in community-acquired pneumonia: a randomised, double-blind, placebo-controlled trial. BMJ Open 2015;5(1):e006251.

98. Root RK, Lodato RF, Patrick W, et al. Multicenter, double-blind, placebo-controlled study of the use of filgrastim in patients hospitalized with pneumonia and severe sepsis. Crit Care Med 2003;31(2):367–73.

99. Alejandria MM, Lansang MAD, Dans LF, et al. Intravenous immunoglobulin for treating sepsis, severe sepsis and septic shock. Cochrane Database Syst Rev 2013;9:CD001090.

100. Kreymann KG, de Heer G, Nierhaus A, et al. Use of polyclonal immunoglobulins as adjunctive therapy for sepsis or septic shock. Crit Care Med 2007;35(12):2677–85.

101. Giamarellos-Bourboulis EJ, Tziolos N, Routsi C, et al. Improving outcomes of severe infections by multidrug-resistant pathogens with polyclonal IgM-enriched immunoglobulins. Clin Microbiol Infect 2016;22(6):499–506.

102. Welte T, Dellinger RP, Ebelt H, et al. Concept for a study design in patients with severe community-acquired pneumonia: a randomised controlled trial with a novel IGM-enriched immunoglobulin preparation - the CIGMA study. Respir Med 2015;109(6):758–67.

103. Gao F, Chiu SM, Motan DAL, et al. Mesenchymal stem cells and immunomodulation: current status and future prospects. Cell Death Dis 2016;7(1):e2062.

104. Ma OK-F, Chan KH. Immunomodulation by mesenchymal stem cells: interplay between mesenchymal stem cells and regulatory lymphocytes. World J Stem Cells 2016;8(9):268–78.

105. Castro-Manrreza ME, Montesinos JJ. Immunoregulation by mesenchymal stem cells: biological aspects and clinical applications. J Immunol Res 2015;2015:394917.

106. Lee JW, Krasnodembskaya A, McKenna DH, et al. Therapeutic effects of human mesenchymal stem cells in ex vivo human lungs injured with live bacteria. Am J Respir Crit Care Med 2013;187(7):751–60.

107. Trabattoni D, Clerici M, Centanni S, et al. Immunomodulatory effects of pidotimod in adults with community-acquired pneumonia undergoing standard antibiotic therapy. Pulm Pharmacol Ther 2017;44:24–9.

Health Care–Associated Pneumonia
Is It Still a Useful Concept?

Grant W. Waterer, MBBS, PhD[a,b],*

KEYWORDS

• Pneumonia • Health care • MRSA • *Pseudomonas* • Antibiotics

KEY POINTS

- Health care–associated pneumonia (HCAP) was introduced into guidelines because of concerns about the increasing prevalence of drug-resistant pathogens, especially methicillin-resistant *Staphylococcus aureus* (MRSA) and *Pseudomonas*, not covered by standard empirical therapy.
- Overall it is now apparent that HCAP risk factors only define a population who are at risk of *Pseudomonas aeruginosa* and MRSA in highly specific locations.
- The predictive power of all of the putative risk factors is highly variable, with the notable exception of a prior culture of one of these pathogens.
- Application of HCAP globally has not resulted in better outcomes and, in most settings, has led to harm through significant overuse of anti-MRSA and antipseudomonal antibiotics.
- A new approach is needed, and it needs to be nuanced by knowledge of local etiologic data and, it is hoped, enhanced by modern point-of-care microbiologic identification platforms.

INTRODUCTION

Community-acquired pneumonia (CAP) is the most common serious infection that physicians encounter in the Western world.[1] Despite all the innovation in medicine over the past few decades, we still do not have a diagnostic platform that is reliable, affordable, and accurate enough to tell us what pathogens we should be treating when we have to make the choice of what antimicrobial agents to prescribe. In the absence of specific data, we have to rely on experience, basing our treatment on etiologic studies of CAP, assuming that what is common elsewhere will also be common in our own patients.

The cause of pneumonia has been changing for decades in response to a multitude of factors, including aging hosts, more vulnerable and chronically ill hosts, antibiotic selection pressure, vaccination strategies (especially conjugate pneumococcal vaccines[2]), and the emergence of new pathogens. Improvements in molecular diagnostic tests have also increased the array of pathogens detected. Examples of new tests changing our knowledge of what causes pneumonia are those for *Legionella spp*[3] and metapneumovirus.[4] It is now more common than not in recent etiologic studies[5,6] to find multiple pathogens being present, although whether these represent true concurrent infection or serial infection remains a matter of contention.

When the American Thoracic Society's (ATS) first guidelines were published 25 years ago,[7] there was a reasonably clear distinction between the pathogens causing CAP and those causing nosocomial pneumonia. Since then, the distinction has become

No conflicts of interest to declare.
[a] University of Western Australia, Royal Perth Hospital, Level 4, MRF Building, GPO Box X2213, Perth 6847, Australia; [b] Northwestern University, Chicago, IL, USA
* University of Western Australia, Level 4 MRF Building, Royal Perth Hospital, Rear 78 Murray Street, Perth 6000, Australia.
E-mail address: grant.waterer@uwa.edu.au

Clin Chest Med 39 (2018) 765–773
https://doi.org/10.1016/j.ccm.2018.07.009

blurred with repeated hospitalization being common in the elderly and those with chronic organ failure, increasing numbers of vulnerable hosts grouped in aged-care facilities enabling the spread of antibiotic-resistant pathogens, and increased uptake of ambulatory care programs blurring the line between hospital care and the home. In the 2005 update on the treatment of nosocomial pneumonias, the ATS and Infectious Diseases Society of America included health care–associated pneumonia (HCAP) as a separate category on the premise that a set of risk factors identified patients at high risk of pathogens not covered by typical CAP empirical therapy.[8] Of particular concern was methicillin-resistant *Staphylococcus aureus* (MRSA) and *Pseudomonas aeruginosa* (PA) that had been identified as becoming increasingly common in patients coming from the community in tertiary centers in the United States.[9,10] The risk factors defining the HCAP population were identified as nursing home residence, recent hospitalization, dialysis, and chronic wound care.[11] Because inadequate empirical antibiotic therapy in CAP is associated with a significantly higher risk of mortality,[12–14] and both MRSA and PA are not covered by standard empirical therapy for CAP, there was a legitimate concern that failure to recognize this population of patients would lead to serious adverse outcomes.

Since the publication of the 2005 guidelines, opinion about the usefulness and/or appropriateness of HCAP as a separate classification of pneumonia has been hotly debated. Several prominent editorialists have called for HCAP to be abandoned as a separate category of pneumonia.[10,15,16] What then is the evidence?

ETIOLOGIC STUDIES OF HEALTH CARE–ASSOCIATED PNEUMONIA

Most pathogens identified in cases of HCAP come from sputum culture. Before considering the etiologic studies of HCAP, it is worth considering whether an organism isolated in sputum truly indicates the pathogen causing pneumonia. Historically, a pathogen isolated from sputum would only be deemed possible rather than definite, the latter category reserved for pathogens isolated from usually sterile sites (eg, blood culture, fine-needle aspiration of a consolidated region or lung abscess, pleural aspiration of an associated empyema, and so forth).

Because there are also gram-negative pathogens other than PA, the author collectively refers to pathogens not covered by standard empirical therapy for CAP as drug-resistant pathogens (DRPs). Several studies have suggested that

DRPs may be cultured in sputum but that they are not the actual pathogens causing pneumonia.[17,18] This idea has long been recognized as a potential issue in hospitalized and elderly patients with gram-negative pathogens.[19] As a previous culture of PA or MRSA is the major risk factor for culturing these pathogens in the setting of HCAP,[20–22] this further raises the finding these organisms may occasionally represent chronic carriage rather than the acute infecting agent. That these pathogens may not be the true cause of pneumonia in some patients may also explain many of the findings outlined in the treatment section later.

The initial publication leading to the adoption of HCAP was that by Kollef and colleagues[23] in 2005. In this analysis of a database of 3209 patients from 59 US hospitals with CAP and a positive culture, 34% of patients had a pathogen resistant to standard empirical therapy, mostly MRSA and PA. A major concern with this study is that *Streptococcus pneumonia* was less prevalent than DRPs, possibly indicating a heavy bias toward culturing patients thought to be at risk of nonstandard pathogens. Nevertheless, for the reasons explained earlier, significant concern was raised that standard CAP regimes may be inappropriate in a significant subset of patients.

Subsequent etiologic studies of CAP have been well reviewed elsewhere,[9,24] but in general few have resembled the high proportion of antibiotic-resistant pathogens reported by Kollef and colleagues.[23] Several studies are worthy of particular mention. Metersky and colleagues[25] reported on 61,000 patients admitted with pneumonia and having HCAP risk factors from the Veterans Affairs database in the United States with only 1.9% of patients having PA and 1.0% having MRSA. The very low prevalence is also consistent with the findings of the Centers for Diseases Control and Prevention CAP cause study whereby only 1% (6 of 568) of those treated empirically for MRSA or PA had these pathogens identified.[26] Jones and colleagues[27] compared the proportion of patients with CAP covered for MRSA with the actual positive identification of MRSA across 128 hospitals in the Veterans Affairs system. Although coverage varied from 8.2% to 42.0%, actual identification was only 0.5% to 3.6%, indicating massive overtreatment. Outside the United States, the prevalence of antibiotic-resistant pathogens in the setting of CAP is typically reported as being substantially lower.[9,10]

TREATMENT OUTCOMES FOR HEALTH CARE–ASSOCIATED PNEUMONIA

If defining HCAP as being separate from CAP is important, then it should be possible to show improved outcomes from doing this. In CAP it has been demonstrated by multiple groups that guideline-discordant therapy is associated with worse patient outcomes.[28–32] In contrast guideline-discordant therapy has not been associated with worse outcomes in patients with HCAP in most studies,[32–38] although there are some exceptions.[39,40]

All studies of HCAP suggest that patients with these risk factors have a higher mortality than patients with standard CAP, but that does not necessarily mean it is due to them having more antibiotic-resistant pathogens.

The overwhelming abundance of data suggest that outcomes are worse in the HCAP population because of the presence of significant comorbidities rather than any difference in the pathogens. For example, Rello and colleagues[41] demonstrated that pneumococcal pneumonia had a much worse outcome in patients with HCAP risk factors. Polverino and colleagues[42] found no difference in pathogens between HCAP and CAP, but the former had much worse outcomes driven by comorbidity. Bjarnason and colleagues[43] studied HCAP mortality in a low-resistance setting. Although there were no multidrug-resistant (MDR) pathogens in their HCAP group of 137 patients, mortality was still much higher than in the CAP population (10% vs 1%). In pooled analysis the higher mortality rates with HCAP compared with CAP are completely accounted for by adjustment for age and comorbidity.[44] The possibility of adverse outcomes from overuse of broad-spectrum antibiotics as outlined later may also impact on outcomes in the total HCAP population when most patients will not have an antibiotic-resistant pathogen present.

ADVERSE IMPACTS OF HEALTH CARE–ASSOCIATED PNEUMONIA CLASSIFICATION

The major concern that has been expressed about the introduction of HCAP is that it has led to a vast overuse of broad-spectrum antibiotics, particularly anti-MRSA antibiotics like vancomycin and linezolid as well as antipseudomonal antibiotics. The use of vancomycin and piperacillin-tazobactam has doubled in the US Veterans Affairs system since 2005.[45] At an individual patient level these antibiotics pose particular risks including renal dysfunction in the case of vancomycin and antipseudomonal aminoglycosides and *Clostridium difficile* infection.[15] Both of these events may be associated with worse patient outcomes.

At a hospital level there is plenty of evidence that the amount of MDR bacteria is directly proportional to total consumption of these antibiotics. At a health-economic level there is substantial increase in cost using these agents rather than conventional CAP therapy. For both of these reasons avoiding unnecessary broad-spectrum antibiotics is important and a major focus of most antibiotic stewardship programs.

IS THERE A BETTER WAY TO DEFINE THE POPULATION REQUIRING EMPIRICAL ANTIBIOTIC COVERAGE FOR ANTIBIOTIC-RESISTANT PATHOGENS?

The problem with HCAP is that in most settings the risk factors do not equate to a significant risk of having an antibiotic-resistant pathogen. Perhaps in part because of this, treating patients with empirical HCAP therapy does not seem to have much impact on outcome, with some evidence there is actual harm. However, in some situations there are high enough rates of DRPs to be concerned about the need to cover these pathogens, particularly in patients with significant sepsis. Is it possible then to better define the group of patients who will have an antibiotic-resistant pathogen?

Multiple different scoring or triage systems for HCAP have emerged over the past decade.[11,21,46,47] None of these scores has been extensively tested and validated across multiple different sites, and those that have lack the specificity to be useful clinically.[48] It is also worth reflecting on whether it is likely that any scoring tool will perform particularly well on an ongoing basis given that the rates of antibiotic-resistant pathogens are constantly changing as a result of population changes, selective antibiotic pressure, antibiotic stewardship programs, and a host of other factors, including health tourism.

Several researchers have focused on individual components of the criteria for HCAP and suggested that some are less robust or are more predictive of MRSA or PA rather than both pathogens. A summary of these risk factors is outlined in **Table 1**. There is enormous similarity between the risk factors for MRSA and PA, which is not surprising given both generally require hosts with compromised immune responses. The only risk factors that stand out are bronchiectasis for PA; however, given reports of increased MRSA in the setting of bronchiectasis,[49] this may also prove to be a nonspecific risk of antibiotic-resistant pathogens and diabetes for MRSA.

Despite the limitations of HCAP criteria, 2 findings are relatively consistent. The first is that prior detection of MRSA or PA predicts a much higher risk of these pathogens at any representation regardless of where the study was conducted.

Table 1
Individual risk factors for methicillin-resistant *Staphylococcus aureus* and multiresistant gram negatives like *Pseudomonas*

Risks for MRSA	Risks for *Pseudomonas* and Other Multiresistant Gram Negatives
Recent hospitalization[20,25,59,60]	Recent hospitalization[25,61]
Residence in aged-care facility[25,62,63]	Residence in aged-care facility[62,64]
Severe chronic obstructive pulmonary disease[25,59]	Severe chronic obstructive pulmonary disease[61,62,65–67]
Antibiotics in the prior 90 d[25]	Antibiotics in the prior 90 d[25,62,66,68]
Prior culture of MRSA[20,21,27,60,70]	Bronchiectasis[61,66,69]
Diabetes[25,60,62,63,71]	Prior culture of PA or multiresistant gram negative[27,64]
Tube feeding[60]	Tube feeding[46,66,72,73]
Cerebrovascular disease[60,63]	Cerebrovascular disease[25]
Chronic wound care[74]	

Physicians should cover empirically for these pathogens if they are known to have been identified in the past. The second consistent finding is that the implications for missing these pathogens empirically is mostly of concern in patients with significant sepsis and/or requiring intensive care. Acknowledgment that the risk is mostly in patients with severe disease, Brito and Niederman[47] suggested it is reasonable to overtreat for antibiotic-resistant pathogens in the critical care setting because of the very different risk versus benefit analysis in this small subgroup of patients.

CAN THE LABORATORY SOLVE THE HEALTH CARE–ASSOCIATED PNEUMONIA DILEMMA?

As outlined in the opening of this article, the primary issue in HCAP, as it is in CAP, is that microbiology has not delivered what we need. Several recent studies suggest that molecular microbiology can now close that gap.

Several studies have looked at nasal screening for MRSA by nucleic acid amplification. Parente and colleagues[50] performed a meta-analysis on 22 studies comprising 5163 patients from studies of CAP, HCAP, and ventilator-associated pneumonia. Overall the pooled sensitivity and specificity for MRSA in the setting of CAP and HCAP was 56.8% and 92.1%, respectively. As some of these studies used older assays and platforms, this is likely an underestimate. On an assumption of a 10% prevalence, the negative predictive value in the CAP and HCAP setting was 98.1%, suggesting that a negative test can be used to withhold anti-MRSA therapy. Incorporating molecular testing may be a very viable strategy clinically and from a health economic standpoint whereby clinicians are empirically covering for MRSA far in excess of what local data suggest is the true prevalence. One study of 100 respiratory tract samples from the United States suggested use of polymerase chain reaction (PCR) screening for MRSA could have safely decreased the use of vancomycin by 68.4% and linezolid by 83%.[51]

Of particular interest are point-of-care testing platforms with rapid turnaround times. To date the best validated is the Gene Xpert system, with apparent excellent performance in nasal swabs as well as respiratory samples for the detection of MRSA.[51–54] Other platforms are, however, in development.[55]

Molecular testing for other DRPs is not as advanced as for MRSA. To date there are no published studies of using PCR on sputum or nasal swabs to determine the clinical utility of this approach.

HOW DO WE MOVE FORWARD WITH HEALTH CARE–ASSOCIATED PNEUMONIA?

So what should physicians do about HCAP? An inescapable conclusion of the data is that physicians must know their local epidemiology of CAP. Reliance on published data from elsewhere may lead to either undertreatment, or more likely overtreatment, for antibiotic-resistant pathogens with potential adverse impacts either way. If molecular screening tests as outlined later are not available, then clinicians treating patients empirically for MRSA or PA need to obtain sputum cultures to allow de-escalation if these pathogens are not present and document the local prevalence of these pathogens. Only with local data can clinicians confidently decide on whether HCAP is a useful concept in their practice.

Fig. 1 outlines a practical approach to the issue of whether to consider treating empirically for DRPs in the setting of CAP, particularly if rapid

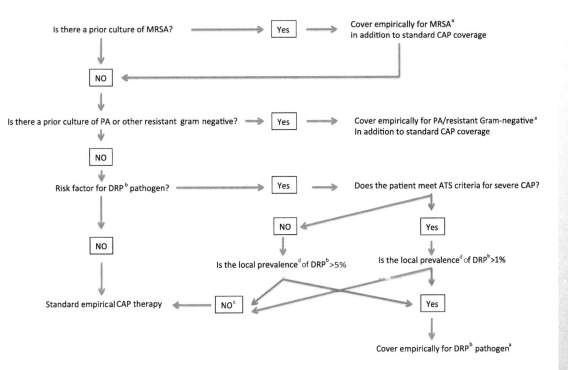

Fig. 1. Suggested management of CAP when rapid MRSA tests are not available. [a] When treating for DRPs, culture is mandatory to allow de-escalation. [b] That is, a pathogen resistant to standard empirical therapy for CAP, the risks for which should be modified by local data. [c] Culture for DRPs to enable coverage if they are detected. [d] Prevalence means the proportion of all cases of CAP caused by these organisms.

MRSA testing as described above is not available to adequately screen for these organisms when appropriate. Although there is legitimate concern about missing an antibiotic-resistant pathogen when choosing empirical antibiotic therapy, the reality is that outside of the setting of severe pneumonia (which the authors defines as pneumonia meeting the ATS's criteria for severe disease[56]), the impact of doing so is very small. Therefore, in the setting of severe pneumonia if there is evidence of DRPs being present locally in any significant amounts (arbitrarily the author defines as >1% of pathogens causing CAP), coverage of DRPs should be considered.

In the setting of less severe pneumonia unless the local prevalence of DRPs is high, empirical coverage should only be given if there is evidence of prior culture of these pathogens. What threshold should be set for high prevalence is very difficult to quantify in the absence of data addressing this issue. The author arbitrarily suggests that if DRPs account for more than 5% of CAP cases, that is sufficient to consider empirical therapy. If coverage for a DRP is selected empirically, then collection of respiratory samples for culture should be mandatory to enable de-escalation if they are not present and to document the local prevalence

of these organisms if they are as well as to identify any site-specific risk factors. Equally, if DRP coverage is not selected but risk factors are present, it is reasonable to obtain cultures in order to switch therapy if they are detected.

De-escalation is often a difficult concept for clinicians, a problem not limited to the pathogens relevant to HCAP or even to pneumonia, as, fundamentally, if patients are doing well why rock the boat? As some reassurance for the de-escalation approach, Boyce and colleagues[57] were able to show in a series of 91 patients with HCAP risk factors that stopping empirical vancomycin if nasal and throat cultures were negative did not alter patient outcomes. Equally, Schlueter and colleagues,[58] in a retrospective analysis of 102 patients with HCAP, found that de-escalation in culture-negative patients led to a shorter length of stay, lower costs, and a trend to improved mortality.

SUMMARY

Overall it is now apparent that HCAP risk factors only define a population who are at risk of PA and MRSA in highly specific locations. The predictive power of all of the putative risk factors is highly variable, with the notable exception of prior culture of one of these pathogens. Application of HCAP globally has not resulted in better outcomes and in most settings has led to harm through significant overuse of anti-MRSA and antipseudomonal antibiotics. A new approach is needed, and it needs to be nuanced by knowledge of local etiologic data and, it is hoped, enhanced by modern point-of-care microbiological identification platforms.

Clinicians cannot rely on published data from other sites but must have an understanding of what pathogens are causing pneumonia in their own hospitals and clinics. The data must also be contemporary, as the frequency of antibiotic-resistant pathogens is constantly changing in response to host, environmental, and pathogen factors. This point does not mean every hospital has to undertake rigorous etiologic studies of pneumonia; but if clinicians are electing to treat empirically with anti-MRSA or antipseudomonal therapy, then there must be culture data justifying these decisions. Clinicians should also de-escalate therapy by dropping anti-MRSA and/or antipseudomonal coverage if adequate cultures (or molecular testing) do not confirm these pathogens.

In summary, asking if HCAP is useful is like asking if wearing a thermal jacket is useful. Depending on your circumstance it may be critical, but for most people it is an unnecessary expense and may, in some circumstances, be harmful. Although it is appealing to have a simple rule that covers all situations, the reality is that pneumonia is complex and cannot be distilled into a one-size-fits-all approach. Although guidelines can help, thankfully for clinicians, clinical skill and knowledge is still required to get the best outcomes for all of our patients.

REFERENCES

1. Organisation WH. The top 10 causes of death. 2016. Available at: http://www.who.int/mediacentre/factsheets/fs310/en/. Accessed May 5, 2016.
2. Griffin MR, Zhu Y, Moore MR, et al. U.S. hospitalizations for pneumonia after a decade of pneumococcal vaccination. N Engl J Med 2013;369(2): 155–63.
3. McDade JE, Shepard CC, Fraser DW, et al. Legionnaires' disease: isolation of a bacterium and demonstration of its role in other respiratory disease. N Engl J Med 1977;297(22):1197–203.
4. van den Hoogen BG, de Jong JC, Groen J, et al. A newly discovered human pneumovirus isolated from young children with respiratory tract disease. Nat Med 2001;7(6):719–24.
5. Jain S, Self WH, Wunderink RG, et al. Community-acquired pneumonia requiring hospitalization among U.S. adults. N Engl J Med 2015;373(5): 415–27.
6. Holter JC, Muller F, Bjorang O, et al. Etiology of community-acquired pneumonia and diagnostic yields of microbiological methods: a 3-year prospective study in Norway. BMC Infect Dis 2015;15:64.
7. Niederman MS, Bass JB Jr, Campbell GD, et al. Guidelines for the initial management of adults with community-acquired pneumonia: diagnosis, assessment of severity, and initial antimicrobial therapy. American Thoracic Society. Medical Section of the American Lung Association. Am Rev Respir Dis 1993;148(5):1418–26.
8. American Thoracic Society, Infectious Diseases Society of America. Guidelines for the management of adults with hospital-acquired, ventilator-associated, and healthcare-associated pneumonia. Am J Respir Crit Care Med 2005;171(4):388–416.
9. Chalmers JD, Rother C, Salih W, et al. Healthcare-associated pneumonia does not accurately identify potentially resistant pathogens: a systematic review and meta-analysis. Clin Infect Dis 2014;58(3):330–9.
10. Dobler CC, Waterer G. Healthcare-associated pneumonia: a US disease or relevant to the Asia Pacific, too? Respirology 2013;18(6):923–32.
11. Shorr AF, Zilberberg MD, Micek ST, et al. Prediction of infection due to antibiotic-resistant bacteria by select risk factors for health care-associated pneumonia. Arch Intern Med 2008;168(20):2205–10.
12. Torres A, Serra-Batlles J, Ferrer A, et al. Severe community-acquired pneumonia. Epidemiology and prognostic factors. Am Rev Respir Dis 1991; 144(2):312–8.
13. Menendez R, Torres A, Zalacain R, et al. Risk factors of treatment failure in community acquired pneumonia: implications for disease outcome. Thorax 2004;59(11):960–5.
14. Bodi M, Rodriguez A, Sole-Violan J, et al. Antibiotic prescription for community-acquired pneumonia in the intensive care unit: impact of adherence to infectious diseases society of America Guidelines on survival. Clin Infect Dis 2005;41(12):1709–16.
15. Ewig S, Welte T, Torres A. Is healthcare-associated pneumonia a distinct entity needing specific therapy? Curr Opin Infect Dis 2012;25(2):166–75.
16. Dean NC, Webb BJ. Health care-associated pneumonia is mostly dead. Long live the acronym PES? Ann Am Thorac Soc 2015;12(2):239–40.
17. Horie H, Ito I, Konishi S, et al. Isolation of ESBL-producing bacteria from sputum in community-acquired pneumonia or healthcare-associated pneumonia does not indicate the need for antibiotics with activity against this class. Intern Med 2018; 57(4):487–95.
18. Enomoto Y, Yokomura K, Hasegawa H, et al. Health-care-associated pneumonia with positive respiratory methicillin-resistant Staphylococcus aureus culture:

predictors of the true pathogenicity. Geriatr Gerontol Int 2017;17(3):456–62.

19. Johanson WG, Pierce AK, Sanford JP. Changing pharyngeal bacterial flora of hospitalized patients. Emergence of gram-negative bacilli. N Engl J Med 1969;281(21):1137–40.

20. Torre-Cisneros J, Natera C, Mesa F, et al. Clinical predictors of methicillin-resistant Staphylococcus aureus in nosocomial and healthcare-associated pneumonia: a multicenter, matched case-control study. Eur J Clin Microbiol Infect Dis 2018;37(1):51–6.

21. Aliberti S, Reyes LF, Faverio P, et al. Global initiative for meticillin-resistant Staphylococcus aureus pneumonia (GLIMP): an international, observational cohort study. Lancet Infect Dis 2016;16(12):1364–76.

22. Sibila O, Laserna E, Maselli DJ, et al. Risk factors and antibiotic therapy in P. aeruginosa community-acquired pneumonia. Respirology 2015;20(4):660–6.

23. Kollef MH, Shorr A, Tabak YP, et al. Epidemiology and outcomes of health-care-associated pneumonia: results from a large US database of culture-positive pneumonia. Chest 2005;128(6):3854–62.

24. Webb BJ, Jones B, Dean NC. Empiric antibiotic selection and risk prediction of drug-resistant pathogens in community-onset pneumonia. Curr Opin Infect Dis 2016;29(2):167–77.

25. Metersky ML, Frei C, Mortensen EM. Predictors of Pseudomonas versus methicillin-resistant Staphylococcus aureus in hospitalized patients with healthcare-associated pneumonia. Respirology 2016;21(1):157–63.

26. Tomczyk S, Jain S, Bramley AM, et al. Antibiotic prescribing for adults hospitalized in the etiology of pneumonia in the community study. Open Forum Infect Dis 2017;4(2):ofx088.

27. Jones BE, Brown KA, Jones MM, et al. Variation in empiric coverage versus detection of methicillin-resistant staphylococcus aureus and pseudomonas aeruginosa in hospitalizations for community-onset pneumonia across 128 US veterans affairs medical centers. Infect Control Hosp Epidemiol 2017;38(8):937–44.

28. Costantini E, Allara E, Patrucco F, et al. Adherence to guidelines for hospitalized community-acquired pneumonia over time and its impact on health outcomes and mortality. Intern Emerg Med 2016;11(7):929–40.

29. McCabe C, Kirchner C, Zhang H, et al. Guideline-concordant therapy and reduced mortality and length of stay in adults with community-acquired pneumonia: playing by the rules. Arch Intern Med 2009;169(16):1525–31.

30. Asadi L, Eurich DT, Gamble JM, et al. Guideline adherence and macrolides reduced mortality in outpatients with pneumonia. Respir Med 2012;106(3):451–8.

31. Frei CR, Attridge RT, Mortensen EM, et al. Guideline-concordant antibiotic use and survival among patients with community-acquired pneumonia admitted to the intensive care unit. Clin Ther 2010;32(2):293–9.

32. Grenier C, Pepin J, Nault V, et al. Impact of guideline-consistent therapy on outcome of patients with healthcare-associated and community-acquired pneumonia. J Antimicrob Chemother 2011;66(7):1617–24.

33. Chen JI, Slater LN, Kurdgelashvili G, et al. Outcomes of health care-associated pneumonia empirically treated with guideline-concordant regimens versus community-acquired pneumonia guideline-concordant regimens for patients admitted to acute care wards from home. Ann Pharmacother 2013;47(1):9–19.

34. Taylor SP, Taylor BT. Health care-associated pneumonia in haemodialysis patients: clinical outcomes in patients treated with narrow versus broad spectrum antibiotic therapy. Respirology 2013;18(2):364–8.

35. Rothberg MB, Zilberberg MD, Pekow PS, et al. Association of guideline-based antimicrobial therapy and outcomes in healthcare-associated pneumonia. J Antimicrob Chemother 2015;70(5):1573–9.

36. Webb BJ, Dangerfield BS, Pasha JS, et al. Guideline-concordant antibiotic therapy and clinical outcomes in healthcare-associated pneumonia. Respir Med 2012;106(11):1606–12.

37. Haessler S, Lagu T, Lindenauer PK, et al. Treatment trends and outcomes in healthcare-associated pneumonia. J Hosp Med 2017;12(11):886–91.

38. Lee H, Park JY, Lee T, et al. Intermediate risk of multidrug-resistant organisms in patients who admitted intensive care unit with healthcare-associated pneumonia. Korean J Intern Med 2016;31(3):525–34.

39. Falcone M, Corrao S, Licata G, et al. Clinical impact of broad-spectrum empirical antibiotic therapy in patients with healthcare-associated pneumonia: a multicenter interventional study. Intern Emerg Med 2012;7(6):523–31.

40. Attridge RT, Frei CR, Restrepo MI, et al. Guideline-concordant therapy and outcomes in healthcare-associated pneumonia. Eur Respir J 2011;38(4):878–87.

41. Rello J, Lujan M, Gallego M, et al. Why mortality is increased in health-care-associated pneumonia: lessons from pneumococcal bacteremic pneumonia. Chest 2010;137(5):1138–44.

42. Polverino E, Torres A, Menendez R, et al. Microbial aetiology of healthcare associated pneumonia in Spain: a prospective, multicentre, case-control study. Thorax 2013;68(11):1007–14.

43. Bjarnason A, Asgeirsson H, Baldursson O, et al. Mortality in healthcare-associated pneumonia in a

low resistance setting: a prospective observational study. Infect Dis (Lond) 2015;47(3):130–6.

44. Chalmers JD, Taylor JK, Singanayagam A, et al. Epidemiology, antibiotic therapy, and clinical outcomes in health care-associated pneumonia: a UK cohort study. Clin Infect Dis 2011;53(2):107–13.

45. Jones BE, Jones MM, Huttner B, et al. Trends in antibiotic use and nosocomial pathogens in hospitalized veterans with pneumonia at 128 medical centers, 2006-2010. Clin Infect Dis 2015;61(9):1403–10.

46. Shindo Y, Ito R, Kobayashi D, et al. Risk factors for drug-resistant pathogens in community-acquired and healthcare-associated pneumonia. Am J Respir Crit Care Med 2013;188(8):985–95.

47. Brito V, Niederman MS. Healthcare-associated pneumonia is a heterogeneous disease, and all patients do not need the same broad-spectrum antibiotic therapy as complex nosocomial pneumonia. Curr Opin Infect Dis 2009;22(3):316–25.

48. Self WH, Wunderink RG, Williams DJ, et al. Comparison of clinical prediction models for resistant bacteria in community-onset pneumonia. Acad Emerg Med 2015;22(6):730–40.

49. Metersky ML, Aksamit TR, Barker A, et al. The prevalence and significance of staphylococcus aureus in patients with non-cystic fibrosis bronchiectasis. Ann Am Thorac Soc 2018;15(3):365–70.

50. Parente DM, Cunha CB, Mylonakis E, et al. The clinical utility of methicillin resistant Staphylococcus aureus (MRSA) nasal screening to rule out MRSA pneumonia: a diagnostic meta-analysis with antimicrobial stewardship implications. Clin Infect Dis 2018;67(1):1–7.

51. Trevino SE, Pence MA, Marschall J, et al. Rapid MRSA PCR on respiratory specimens from ventilated patients with suspected pneumonia: a tool to facilitate antimicrobial stewardship. Eur J Clin Microbiol Infect Dis 2017;36(5):879–85.

52. Yarbrough ML, Warren DK, Allen K, et al. Multicenter evaluation of the Xpert MRSA NxG assay for detection of methicillin-resistant Staphylococcus aureus in nasal swabs. J Clin Microbiol 2018;56(1) [pii: e01381-17].

53. Lepainteur M, Delattre S, Cozza S, et al. Comparative evaluation of two PCR-based methods for detection of methicillin-resistant Staphylococcus aureus (MRSA): Xpert MRSA Gen 3 and BD-Max MRSA XT. J Clin Microbiol 2015;53(6):1955–8.

54. Dangerfield B, Chung A, Webb B, et al. Predictive value of methicillin-resistant Staphylococcus aureus (MRSA) nasal swab PCR assay for MRSA pneumonia. Antimicrob Agents Chemother 2014;58(2):859–64.

55. Mehta SR, Estrada J, Ybarra J, et al. Comparison of the BD MAX MRSA XT to the Cepheid Xpert(R) MRSA assay for the molecular detection of methicillin-resistant Staphylococcus aureus from nasal swabs. Diagn Microbiol Infect Dis 2017;87(4):308–10.

56. Mandell LA, Wunderink RG, Anzueto A, et al. Infectious Diseases Society of America/American Thoracic Society consensus guidelines on the management of community-acquired pneumonia in adults. Clin Infect Dis 2007;44(Suppl 2):S27–72.

57. Boyce JM, Pop OF, Abreu-Lanfranco O, et al. A trial of discontinuation of empiric vancomycin therapy in patients with suspected methicillin-resistant Staphylococcus aureus health care-associated pneumonia. Antimicrob Agents Chemother 2013;57(3):1163–8.

58. Schlueter M, James C, Dominguez A, et al. Practice patterns for antibiotic de-escalation in culture-negative healthcare-associated pneumonia. Infection 2010;38(5):357–62.

59. Wooten DA, Winston LG. Risk factors for methicillin-resistant Staphylococcus aureus in patients with community-onset and hospital-onset pneumonia. Respir Med 2013;107(8):1266–70.

60. Minejima E, Lou M, Nieberg P, et al. Patients presenting to the hospital with MRSA pneumonia: differentiating characteristics and outcomes with empiric treatment. BMC Infect Dis 2014;14:252.

61. Arancibia F, Bauer TT, Ewig S, et al. Community-acquired pneumonia due to gram-negative bacteria and pseudomonas aeruginosa: incidence, risk, and prognosis. Arch Intern Med 2002;162(16):1849–58.

62. Prina E, Ranzani OT, Polverino E, et al. Risk factors associated with potentially antibiotic-resistant pathogens in community-acquired pneumonia. Ann Am Thorac Soc 2015;12(2):153–60.

63. Shorr AF, Myers DE, Huang DB, et al. A risk score for identifying methicillin-resistant Staphylococcus aureus in patients presenting to the hospital with pneumonia. BMC Infect Dis 2013;13:268.

64. Gross AE, Van Schooneveld TC, Olsen KM, et al. Epidemiology and predictors of multidrug-resistant community-acquired and health care-associated pneumonia. Antimicrob Agents Chemother 2014;58(9):5262–8.

65. Rodrigo-Troyano A, Sibila O. The respiratory threat posed by multidrug resistant Gram-negative bacteria. Respirology 2017;22(7):1288–99.

66. von Baum H, Welte T, Marre R, et al. Community-acquired pneumonia through Enterobacteriaceae and Pseudomonas aeruginosa: diagnosis, incidence and predictors. Eur Respir J 2010;35(3):598–605.

67. Pifarre R, Falguera M, Vicente-de-Vera C, et al. Characteristics of community-acquired pneumonia in patients with chronic obstructive pulmonary disease. Respir Med 2007;101(10):2139–44.

68. Cilloniz C, Gabarrus A, Ferrer M, et al. Community-acquired pneumonia due to multidrug- and non-multidrug-resistant Pseudomonas aeruginosa. Chest 2016;150(2):415–25.

69. Polverino E, Cilloniz C, Menendez R, et al. Microbiology and outcomes of community acquired pneumonia in non cystic-fibrosis bronchiectasis patients. J Infect 2015;71(1):28–36.

70. Jung WJ, Kang YA, Park MS, et al. Prediction of methicillin-resistant Staphylococcus aureus in patients with non-nosocomial pneumonia. BMC Infect Dis 2013;13:370.

71. Wu HP, Chu CM, Lin CY, et al. Liver cirrhosis and diabetes mellitus are risk factors for staphylococcus aureus infection in patients with healthcare-associated or hospital-acquired pneumonia. Pulm Med 2016;2016:4706150.

72. Jung JY, Park MS, Kim YS, et al. Healthcare-associated pneumonia among hospitalized patients in a Korean tertiary hospital. BMC Infect Dis 2011; 11:61.

73. Falcone M, Russo A, Giannella M, et al. Individualizing risk of multidrug-resistant pathogens in community-onset pneumonia. PLoS One 2015; 10(4):e0119528.

74. Wang PH, Wang HC, Cheng SL, et al. Selection of empirical antibiotics for health care-associated pneumonia via integration of pneumonia severity index and risk factors of drug-resistant pathogens. J Formos Med Assoc 2016;115(5):356–63.

Airway Devices in Ventilator-Associated Pneumonia Pathogenesis and Prevention

Anahita Rouzé, MD[a], Ignacio Martin-Loeches, MD, PhD[b], Saad Nseir, MD, PhD[a,c,*]

KEYWORDS

- Ventilator-associated pneumonia • Prevention • Device • Tracheal tube
- Subglottic secretion drainage

KEY POINTS

- Airway devices play a major role in the pathogenesis of microaspiration of contaminated secretions and VAP occurrence.
- Subglottic secretion drainage is an effective measure for VAP prevention, and no routine change of ventilator circuit.
- Continuous control of cuff pressure, silver-coated tracheal tubes, low-volume low-pressure tracheal tubes, and the mucus shaver are promising devices that should be further evaluated.
- Polyurethane-cuffed, conical-shaped cuff, and closed tracheal suctioning system are not effective and should not be used for VAP prevention.

INTRODUCTION

Ventilator-associated pneumonia (VAP) is the most common intensive care unit (ICU)-acquired infection. It is associated with increased mortality, duration of mechanical ventilation, and cost.[1,2] Prevention of VAP has become a major issue in the ICU. During the last two decades, several studies on VAP prevention allowed improvement of quality of care and reducing VAP incidence. Although a large percentage of VAP episodes could be prevented, zero VAP rate is probably not realistic. In fact, some episodes are related to comorbidities and prolonged invasive mechanical ventilation.[3]

Better understanding of the pathophysiology of VAP is a major issue to improve VAP prevention in critically ill patients. This article discusses recent clinical data on the relationship between airway devices and VAP.

PATHOGENESIS

In patients receiving invasive mechanical ventilation, colonization of the lower respiratory tract occurs rapidly after intubation. The pathogens colonizing the lower respiratory tract are mainly endogenous, coming from contaminated oropharyngeal secretions and gastric contents. However, the exogenous route has also been described, resulting from contamination during tracheal suctioning, fiberoptic bronchoscopy, or ventilator circuit disconnection for aerosols or patient

Conflicts of Interest: S. Nseir: MSD (lecture) and CielMedical (advisory board). I. Martin-Loeches and A. Rouzé: none.
Funding: None.
[a] CHU Lille, Critical Care Center, bd du Pr Leclercq, Lille F-59000, France; [b] Department of Clinical Medicine, Trinity College, Welcome Trust-HRB Clinical Research Facility, St James Hospital, Dublin 94568, Ireland; [c] Lille University, Medicine School, 1 Place de Verdun, Lille F-59000, France
* Corresponding author. Centre de Réanimation, Hôpital Salengro, CHRU Lille, Lille Cedex 59037, France.
E-mail address: s-nseir@chru-lille.fr

Clin Chest Med 39 (2018) 775–783
https://doi.org/10.1016/j.ccm.2018.08.001
0272-5231/18/© 2018 Elsevier Inc. All rights reserved.

transport.[4,5] Microaspiration of contaminated secretions from the subglottic area, above the tracheal cuff, to the lower respiratory tract is common. Several factors increase microaspiration in intubated critically ill patients, including the tracheal tube, ventilator settings, enteral nutrition, and other patient-related factors.[6,7]

A multicenter study was performed in 604 intubated patients to determine the best cuff material and shape in preventing tracheobronchial colonization.[8] The results of this study provide valuable information on the incidence of colonization of the lower respiratory tract, which was diagnosed ($>10^3$ CFU/mL[1]) at Day 2 after intubation, regardless of randomization group, in approximately two-thirds of study patients. However, only 14.4% of study patients developed subsequent VAP. Previous studies suggested a continuum between lower respiratory tract colonization and subsequent ventilator-associated lower respiratory tract infections.[9,10] Progression from colonization to ventilator-associated tracheobronchitis and VAP is related to quantity and virulence of bacteria. In addition, local and general host defense also play an important role in the development of ventilator-associated tracheobronchitis and VAP in colonized patients.

Biofilm formation around the tracheal tube is one mechanism for VAP occurrence, and recurrence. Clinical studies showed a close relationship between bacteria isolated in the biofilm and those responsible for VAP,[11] and suggested that biofilm stands as a pathogenic mechanism for microbial persistence, and impaired response to treatment in VAP.[12]

SUBGLOTTIC SECRETION DRAINAGE

Subglottic secretion drainage (SSD) is the most frequently studied measure for VAP prevention. More than 20 randomized controlled trials, and six meta-analyzes were conducted to determine the efficiency of this measure in reducing VAP rate. Caroff and colleagues[13] conducted a meta-analysis of 17 randomized controlled trials, including 3369 patients, and reported a significant reduction of VAP incidence in patients with SSD, compared with those with no SDD (risk ratio [RR], 0.58; 95% confidence interval [CI], 0.51–0.67; $I^2 = 0$%). No significant difference was found in duration of mechanical ventilation, ICU length of stay, or mortality between the two groups. Another recent meta-analysis,[14] including three additional randomized controlled trials, with a total of 3544 patients, reported similar results on efficacy. SSD was associated with reduction of VAP incidence in four high-quality trials (RR, 0.54; 95% CI, 0.40–0.74; $P<.00001$; $I^2 = 0$%), and in all trials

(RR, 0.55; 95% CI, 0.48–0.63; $P<.00001$; $I^2 = 0$%). SSD also significantly reduced the duration of mechanical ventilation (-1.17 d [-2.28 to -0.06]; $P = .006$). However, heterogeneity was apparent ($I^2 = 54$%) in SSD effect size across trials. Damas and colleagues[15] performed a randomized controlled trial to determine the impact of SSD on VAP incidence. A total of 352 adult patients intubated with a tracheal tube allowing subglottic secretion suctioning were randomly assigned to undergo suctioning (n = 170) or not (n = 182). The incidence rate of VAP was substantially reduced (9.6 of 1000 ventilator days vs 19.8 of 1000 ventilator days, in SSD vs control groups, respectively; $P = .0076$). In addition, the total number of antibiotic days was also significantly reduced (1696, representing 61.6% of the 2754 ICU days; and 1965, representing 68.5% of the 2868 ICU days; $P<.0001$).

To evaluate cost-effectiveness of SSD, Shorr and O'Malley[16] used a decision model with reduction of VAP prevalence, among patients requiring more than 72 hours of mechanical ventilation, as the primary outcome. Assuming a baseline 25% prevalence of VAP along with a 30% relative reduction in the SSD group, a nearly US$5000 savings per one case of prevented VAP was reported, despite a substantially higher acquisition cost for the SSD tracheal tube. Hallais and colleagues[17] performed a cost-benefit analysis, based on hypothetical replacement of conventional endotracheal tubes by continuous SSD. They reported that assuming a VAP cost of €4,387, a total of three averted VAP episodes would neutralize the additional cost, and that continuous SSD was cost-effective even when assuming the most pessimistic scenario of VAP incidence and cost. More recently, Branch-Elliman and colleagues[2] performed a cost-benefit decision model, and constructed a Markov model to determine the preferred VAP prevention strategy. They suggested that the use of SSD and probiotics were cost-effective for VAP prevention.

An animal study raised concern on the possible tracheal ischemic lesions related to SSD.[18] In addition, a recent case series of six patients reported that automated intermittent subglottic aspiration may result in significant and potential harmful invagination of tracheal mucosa into the suction lumen.[19] However, SSD is widely used in Europe and no significant concern on side effects was reported. A large randomized controlled multicenter trial reported similar rates of postextubation laryngeal dyspnea in patients with SSD, as compared with control subjects.[20] Vallés and colleagues[21] recently studied 86 consecutive adult patients with continuous SSD, and prospectively recorded clinical airway complications during the period after extubation. Six (6.9%) patients had transient dyspnea, seven (8.1%) had upper airway obstruction, and 18 (20.9%) had dysphonia at extubation. Multidetector computed tomography was performed in 37 patients following extubation, and injuries were observed in nine patients (24.3%) and classified as tracheal injuries in two patients (one cartilage thickening and one mild stenosis with cartilage thickening) and as subglottic mucosal thickenings in seven patients. These data suggest that SSD could be safely used in critically ill patients.

Although SSD is recommended (moderate level of evidence) by the recent Infectious Diseases Society of America/Society for healthcare epidemiology of America guidelines on VAP prevention[22] and other national guidelines,[23] further studies are required to better evaluate the cost-effectiveness of this preventive measure. In routine practice, the major limitation for its use is that many patients are intubated before ICU admission with tracheal tubes with no additional channel for SSD. A new device allowing performance of SSD in patients intubated with standard tracheal tubes has been developed and commercialized in the United States and recently in Europe.[24] However, further clinical evaluation is required to determine its efficiency in drainage of subglottic secretions, and VAP prevention. SSD is an interesting preventive measure in patients requiring invasive mechanical ventilation greater than 48 hours. However, identifying these patients before intubation could be a difficult task. To overcome this difficulty, some authors evaluated the efficiency of SSD in all patients requiring intubation.[25] However, the cost-effectiveness would probably be better in targeted patients with expected duration of mechanical ventilation greater than 48 hours. Although physicians could sometimes easily identify these patients, better predictive scores should be developed to accurately select this population.

CONTINUOUS CONTROL OF CUFF PRESSURE

Underinflation of the tracheal cuff was identified as a risk factor for VAP by an observational study.[26] Despite intermittent control of cuff pressure (P_{cuff}), using a manometer, intubated critically ill patients spend a large amount of time with underinflation (<20 cm H_2O) or overinflation (>30 cm H_2O) of P_{cuff}.[27] Underinflation and overinflation of P_{cuff} were identified as risk factors for short-term complications, such as microaspiration of contaminated secretions, VAP, and tracheal ischemic lesions.[28] Several devices aiming at continuously controlling P_{cuff} are available,[29–32] but only a few of them were validated by clinical studies.[7,29,33] In fact, only two available devices, one pneumatic and one electronic, were validated by clinical studies. A third available device was studied recently in 18 critically ill patients, and performed worse than manometer. This raises the important question of why medical devices, such as tracheal tubes or P_{cuff} controllers, can obtain the Food and Drug Administration or CE mark and be used in critically ill patients without any published clinical data proving their efficacy.

Two randomized controlled trials were conducted to determine the impact of continuous control of P_{cuff} on intubation-related complications.[33,34] The study conducted by Valencia and colleagues[34] did not show any significant impact of continuous control of P_{cuff} on VAP incidence. The subsequent study, conducted by our group,[33] found a significant reduction in abundant microaspiration of gastric contents, and a substantial decrease in VAP rate (62%) in patients who received continuous control of P_{cuff}, compared with control group. However, no significant impact was found on tracheal ischemic lesions. Several factors might explain the different results of these trials, including the difference in devices used for P_{cuff} control, study population, and VAP rate in the control group.

Recently, a quasi-randomized controlled study was conducted to determine the impact of continuous control of P_{cuff}, using an electronic device, on VAP incidence in critically ill patients.[35] The authors reported a significant reduction (51%) in VAP rate in patients who received continuous control of P_{cuff}, compared with those who received routine care with a manometer.

A meta-analysis of the individual data of patients (n = 543) included in the three previously discussed single-center trials was performed.[36] Thirty-six (13.6%) VAPs were diagnosed in the continuous control group, and 72 (25.7%) in the routine care group (hazard ratio, 0.47; 95% CI, 0.31–0.71; $P<.001$). However, heterogeneity was apparent in continuous control effect size across trials ($I^2 = 58\%$; $P = .085$). The number of patients needed to treat to prevent one VAP episode was eight. No significant impact of continuous control of P_{cuff} was found on duration of mechanical ventilation, ICU length of stay, or mortality.

Further large multicenter studies are required to confirm the impact of continuous control of P_{cuff} on VAP rate, and to evaluate its cost-effectiveness. The results of the currently conducted French multicenter PAV-PROTECT and AGATE studies[37,38] will give further insights on this issue.

CUFF SHAPE AND MATERIAL
Polyurethane-Cuffed Tracheal Tubes

Polyurethane is 40-fold thinner than polyvinyl chloride (PVC), resulting in reduced channel formation between the tracheal cuff and the tracheal wall.[39] Several in vitro and preliminary clinical reports suggested that polyurethane-cuffed tracheal tube might reduce microaspiration of contaminated secretions, and VAP incidence.[40–42] In addition, two before-after studies suggested beneficial effects of these tubes on microaspiration and VAP incidence.[43,44]

Lucangelo and colleagues[45] randomized 40 critically ill patients to be intubated with polyurethane or PVC cuffed tracheal tubes. The effect of a 5 cm H_2O positive end-expiratory pressure aspiration of blue dye was also evaluated. Polyurethane and positive end-expiratory pressure significantly protected patients from aspiration of blue dye.

Poelaert and colleagues[46] performed a randomized controlled open-label study to determine the impact of polyurethane-cuffed tracheal tube on postoperative pneumonia rate. A total of 134 patients scheduled for cardiac surgery were included, and the rate of early postoperative pneumonia was significantly lower in the polyurethane group than the PVC group (23% vs 42%; $P = .026$). Two other randomized controlled trials reported reduced incidence of VAP in patients intubated with polyurethane-cuffed tracheal tubes compared with PVC-cuffed tracheal tubes.[47,48] However, in these studies SSD was only used in the intervention group, resulting in difficult interpretation of the results. In fact, whether the reduced rate of VAP in the intervention group is related to the polyurethane cuff or to SSD is unknown.

The TOP-CUFF study[8] carefully evaluated the impact of polyurethane/tapered shape cuffed tracheal tubes versus PVC/conical shape tubes. A total of 621 patients were randomized to receive cylindrical-PVC, cylindrical-polyurethane, tapered-PVC, or tapered-polyurethane tracheal tubes. The percentage of patients with tracheobronchial colonization at Day 3, which was the primary objective of the study, was similar ($P = .55$) in the four study groups (66%, 61%, 67%, and 62%, respectively). Similarly, no significant difference was found in time to VAP occurrence in different study groups (log rank, $P = .28$). Some study limitations should be outlined. First, a large proportion of study patients received antibiotic treatment during their ICU stay, which might have been a confounder regarding the results on colonization rate. Second, tracheobronchial colonization is probably not an excellent marker for microaspiration because it could also result from exogenous contamination.

One drawback of the use of polyurethane-cuffed tracheal tubes is the difficult measurement of P_{cuff} in patients intubated with these tubes. Because of physical and chemical features of polyurethane, condensation is generated by this material resulting in water presence in the pilot balloon, precluding any accurate P_{cuff} measurement. This phenomenon was described by in vitro and clinical studies.[49,50]

Tapered-Cuff Tracheal Tubes

Tracheal cuff shape might play an important role in the occurrence of microaspiration in intubated patients.[51,52] Previous bench studies suggested a beneficial effect of tapered-cuff tracheal tubes in reducing leakage around the cuff, by providing a permanent sealing zone between the cuff and the tracheal wall.[41,53] An animal study also reported significant reduction of leakage using PVC tapered cuffs versus cylindrical cuffs.[54] However, other in vitro and animal studies did not confirm these findings.[24,55] Recent clinical studies reported conflicting results on the impact of tapered-cuff tracheal tube on microaspiration, tracheobronchial colonization, early onset postoperative pneumonia, and VAP.[8,43,50,56–58]

Three randomized controlled trials[6,8,57] evaluated the impact of tapered-shaped tracheal cuff on microaspiration, tracheobronchial colonization, early postoperative pneumonia, and VAP in critically ill patients. In the previously discussed TOP-CUFF trial,[8] no significant impact was found of tapered-cuff shape on tracheobronchial colonization, or VAP incidence. In the single-center randomized controlled TETRIS study, Monsel and colleagues[57] aimed at evaluating the impact of tapered-cuff, compared with standard-cuff tracheal tube, on postoperative pneumonia, and microaspiration. No significant impact of this intervention was found on primary or secondary outcomes. As acknowledged by the authors, the single-center design, and inclusion of only patients after major vascular surgery, preclude definite conclusions. In addition, pepsin and alpha amylase were only measured at two time-points. Our group performed a multicenter cluster crossover randomized controlled study to determine the impact of tapered-cuff tracheal tube, compared with standard (barrel)-cuff tracheal tube on abundant microaspiration of gastric contents.[59] A total of 326 patients were included (162 and 164 in tapered- and standard-cuff groups, respectively). The percentage of patients with abundant microaspiration of gastric contents was 53.5% in tapered-cuff and 51.0% in standard-cuff groups (odds ratio, 1.14; 95% CI, 0.72–1.82). Percentage of patients with tracheobronchial colonization was significantly lower in tapered-cuff compared with standard-cuff group. However, no significant difference was found in other secondary outcomes, including abundant microaspiration of oropharyngeal secretions, ventilator-associated events, and VAP, between the two groups. The results of these studies suggest that tapered-cuff should not be used to prevent VAP in critically ill patients.

A recent meta-analysis[60] analyzed six randomized controlled clinical trials with 1324 patients from ICU and postoperative wards. No significant difference in hospital-acquired pneumonia incidence per patient was found when tapered cuffs were compared with standard cuffs (odds ratio, 0.97; 95% CI, 0.73–1.28; $P = .81$). There were likewise no differences in secondary outcomes.

OTHER DEVICES
Silver-Coated Tracheal Tubes

In vitro, animal, and preliminary clinical studies suggested a beneficial effect of silver-coated tracheal tubes in reducing biofilm formation and lower respiratory tract colonization.[61–63] A large multicenter randomized controlled study was performed to determine the impact of silver-coated tracheal tubes on VAP incidence.[64] Among patients intubated for 24 hours or longer, rates of microbiologically confirmed VAP were significantly lower in the group receiving the silver-coated tube than the group receiving the uncoated tube (4.8% vs 7.5; $P = .03$). The silver-coated tracheal tube was associated with delayed occurrence of VAP ($P = .005$). However, the beneficial effect of this measure was only obvious during the first 10 days of mechanical ventilation. Furthermore, a significantly higher rate of chronic obstructive pulmonary disease was reported in the control group, resulting in difficult interpretation of the results. Chronic obstructive pulmonary disease was repeatedly identified as risk factor for VAP.[65] Further large randomized controlled trials are needed to determine the impact of silver-coated tracheal tubes on VAP incidence.

Circuit Change

A meta-analysis of 10 studies[66] including 19,169 patients reported that compared with patients exposed to circuit changes every 7 days, patients who received circuit changes every 2 days had a higher risk of VAP (odds ratio, 1.9; 95% CI, 1.08–3.4). In addition, compared with no routine circuit change, changing the ventilator circuit at a 2-day

or 7-day interval was associated with an odds ratio of 1.13 (95% CI, 0.79–1.6). Therefore, no routine circuit change is safe and justified.

Closed Tracheal Suctioning System

Kuriyama and colleagues[67] conducted a meta-analysis of 16 trials including 1929 patients to determine the effect of closed tracheal suctioning system on VAP incidence. This intervention was associated with significantly reduced VAP rates (odds ratio, 0.69; 95% CI, 0.54–0.88). However, no significant impact was found on other outcomes, such as duration of mechanical ventilation, or mortality. Furthermore, trial sequential analysis suggested a lack of firm evidence for 20% relative risk reduction in the incidence of VAP, and most included trials were of low quality with variations in procedures and characteristics.

Low-Volume Low-Pressure Cuff

The use of tracheal tubes with low-volume low-pressure cuff was suggested to reduce microaspiration and VAP. Several small clinical trials reported improved sealing, and lower VAP rates in patients intubated with these tubes.[68,69] The PneuX System incorporates several strategies to minimize the aspiration of oropharyngeal secretions. These include a securing flange, a low-volume low-pressure cuff, multiple SSD ports, a tracheal seal monitor, and a coated tube lumen. Recently, a randomized controlled single-center open label study was performed to determine the impact of the PneuX system on postoperative pneumonia rate in high-risk patients undergoing cardiac surgery.[70] A total of 240 patients were included, and the rate of pneumonia was significantly lower in the PneuX group compared with control group (10.8% vs 21%; $P = .03$). However, the single-center design, and the short duration of mechanical ventilation in study patients (15 vs 13 hours in PneuX and standard tube groups, respectively) preclude any definite conclusions regarding the interest of using the PneuX tube for VAP prevention. In addition, it is difficult, if not impossible, to determine which of the tested measures, that is, low-volume low-pressure, continuous control of P_{cuff}, or SSD, was responsible for the positive results obtained on postoperative pneumonia rate.

Mucus Shaver

A novel device for tracheal tube cleaning was recently evaluated in a small randomized controlled trial.[71] Treated tubes showed reduced mucus accumulation (0.56 ± 0.12 mL vs 0.71 ± 0.28 mL; $P = .004$) and reduced occlusion

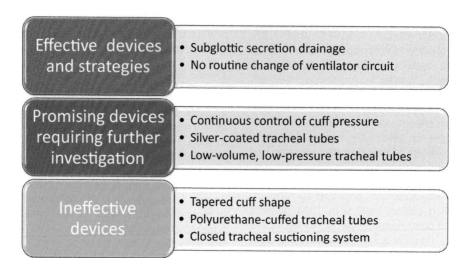

Fig. 1. Effectiveness of airway devices for prevention of ventilator-associated pneumonia.

(6.3 ± 1.7% vs 8.9 ± 7.6%; *P* = .039). The high-resolution computed tomography slice showing the narrowest lumen within each tracheal tube exhibited less occlusion in cleaned tubes (10.6 ± 8.0% vs 17.7 ± 13.4%; 95% CI, 2–12.1; *P* = .007). However, the device had no significant impact on tracheal colonization or VAP rates. Further studies are required to determine the impact of this device on VAP incidence.

The different devices and strategies discussed in this review are summarized in **Fig. 1** and **Table 1**.

Table 1
Devices and strategies for VAP prevention

Device	Efficacy	Level of Evidence	Studies	Ref #
Subglottic secretion drainage	Yes	High	23 RCT, and 2 meta-analyses	Caroff et al,[13] 2016; Mao et al, 2016[14]
No routine change of ventilator circuit	Yes	High	RCT, and 1 meta-analysis	Han & Liu,[66] 2010
Continuous control of cuff pressure	Yes	Moderate/low	3 small single-center RCT, and 1 patient-based meta-analysis	[33–36]
Silver-coated tracheal tubes	Yes	Moderate/low	One large RCT	Kollef et al,[64] 2008
Low-volume low-pressure	Yes	Low	2 single-center RCT	Young et al,[69] 2006; Gopal et al,[70] 2015
Tapered cuff shape	No	High	3 RCT, and one meta-analysis	Jaillette et al,[6] 2017; Philippart et al,[8] 2015; Monsel et al,[57] 2016
Polyurethane-cuffed tracheal tubes	No	Moderate/low	One negative large multicenter RCT	Philippart et al,[8] 2015
Closed tracheal suctioning system	Indeterminate	Low	One meta-analysis	Kuriyama et al,[67] 2014

Abbreviation: RCT, randomized controlled trial.

SUMMARY

Airway devices play a major role in the pathogenesis of microaspiration of contaminated secretions and VAP occurrence. SSD is an efficient measure for VAP prevention, and no routine change of ventilator circuit. Continuous control of cuff pressure, silver-coated tracheal tubes, low-volume low-pressure tracheal tubes, and the mucus shaver are promising devices that should be further evaluated. Polyurethane-cuffed, conical-shape cuff, and closed tracheal suctioning system are not efficient and should not be used for VAP prevention.

REFERENCES

1. Moreau A-S, Martin-Loeches I, Povoa P, et al. Impact of immunosuppression on incidence, aetiology and outcome of ventilator-associated lower respiratory tract infections. Eur Respir J 2018;51:1701656.

2. Branch-Elliman W, Wright SB, Howell MD. Determining the ideal strategy for ventilator-associated pneumonia prevention. Cost–benefit analysis. Am J Respir Crit Care Med 2015;192:57–63.

3. Torres A, Niederman MS, Chastre J, et al. International ERS/ESICM/ESCMID/ALAT guidelines for the management of hospital-acquired pneumonia and ventilator-associated pneumonia. Eur Respir J 2017;50:1700582.

4. Nseir S, Ader F, Lubret R, et al. Pathophysiology of airway colonization in critically ill COPD patient. Curr Drug Targets 2011;12:514 20.

5. Nseir S, Zerimech F, Jaillette E, et al. Microaspiration in intubated critically ill patients: diagnosis and prevention. Infect Disord Drug Targets 2011;11: 413–23. Available at: http://eutils.ncbi.nlm.nih.gov/entrez/eutils/elink.fcgi?dbfrom=pubmed&id=21679139&retmode=ref&cmd=prlinks. Accessed January 26, 2013.

6. Jaillette E, Girault C, Brunin G, et al. Impact of tapered-cuff tracheal tube on microaspiration of gastric contents in intubated critically ill patients: a multicenter cluster-randomized cross-over controlled trial. Intensive Care Med 2017;43: 1562–71.

7. Rouzé A, De Jonckheere J, Zerimech F, et al. Efficiency of an electronic device in controlling tracheal cuff pressure in critically ill patients: a randomized controlled crossover study. Ann Intensive Care 2016;6:93.

8. Philippart F, Gaudry S, Quinquis L, et al. Randomized intubation with polyurethane or conical cuffs to prevent pneumonia in ventilated patients. Am J Respir Crit Care Med 2015;191:637–45.

9. Riera J, Caralt B, López I, et al. Ventilator-associated respiratory infection following lung transplantation. Eur Respir J 2015;45:726–37.

10. Nseir S, Povoa P, Salluh J, et al. Is there a continuum between ventilator-associated tracheobronchitis and ventilator-associated pneumonia? Intensive Care Med 2016;42:1190–2.

11. Adair CG, Gorman SP, Feron BM, et al. Implications of endotracheal tube biofilm for ventilator-associated pneumonia. Intensive Care Med 1999;25:1072–6. Available at: http://www.ncbi.nlm.nih.gov/pubmed/10551961. Accessed January 2, 2017.

12. Gil-Perotin S, Ramirez P, Marti V, et al. Implications of endotracheal tube biofilm in ventilator-associated pneumonia response: a state of concept. Crit Care 2012;16:R93.

13. Caroff DA, Li L, Muscedere J, et al. Subglottic secretion drainage and objective outcomes: a systematic review and meta-analysis. Crit Care Med 2016;44: 830–40.

14. Mao Z, Gao L, Wang G, et al. Subglottic secretion suction for preventing ventilator-associated pneumonia: an updated meta-analysis and trial sequential analysis. Crit Care 2016;20:353.

15. Damas P, Frippiat F, Ancion A, et al. Prevention of ventilator-associated pneumonia and ventilator-associated conditions. Crit Care Med 2015;43: 22–30.

16. Shorr AF, O'Malley PG. Continuous subglottic suctioning for the prevention of ventilator-associated pneumonia: potential economic implications. Chest 2001;119:228–35. Available at: http://www.ncbi.nlm.nih.gov/pubmed/11157609. Accessed April 5, 2017.

17. Hallais C, Merle V, Guitard P-G, et al. Is continuous subglottic suctioning cost-effective for the prevention of ventilator-associated pneumonia? Infect Control Hosp Epidemiol 2011;32:131–5.

18. Berra L, De Marchi L, Panigada M, et al. Evaluation of continuous aspiration of subglottic secretion in an in vivo study. Crit Care Med 2004;32:2071–8.

19. Suys E, Nieboer K, Stiers W, et al. Intermittent subglottic secretion drainage may cause tracheal damage in patients with few oropharyngeal secretions. Intensive Crit Care Nurs 2013;29:317–20.

20. Lacherade J-C, De Jonghe B, Guezennec P, et al. Intermittent subglottic secretion drainage and ventilator-associated pneumonia: a multicenter trial. Am J Respir Crit Care Med 2010;182:910–7.

21. Vallés J, Millán S, Díaz E, et al. Incidence of airway complications in patients using endotracheal tubes with continuous aspiration of subglottic secretions. Ann Intensive Care 2017;7:109.

22. Klompas M, Branson R, Eichenwald EC, et al. Strategies to prevent ventilator-associated pneumonia in acute care hospitals: 2014 update. Infect Control Hosp Epidemiol 2014;35:915–36.

23. Leone M, Bouadma L, Bouhemad B, et al. Hospital-acquired pneumonia in ICU. Anaesth Crit Care Pain Med 2018;37(1):83–98.

24. Li Bassi G, Ranzani OT, Marti JD, et al. An in vitro study to assess determinant features associated with fluid sealing in the design of endotracheal tube cuffs and exerted tracheal pressures. Crit Care Med 2013;41:518–26.

25. Deem S, Yanez D, Sissons-Ross L, et al. Randomized pilot trial of two modified endotracheal tubes to prevent ventilator-associated pneumonia. Ann Am Thorac Soc 2016;13:72–80.

26. Vallés J, Artigas A, Rello J, et al. Continuous aspiration of subglottic secretions in preventing ventilator-associated pneumonia. Ann Intern Med 1995;122: 179–86. Available at: http://www.ncbi.nlm.nih.gov/pubmed/7810935. Accessed December 8, 2015.

27. Nseir S, Brisson H, Marquette C-H, et al. Variations in endotracheal cuff pressure in intubated critically ill patients: prevalence and risk factors. Eur J Anaesthesiol 2009;26:229–34.

28. Rouzé A, Nseir S. Continuous control of tracheal cuff pressure for the prevention of ventilator-associated pneumonia in critically ill patients: where is the evidence? Curr Opin Crit Care 2013;19:440–7.

29. Duguet A, D'Amico L, Biondi G, et al. Control of tracheal cuff pressure: a pilot study using a pneumatic device. Intensive Care Med 2007;33:128–32.

30. Weiss M, Doell C, Koepfer N, et al. Rapid pressure compensation by automated cuff pressure controllers worsens sealing in tracheal tubes. Br J Anaesth 2009;102:273–8.

31. Chenelle CT, Oto J, Sulemanji D, et al. Evaluation of an automated endotracheal tube cuff controller during simulated mechanical ventilation. Respir Care 2015;60:183–90.

32. Nseir S, Rodriguez A, Saludes P, et al. Efficiency of a mechanical device in controlling tracheal cuff pressure in intubated critically ill patients: a randomized controlled study. Ann Intensive Care 2015;5:54.

33. Nseir S, Zerimech F, Fournier C, et al. Continuous control of tracheal cuff pressure and microaspiration of gastric contents in critically ill patients. Am J Respir Crit Care Med 2011;184:1041–7.

34. Valencia M, Ferrer M, Farre R, et al. Automatic control of tracheal tube cuff pressure in ventilated patients in semirecumbent position: a randomized trial. Crit Care Med 2007;35:1543–9.

35. Lorente L, Lecuona M, Jiménez A, et al. Continuous endotracheal tube cuff pressure control system protects against ventilator-associated pneumonia. Crit Care 2014;18:R77.

36. Nseir S, Lorente L, Ferrer M, et al. Continuous control of tracheal cuff pressure for VAP prevention: a collaborative meta-analysis of individual participant data. Ann Intensive Care 2015;5:43.

37. Mégarbane B. Simple mechanical device to control pressure in the balloon of the endotracheal tube to prevent ventilator-acquired pneumonia - full text view - ClinicalTrials.gov. ClinicalTrials.gov

Identifier: NCT02514655. :ClinicalTrials.gov Identifier: NCT02514655. Available at: https://clinical trials.gov/ct2/show/NCT02514655. Accessed January 2, 2017.

38. Marjanovic N, Frasca D, Asehnoune K, et al. Multicentre randomised controlled trial to investigate the usefulness of continuous pneumatic regulation of tracheal cuff pressure for reducing ventilator-associated pneumonia in mechanically ventilated severe trauma patients: the AGATE study protocol. BMJ Open 2017;7:e017003.

39. Blot SI, Rello J, Koulenti D. The value of polyurethane-cuffed endotracheal tubes to reduce microaspiration and intubation-related pneumonia: a systematic review of laboratory and clinical studies. Crit Care 2016;20:203.

40. Dullenkopf A, Gerber A, Weiss M. Fluid leakage past tracheal tube cuffs: evaluation of the new Microcuff endotracheal tube. Intensive Care Med 2003;29: 1849–53.

41. Dave MH, Frotzler , Spielmann N, et al. Effect of tracheal tube cuff shape on fluid leakage across the cuff: an in vitro study. Br J Anaesth 2010;105: 538–43.

42. Ouanes I, Lyazidi A, Danin PE, et al. Mechanical influences on fluid leakage past the tracheal tube cuff in a benchtop model. Intensive Care Med 2011;37: 695–700.

43. Nseir S, Zerimech F, De Jonckheere J, et al. Impact of polyurethane on variations in tracheal cuff pressure in critically ill patients: a prospective observational study. Intensive Care Med 2010;36:1156–63.

44. Miller MA, Arndt JL, Konkle MA, et al. A polyurethane cuffed endotracheal tube is associated with decreased rates of ventilator-associated pneumonia. J Crit Care 2011;26:280–6.

45. Lucangelo U, Zin WA, Antonaglia V, et al. Effect of positive expiratory pressure and type of tracheal cuff on the incidence of aspiration in mechanically ventilated patients in an intensive care unit. Crit Care Med 2008;36:409–13.

46. Poelaert J, Depuydt P, De Wolf A, et al. Polyurethane cuffed endotracheal tubes to prevent early postoperative pneumonia after cardiac surgery: a pilot study. J Thorac Cardiovasc Surg 2008;135:771–6.

47. Lorente L, Lecuona M, Jiménez A, et al. Influence of an endotracheal tube with polyurethane cuff and subglottic secretion drainage on pneumonia. Am J Respir Crit Care Med 2007;176:1079–83.

48. Mahmoodpoor A, Hamishehkar H, Hamidi M, et al. A prospective randomized trial of tapered-cuff endotracheal tubes with intermittent subglottic suctioning in preventing ventilator-associated pneumonia in critically ill patients. J Crit Care 2017;38:152–6.

49. Spapen H, Moeyersons W, Stiers W, et al. Condensation of humidified air in the inflation line of a polyurethane cuff precludes correct continuous pressure

monitoring during mechanical ventilation. J Anesth 2014;28:949–51.

50. Jaillette E, Zerimech F, De Jonckheere J, et al. Efficiency of a pneumatic device in controlling cuff pressure of polyurethane-cuffed tracheal tubes: a randomized controlled study. BMC Anesthesiol 2013;13:50.

51. Branson RD, Hess DR. Lost in translation: failure of tracheal tube modifications to impact ventilator-associated pneumonia. Am J Respir Crit Care Med 2015;191:606–8.

52. Haas CF, Eakin RM, Konkle MA, et al. Endotracheal tubes: old and new. Respir Care 2014;59:933–52 [discussion: 952–5].

53. Madjdpour C, Mauch J, Dave MH, et al. Comparison of air-sealing characteristics of tapered- vs. cylindrical-shaped high-volume, low-pressure tube cuffs. Acta Anaesthesiol Scand 2012;66:230–5

54. Lichtenthal P, Borg U, Maul D. Do endotracheal tubes prevent microaspiration? Crit Care 2010; 14(Suppl 1):P229.

55. Li Bassi G, Luque N, Martí JD, et al. Endotracheal tubes for critically ill patients. Chest 2015;147: 1327–35.

56. D'Haese J, De Keukeleire T, Remory I, et al. Assessment of intraoperative microaspiration: does a modified cuff shape improve sealing? Acta Anaesthesiol Scand 2013;57:873–80.

57. Monsel A, Lu Q, Le Corre M, et al. Tapered-cuff endotracheal tube does not prevent early postoperative pneumonia compared with spherical-cuff endotracheal tube after major vascular surgery: a randomized controlled trial. Anesthesiology 2016; 124:1041–52.

58. Bowton DL, Hite RD, Martin RS, et al. The impact of hospital-wide use of a tapered-cuff endotracheal tube on the incidence of ventilator-associated pneumonia. Respir Care 2013;58:1582–7.

59. Jaillette E, Brunin G, Girault C, et al. Impact of tracheal cuff shape on microaspiration of gastric contents in intubated critically ill patients: study protocol for a randomized controlled trial. Trials 2015; 16:429.

60. Maertens B, Blot K, Blot S. Prevention of ventilator-associated and early postoperative pneumonia through tapered endotracheal tube cuffs. Crit Care Med 2018;46:316–23.

61. Olson ME, Harmon BG, Kollef MH. Silver-coated endotracheal tubes associated with reduced bacterial burden in the lungs of mechanically ventilated dogs. Chest 2002;121:863–70. Available at: http://www.ncbi.nlm.nih.gov/pubmed/11888974. Accessed January 2, 2017.

62. Rello J, Kollef M, Diaz E, et al. Reduced burden of bacterial airway colonization with a novel silver-coated endotracheal tube in a randomized multiple-center feasibility study. Crit Care Med 2006;34:2766–72.

63. Rello J, Afessa B, Anzueto A, et al. Activity of a silver-coated endotracheal tube in preclinical models of ventilator-associated pneumonia and a study after extubation. Crit Care Med 2010;38: 1135–40.

64. Kollef MH, Afessa B, Anzueto A, et al. Silver-coated endotracheal tubes and incidence of ventilator associated pneumonia: the NASCENT randomized trial. JAMA 2008;300:805–13.

65. Rouzé A, Cottereau A, Nseir S. Chronic obstructive pulmonary disease and the risk for ventilator-associated pneumonia. Curr Opin Crit Care 2014; 20:525–31.

66. Han J, Liu Y. Effect of ventilator circuit changes on ventilator-associated pneumonia: a systematic review and meta-analysis. Respir Care 2010;55: 467–74. Available at: http://www.ncbi.nlm.nih.gov/pubmed/20406515. Accessed April 11, 2017.

67. Kuriyama A, Umakoshi N, Fujinaga J, et al. Impact of closed versus open tracheal suctioning systems for mechanically ventilated adults: a systematic review and meta-analysis. Intensive Care Med 2014;41: 402–11.

68. Doyle A, Flotcher A, Carter J, et al. The incidence of ventilator-associated pneumonia using the PneuX System with or without elective endotracheal tube exchange: a pilot study. BMC Res Notes 2011;4:92.

69. Young PJ, Pakeerathan S, Blunt MC, et al. A low-volume, low-pressure tracheal tube cuff reduces pulmonary aspiration. Crit Care Med 2006;34:632–9.

70. Gopal S, Luckraz H, Giri R, et al. Significant reduction in ventilator-associated pneumonia with the Venner-PneuX System in high-risk patients undergoing cardiac surgery: the Low Ventilator-Associated-Pneumonia study. Eur J Cardiothorac Surg 2015; 47:e92–6.

71. Pinciroli R, Mietto C, Piriyapatsom A, et al. Endotracheal tubes cleaned with a novel mechanism for secretion removal: a randomized controlled clinical study. Respir Care 2016;61:1431–9.

How Can We Distinguish Ventilator-Associated Tracheobronchitis from Pneumonia?

Sean Keane, MD[a], Maria Sole Vallecoccia, MD[a,b], Saad Nseir, MD, PhD[c,d], Ignacio Martin-Loeches, MD, PhD[a,e,f,*]

KEYWORDS

• Pneumonia • Sepsis • Tracheobronchitis • VAP • VAT • ICU • MDR • Stewardship

KEY POINTS

- There is no gold standard clinical and microbiological definition of ventilator-associated tracheobronchitis (VAT).
- Chest radiograph has been shown to be less reliable than computed tomography or lung ultrasound in detecting pulmonary infiltrates, and it may be assumed that a percentage of critically ill patients with ventilator-associated pneumonia (VAP) are mistakenly diagnosed as having VAT according to current diagnostic criteria.
- VAT has been proposed as a distinct intermediate entity between colonization of the lower respiratory tract and pneumonia.
- VAT has been shown to prolong the duration of invasive mechanical ventilation, increase the length of intensive care unit stay, and predispose the patient to subsequent episodes of VAP, without an increase in mortality, when compared with intubated mechanically ventilated patients without VAT.
- Future studies should determine the interest of the Pao_2 to fraction of inspired oxygen (Fio_2) ratio and the modified Clinical Pulmonary Infection Score in differentiating VAT from VAP.

INTRODUCTION

When a patient is critically ill, mechanical ventilation is often provided and is the most common artificial assistance used in intensive care units (ICUs). Ventilator-associated pneumonia (VAP) is linked to significantly enhanced patient morbidity and mortality globally. Data from Europe are scarce; in the United States, it is estimated that VAP annually consumes $1.2 billion of critical care resources.[1]

Mechanical ventilation is a cornerstone of supportive therapy in intensive care worldwide.

Contributions of Authors: Recognition of the need to undertake this work: S. Keane, M.S. Vallecoccia, S. Nseir, and I. Martin-Loeches. Preparation of the article: S. Keane, M.S. Vallecoccia, S. Nseir, and I. Martin-Loeches. Disclosure Statement: Nil (S. Keane, M.S. Vallecoccia, and I. Martin-Loeches). Bayer (advisory board) and MSD (lecture) (S. Nseir).
[a] Department of Anaesthesia and Critical Care Medicine, St. James's Hospital, James's Street, Dublin 8, Ireland; [b] Department of Anesthesia and Intensive Care Medicine, Università Cattolica del Sacro Cuore—Fondazione Policlinico Universitario A.Gemelli, Largo Agostino Gemelli 8, Rome 00168, Italy; [c] CHU Lille, Centre de Réanimation, 2 Avenue Oscar Lambret, Lille 59000, France; [d] Lille University, Faculté de Médecine, 2 Avenue Eugène Avinée, Lille 59120, France; [e] Multidisciplinary Intensive Care Research Organization (MICRO), St James's Hospital, James's Street, Dublin 8, Ireland; [f] Trinity Centre for Health Sciences, James's Street, Dublin 8, Ireland
* Corresponding author. Department of Anaesthesia and Critical Care Medicine, St James's Hospital, Dublin 8, Ireland.
E-mail address: drmartinloeches@gmail.com

Clin Chest Med 39 (2018) 785–796
https://doi.org/10.1016/j.ccm.2018.08.003
0272-5231/18/© 2018 Elsevier Inc. All rights reserved.

Studies have estimated that more than 300,000 patients receive mechanical ventilation in the United States each year; ventilator-associated complications (VACs) are those complications that develop during a period of mechanical ventilation. The most frequent VACs are ventilator-associated infections (VAIs), namely VAP and ventilator-associated tracheobronchitis (VAT).[2] The problem that VAC and VAI present for health care systems is of such magnitude that in the United States the Critical Care Societies Collaborative agreed with the Department of Health and Human Services to address the challenging problem of VAIs.[3] Significant published work exists on the diagnosis, treatment, and impact of VAP on the outcome of critically ill patients, with a recent CDC algorithm that outlines an optimal approach to care.[3] However, similar levels of research work and clinical guidelines are lacking in VAT.[4]

DIFFICULTY IN DEFINING VENTILATOR-ASSOCIATED TRACHEOBRONCHITIS AND RESULTING DIFFERENCES IN EPIDEMIOLOGY

There is no gold standard clinical and microbiological definition of VAT, making it difficult to accurately evaluate the global epidemiologic picture. Elements that affect reported VAT incidence include the definition used, diagnostic uncertainty surrounding overlap with VAP, and ongoing controversy regarding the recognition of VAT as a separate clinical entity to VAP. The point in time during which a piece of research was conducted, along with the investigator's attitude on the relationship between VAT and VAP, may ultimately have the greatest impact on the reported incidence. As VAT is increasingly accepted as a distinct process, and the international research community recognizes a unifying definition, historical differences in epidemiologic patterns will conceivably harmonize. Due to these ongoing controversies, the reported incidence of VAT can vary between 0% and 16.5%.[5–9] Epidemiologic variances are likely to continue until an international consensus is reached on a clinical and microbiological definition for VAT. Whereas VAP is an accepted entity that has a very clear algorithm for diagnosis and treatment, VAT is a neglected entity by many researchers.

VAT has been defined differently in recent years. The Centers for Disease Control and Prevention (CDC) define VAT as the radiological absence of pneumonia in a chest radiograph (CXR) and at least 2 of the following: fever (>38°C), cough, new or increased production of sputum, rhonchi and wheezing, and bronchospasm. In addition, a culture of bronchial secretions obtained by endotracheal aspirate (ETA) or bronchoscopic technique should be positive.[10] More recently, an updated definition has been commonly used. Along with an absence of new or progressive pulmonary infiltrates on CXR, a diagnosis of VAT requires at least 2 of the following: body temperature greater than 38.5°C or less than 36.5°C, leukocyte count greater than 12,000 cells per microliter or less than 4000 cells per microliter, and purulent ETA or bronchoalveolar lavage (BAL). In addition, VAT must be microbiologically confirmed by the growth of a potentially pathogenic microorganism in the ETA of equal to or greater than 10^5 colony forming units (CFUs) per milliliter, or BAL of equal to or greater than 10^4 CFUs per milliliter.[5,8,9,11] The combination of clinical findings and microbiological confirmation leads to a diagnosis of VAT but not when they occur independently of each another (**Table 1**).

Table 1
Centers for Disease Control and Prevention versus Martin-Loeches and Nseir's criteria for diagnosing ventilator-associated tracheobronchitis

	CDC Criteria	Martin-Loeches and Nseir's Criteria
Clinical	At least 2 of: fever >38°C, cough, new or increased production of sputum, rhonchi and wheezing, or bronchospasm	At least 2 of: body temperature >38.5°C or <36.5°C, leukocyte count >12,000 cells/μL or <4000 cells/μL, and purulent ETA or BAL
Microbiology	Positive culture of bronchial secretions (ETA or bronchoscopic)	Positive culture of potentially pathogenic microorganism on ETA of ≥10^5 CFU/mL, or BAL of ≥10^4 CFU/mL
CXR	Absence of new or progressive pulmonary infiltrates	Absence of new or progressive pulmonary infiltrates

Diagnosis requires clinical, microbiological, and CXR findings.
From Martin-Loeches I, Povoa P, Rodríguez A, et al. Incidence and prognosis of ventilator-associated tracheobronchitis (TAVeM): a multicentre, prospective, observational study. Lancet Respir Med 2015;3:859–68; with permission.

DIAGNOSING VENTILATOR-ASSOCIATED TRACHEOBRONCHITIS VERSUS VENTILATOR-ASSOCIATED PNEUMONIA

The definition of VAP is generally accepted as pneumonia occurring 48 hours or longer after mechanical ventilation, characterized by new or progressive infiltrates on radiographic imaging, and the presence of at least 2 of the following criteria: body temperature greater than 38.5°C or less than 36.5°C, leukocyte count greater than 12,000 cells per microliter or less than 4000 cells per microliter, and purulent sputum. New or progressive radiographic chest infiltrates represent infection-induced neutrophil infiltration, fibrinous exudates, and cellular debris in the intraalveolar spaces that was not incubating or present at the onset of mechanical ventilation.[12–14]

The definition of VAP is, therefore, similar to the updated criteria for that of VAT, aside from radiographic infiltrates representative of infective intraalveolar infiltration. CXR is mandatory for making a diagnosis of VAP and sometimes is difficult to interpret in a patient in the supine position with potential multiple artifacts for an accurate diagnosis.

CXR has been shown to be less reliable than computed tomography (CT) or lung ultrasound (LUS) in detecting pulmonary infiltrates.[15–19] It may be assumed that a percentage of critically ill patients with VAP are mistakenly diagnosed as having VAT according to current diagnostic criteria.

When radiographic uncertainty is combined with clinical and laboratory similarities, it is clear the physician faces a diagnostic challenge in accurately distinguishing VAT from VAP.

DIAGNOSTIC DIFFICULTIES IN CLEARLY DEFINING VENTILATOR-ASSOCIATED TRACHEOBRONCHITIS VERSUS VENTILATOR-ASSOCIATED PNEUMONIA

VAT has been proposed as a distinct intermediate entity between colonization of the lower respiratory tract and pneumonia by some investigators[20–22]; others suggest that distinguishing VAT from VAP is futile in clinical practice.[14]

VAT has been shown to prolong the duration of invasive mechanical ventilation, increase the length of ICU stay, and predispose the patient to subsequent episodes of VAP, without an increase in mortality, when compared with intubated mechanically ventilated patients without VAT.[9,11,20,23] In contrast, VAP is a well-recognized independent risk factor for increased mortality[24,25] and carries a higher mortality rate than VAT.[26] This makes it a challenging proposition to merge VAT and VAP as the unified clinical entity, ventilator-associated lower respiratory infections (VA-LRTIs),[22] and physicians must acknowledge them as separate conditions.

Infective intraalveolar infiltrates are the cardinal feature delineating VAT from VAP, and the challenge in applying radiographic imaging to make this distinction has been identified. To complicate matters further, studies on patients with acute respiratory distress syndrome (ARDS), atelectasis, and pulmonary edema demonstrate that most VAP cases develop in previously injured lung regions.[27–29] Therefore, radiographic progression in the appearance of pulmonary infiltrates cannot be used to differentially diagnose VAT from VAP in this setting. As a result of these diagnostic challenges, physicians may require additional investigations to reach a differential diagnosis in a certain proportion of cases.

Culture of respiratory secretions may aid the differentiation between VAT and VAP, and should ideally be collected before commencing antimicrobial therapy. Cultures may be analyzed quantitatively or semiquantitatively and/or qualitatively, and the most appropriate technique for diagnosing VA-LRTI remains an area of active debate. A recent Cochrane review of 1240 participants across 3 randomized controlled trials compared invasive quantitative versus noninvasive qualitative cultures of respiratory secretions in subjects with VAP. No significant difference was demonstrated in 28-day mortality, days on mechanical ventilation, length of ICU stay, or changes in antimicrobial therapy.[30] Most of the literature in relation to quantitative versus qualitative culture analysis relates to VAP, though it is reasonable to apply the considerations, conclusions, and controversies described to patients with VAT. Quantitative versus qualitative culture in itself does not have a current role in distinguishing VAT from VAP.

Quantitative culture of respiratory samples determines a threshold count to differentiate between colonization and infection of the lower airways. Infection is accepted as growth of a potentially pathogenic microorganism in the ETA of equal to or greater than 10^5 CFUs per milliliter, BAL of equal to or greater than 10^4 CFUs per milliliter, and protected specimen brush (PSB) of equal to or greater than 10^3 CFUs per milliliter.[8,9,12,31–35] A quantitative ETA of equal to or greater than 10^6 CFUs per milliliter has also been advocated because it is more specific, although less sensitive, than equal to or greater than 10^5 CFUs per milliliter[11,36] (**Table 2**). Semiquantitative analysis is considered an acceptable alternative, and cultures with at least moderate growth have been

Table 2
Threshold count to differentiate between colonization and infection of the lower airways

Type of Culture	Threshold
BAL	$\geq 10^4$ CFUs/mL
ETA	$\geq 10^5$ CFUs/mL
PSB	$\geq 10^3$ CFUs/mL

shown to correlate with quantitative counts diagnostic of infection.[8,37]

Quantitative culture thresholds for VAP have been correlated with histologic postmortem analysis,[36,38] though no investigators have performed similar research for VAT. This means consensus culture threshold values for VAT are somewhat theoretic and a patient-specific approach should be taken in each case.[39,40] The key role of quantitative culture threshold is to distinguish colonization from infection in the lower respiratory tract. The acceptance of VAT as a distinct intermediate infectious entity between colonization and VAP renders null the ability of a quantitative culture threshold to make a differential diagnosis between VAT and VAP.

BIOMARKERS AND INFLAMMATORY RESPONSE

Impaired immunity and a relative antiinflammatory state are hypothesized to contribute to critically ill patients developing VAT or VAP.[41] The absence of clinically useful biomarkers that identify respiratory infection in mechanically ventilated patients and that can predict the severity of such infections on an individual basis is a significant unmet need.[42,43] In the absence of these biomarkers, therapy becomes empirical: there is no attempt to individualize therapy, patients are treated by protocol, and there is unrestricted overuse of antimicrobials with inevitable emergence of resistant pathogens.[44] However, the absence of these biomarkers is underpinned by fundamental ignorance of patient immune and inflammatory response in this area of medicine.

The accuracy of several biomarkers in diagnosing VAP has been evaluated across a range of studies.[45–49] The most frequently investigated are C-reactive protein (CRP), procalcitonin (PCT), and soluble triggering receptor expressed on myeloid cells-1. Conclusions reached across studies are often contradictory, due in part to varying methodologies and subject recruitment strategies.[48–51]

Research focuses almost exclusively on VAP, with no studies specifically looking at the application of biomarkers to distinguish VAT from VAP. However, some inferred conclusions can be made. Ramirez and colleagues[49] analyzed serial CRP and PCT in mechanically ventilated subjects from 48 hours or more to the development of VAP. Infective symptoms consistent with VAT before a diagnosis of VAP were demonstrated in 43 subjects. Results showed no significant difference in CRP between the VAT stage and the subsequent development of VAP (159 vs 132 mg/dL; $P = .502$), whereas PCT increased significantly (0.9 vs 1.42 ng/dL; $P = .008$). This implies CRP is raised throughout the continuum of VAT and VAP, and cannot be used to differentiate. PCT may have some promise, and this conclusion is supported by a study in chronic obstructive pulmonary disease subjects showing PCT was independently associated with community-acquired bacterial bronchitis.[52] Recently, Suberviola and colleagues[53] found that after lung transplantation PCT can be useful in detecting infections during the first postoperative week and was superior to CRP. Dedicated studies are needed to investigate the utility of biomarkers in diagnosing VAT, and the potential application in distinguishing VAT and VAP.

BRONCHOSCOPY IN DISTINGUISHING VENTILATOR-ASSOCIATED TRACHEOBRONCHITIS VERSUS VENTILATOR-ASSOCIATED PNEUMONIA

Flexible fiberoptic bronchoscopy (FFB) can be useful in distinguishing VAT from VAP. One of the key roles is invasive sampling, with BAL or PSB, for culture. BAL and PSB are comparable invasive FFB sampling techniques[54]; ETA is the recognized noninvasive standard. Invasive samples are considered more specific for diagnosis[12] and facilitate antimicrobial stewardship initiatives.[55] On the other hand, major review articles found no evidence of reduced mortality in patients with VAP when comparing invasive with noninvasive sampling.[30,56]

Interpreting the evidence is challenging, and recent expert international guidelines offer an astute overview.[4] To accurately guide future therapy, invasive quantitative samples are recommended in stable patients before commencing antimicrobials (weak recommendation, low quality of evidence), with any subsequent samples being invasive quantitative or non-invasive quantitative or qualitative cultures (strong recommendation, low quality of evidence).[4] The potential benefits of reduced antimicrobial exposure are deemed to outweigh potential complications of invasive techniques in stable patients, particularly if collected before commencing new antimicrobials.

FFB is generally considered safe, and acute severe complications occur rarely. Cardiorespiratory disturbances may be exacerbated in critically ill patients.[57] FFB may induce mesenteric ischemia and gastrointestinal bacterial translocation through a mechanism of reduced mesenteric blood flow.[58] In addition, low-grade pyrexias occur in up to one-third of cases, probably due to induced cytokine activity, whereas transient radiographic abnormalities may reflect retained saline. These features may mimic those of VAT or VAP, leading to diagnostic challenges in the postprocedural phase.[59]

Interestingly, it has been proposed that FFB in combination with CXR can enhance clinical accuracy in diagnosing VA-LRTI in select cases.[34] VAT is considered when purulent secretions are surrounding the endotracheal tube and not coming from deep lung regions, whereas VAP is considered if they are coming from deep lung regions (**Fig. 1**). Although simple and not part of current diagnostic criteria, it may help identify those with VAT at high risk of progression to VAP. In other words, FFB facilitates invasive sampling techniques and may help predict which patients with VAT are at high risk of progressing to VAP. However, in terms of distinguishing VAT from VAP, FFB does not have a defining role.

IS CHEST RADIOGRAPH A RELIABLE DIAGNOSTIC TOOL?

The presence of a new or progressive infiltrate on CXR or CT is required to diagnose VAP, although the quality of a portable CXR can be highly variable. It is challenging for the technologist in the ICU to obtain diagnostic-quality studies on unstable, uncooperative patients, or patients who have numerous support devices. There is accumulating evidence about the low reliability of CXR in ventilated patients, even after having reviewed previous images.[27,60,61] CXRs are also difficult to interpret because ICU patients frequently have abnormal CXRs at the time of admission; for example, preexisting infiltrates or concurrent disease, such as congestive heart failure, atelectasis, prior pneumonia, or ARDS.[11,61] It is important to note that the CXR in ICU is not always clear-cut because many clinical patterns can produce identical findings, such as pulmonary edema, ARDS, VAP, and atelectasis. The anteroposterior portable CXR is the most frequent radiologic test performed in the ICU. However, pulmonary infiltrates on CXR are often the result of fluid, pus, or lung consolidation due to the host inflammatory response. In a necropsy study about proven VAP, Wunderink and colleagues[62] could not find any radiographic sign that correlated well with pneumonia except air bronchogram; however, its low sensitivity (17%) suggests that this sign is infrequently found. Moreover, they proved that pneumonia could be radiologically confused with most of the pathologic conditions found in autopsies of mechanically ventilated patients, such as lobar or subsegmental atelectasis, ARDS, alveolar hemorrhage, or infarction.

LUS has a consolidated role in the diagnosis of community-acquired pneumonia. Nevertheless, its utility for VAP is limited by the common presence of lung infiltrates in ventilated patients.

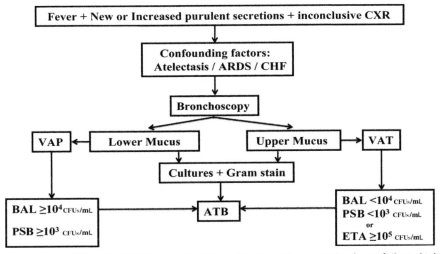

Fig. 1. Bronchoscopy to distinguish VAT from VAP. ATB, antibiotic; CHF, congestive heart failure. (*Adapted from* Martin-Loeches I, Pobo A. What is new in ventilator-associated tracheobronchitis? Clin Pulm Med 2010;17:119; with permission.)

Several patterns have been proposed: consolidation, multiple irregularly spaced B-lines, multiple abutting so-called comets issued from the pleural line, or a small subpleural consolidation.[63] A recent meta-analysis about this topic suggests that the most accurate and useful sonographic signs to diagnose VAP are consolidations with dynamic air bronchograms or fluid bronchograms (linear or arborescent anechoic images within a consolidation) and small subpleural consolidations[64] (Fig. 2). It was suggested that a combination of LUS findings, clinical parameters, and microbiological results could increase the diagnostic accuracy of VAP.[65]

IS COMPUTED TOMOGRAPHY THE GOLD STANDARD?

Due to the inherent subjectivity and shortcomings of the CXR, CT was proposed to be the gold standard for chest imaging. CT is a more precise technique, allowing detection of small opacities and enhanced visualization of chest cavity regions, such as lung bases and lingual areas. There are data suggesting a real risk of missing pneumonia in CXRs if the pneumonic infiltrates are located in the upper and lower lobes of the lungs or the lingula, which may lead to an erroneous treatment decision.[15] Studies that compared CT and CXR in community-acquired pneumonia showed that CT is likely to be a more sensitive and specific tool for diagnosing pneumonia.[16,17] Unfortunately, CT is not routinely used due to greater cost, increased time required to obtain images, and higher radiation exposure. It could become the gold standard in cases in which infiltrates suggestive of VAP may be difficult to confirm, such as in patients with diffuse infiltrates, ARDS, pleural effusions, or prior surgery. In this type of patient, the risk-to-benefit ratio may favor using CT.

ARE DANGERS IN TRANSFER FOR COMPUTED TOMOGRAPHY WORTH THE RISK?

The intrahospital transport (IHT) of a critically ill patient to radiology department is associated with an important risk of complications. Airway problems, such as accidental extubation, bronchospasm, atelectasis, and pneumothorax, are frequent. Hospital staff should confirm the correct position of endotracheal tube and secure it. Patients should be adequately sedated, suctioned, and auscultated. Basic resuscitation drugs should be carried to treat cardiovascular complications, such as tachycardia, hypotension, hypertension, arrhythmia, and cardiac arrest, which can occur up to 1.6% of patient transports.[66,67] Other

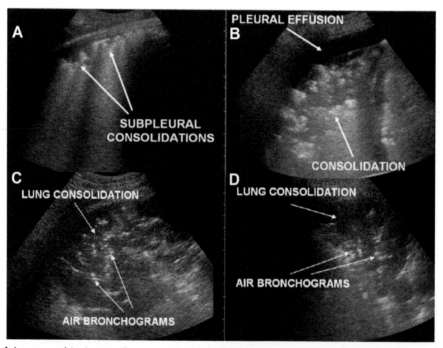

Fig. 2. Useful sonographic signs to diagnose VAP. (A) Subpleural consolidations. (B) Consolidation with an associated effusion. (C, D) Consolidations and air bronchograms. (Data from Staub LJ, Biscaro RR, Maurici R. Accuracy and applications of lung ultrasound to diagnose ventilator-associated pneumonia: a systematic review. J Intensive Care Med 2018;33(8):447–55.)

complications that can increase the morbidity and mortality are disconnection of ventilation or peripheral or central catheter lines, kink or obstruction of lines, or changes in speed of fluid infusion.

Interestingly, some studies show that IHT is a risk factor for developing VAP. In a multicenter study about IHT that included 6242 subjects, IHT was associated with a 1.4-fold increase in odds of VAP and with a longer ICU length of stay. It is noteworthy that in this study IHT had no significant impact on mortality.[68] The prolonged supine position, the frequent manipulation of ventilator circuits, and possible aspiration of contaminated secretions or gastric content during IHT could be determining factors of this increased risk of VAP. Moreover, multiple routes and destinations could increase the patient colonization with pathogens. In conclusion, the weight of evidence suggests that IHT can be a risk factor of VAP; however, it must not prevent ordering a CT for critically ill patients when it is needed.

CAN THE CLINICAL PULMONARY INFECTIVE SCORE BE USED IN THE DIAGNOSIS OR DECISION TO TREAT?

A major problem for the physicians caring for critically ill patients is that a clinically relevant gold standard for the diagnosis of VAP is not clearly established. The Clinical Pulmonary Infective Score (CPIS) was created by Pugin and colleagues[69] as a clinical marker for VAP. The primary outcome of the study was to validate a new blind BAL technique for diagnosing VAP in medically ill patients, compared with the gold standard FFB BAL. To compare the two methods, the investigators used six clinical and laboratory variables to develop a clinical score for pneumonia, ranging from 0 to 12 (**Table 3**). The investigators found a good correlation between this score and quantitative bacteriology, and further noted that a CPIS greater than 6 had a sensitivity of 93% and a specificity of 96% for diagnosing VAP, which corresponded to an area under the receiver operating characteristic curve of 0.95. However, clinicians who initially assess a mechanically ventilated patient should be aware that the investigators did not retrospectively evaluate the original data to refine the score accuracy and that the original score included culture results, which are not initially available when VAP is only suspected. Subsequent studies demonstrated that a modified version of CPIS excluding culture results has low sensitivity and specificity.[70–72] It was also proved that this score has a low accuracy when it is used in polytrauma,[73] surgical,[74] or burn patients[75] because it is not helpful in differentiating VAP from noninfectious causes of lung injury. Moreover, none of the studies that attempted to validate CPIS enrolled high-risk population groups, such as patients with ARDS.

Overdiagnosis of VAP could lead to inappropriate antimicrobial use, favoring the increase of multidrug-resistant germs, fungal, and *Clostridium difficile* infection. Conversely, inadequate treatment of VAP increases mortality. Because of the important consequences of this pathologic condition, physicians should not rely heavily on CPIS but should consider additional tests to diagnose VAP or to find a differential diagnosis. Nevertheless, CPIS could still have a role during daily practice in the decision-making regarding antimicrobial therapy. According to the international panel from the European Respiratory Society (ERS), European Society of Intensive Care Medicine (ESICM), European Society of Clinical Microbiology and Infectious Diseases (ESCMID), and Asociación Latinoamericana del Tórax (ALAT)

Table 3
Variables of the Clinical Pulmonary Infective Score

CPIS Point	0	1	2
Temperature (°C)	$\geq$36.5 and $\leq$38.4	$\geq$38.5 and $\leq$38.8	$\geq$39 or $\leq$36
Blood leukocytes (cubic millimeter)	$\geq$4000 and $\leq$11,000	$\leq$4000 and $\geq$11,000	$\leq$4000 and $\geq$11,000 plus band forms $\geq$500
Tracheal secretions	Absent	Present	Present and purulent
Oxygenation: P_{AO_2} to fraction of inspired oxygen (FIO_2) (millimeters of mercury)	>240	—	$\leq$240 and no evidence of ARDS
Pulmonary radiography	No infiltrate	Diffuse (or patchy) infiltrate	Localized infiltrate
Culture of tracheal aspirate	Negative	—	Positive

guidelines for the management of hospital-acquired pneumonia (HAP) and VAP, a low CPIS (eg, ≤6) could be used to evaluate patients with a low probability of HAP. In these patients, provided they are clinically stable, the treatment should not be extended for more than 3 days.[4] This is a weak recommendation based on a single study that showed that a short-course therapy for HAP seems not to be associated with worse clinical outcome and may reduce the risk of subsequent infection or the emergence of resistant organisms.[76]

SUMMARY

In the United States, VAC surveillance is publicly reported for each institution and is linked with remuneration based on pay-for-performance. Unfortunately, Europe does not have adequate implementation or data related to complications associated with mechanical ventilation. This is a rather blunt approach with significant limitations.[77] The clinical diagnosis of VAP, based on the aspiration of purulent tracheobronchial secretions and signs of systemic inflammation, is often inaccurate because purulent tracheobronchial secretions are invariably present in patients receiving prolonged mechanical ventilation, even in the absence of either VAT or VAP. In addition, the systemic signs of inflammation, such as fever, tachycardia, and leukocytosis, are nonspecific. Clinical diagnosis is further undermined because the criteria for VAP include both subjective and objective components.

Prior reports, including a recent multicenter study, have shown that VAP can develop in patients with VAT when antimicrobial therapy is inappropriate.[9] However it is also plausible that VAT might represent an intermediate process between lower respiratory tract colonization and VAP, or even a less severe spectrum of VAP.[21] Thus the continuum from colonization to VAT and then VAP in ventilated patients does exist (**Fig. 3**). There is an urgent need for new concepts in the arena of VAIs. Ideally the gold standard of care should be based on prevention rather than treatment of respiratory infection in ventilated patients. Currently, there is a wide range of clinical measures that generally involve some physical patient manipulation aimed at reducing the incidence of respiratory infection in mechanically ventilated patients. However, despite numerous and sometimes imaginative efforts to validate the benefit of these measures, most clinicians now accept that currently available measures have failed to eradicate VA-LRTI.[78]

Contemporary therapy for ventilator-associated respiratory infection emphasizes the importance of prompt antimicrobial therapy with broad-spectrum antimicrobial therapy.[79] There is an

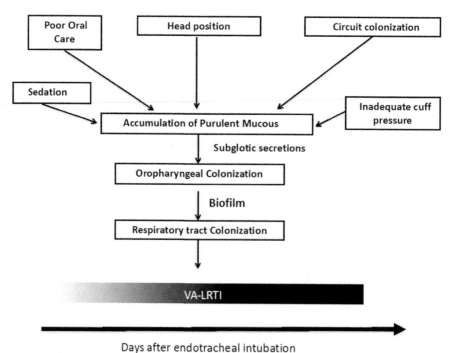

Fig. 3. The continuum from colonization to VA-LRTI.

mplicit risk within this strategy that liberal use of antimicrobial combinations will encourage the emergence of polymicrobial-resistant organisms and generate untreatable infections.[80,81] Given the more recent significant decrease in the discovery of next-generation novel antibacterial agents by the pharmaceutical industry, the emergence of antibiotic resistant pathogens has led global leaders to warn of a future in which common bacterial infections become untreatable and often fatal.[82] The development of antibiotic resistance represents a global public health challenge that is causing widespread concern as expressed by Dame Sally Davies, England's Chief Medical Officer, who opined in 2013 that "…untreatable infection caused by antibiotic-resistant bacteria 'poses a catastrophic threat' to humans and has urged immediate global action."[83] Only by early recognition and preventing progression of VAT to VAP, will there be an opportunity to consider VA-LRTIs as a whole.

REFERENCES

1. Weber DJ, Sickbert-Bennett EE, Brown V, et al. Completeness of surveillance data reported by the National Healthcare Safety Network: an analysis of healthcare-associated infections ascertained in a tertiary care hospital, 2010. Infect Control Hosp Epidemiol 2012;33:94–6.

2. Magill SS, Klompas M, Balk R, et al. Developing a new, national approach to surveillance for ventilator-associated events. Am J Crit Care 2013; 22:469–73.

3. Klompas M. Complications of mechanical ventilation—the CDC's new surveillance paradigm. N Engl J Med 2013;368:1472–5.

4. Torres A, Niederman MS, Chastre J, et al. International ERS/ESICM/ESCMID/ALAT guidelines for the management of hospital-acquired pneumonia and ventilator-associated pneumonia. Eur Respir J 2017;50:1700582.

5. Malacarne P, Langer M, Nascimben E, et al. Building a continuous multicenter infections surveillance system in the intensive care unit: finding from initial date set of 9493 patients from 71 Italian intensive care units. Crit Care Med 2008;36:1105–13.

6. Agrafiotis M, Siempos II, Falagas ME. Frequency, prevention, outcome and treatment of ventilator-associated tracheobronchitis: systematic review and meta-analysis. Respir Med 2010;104:325–36.

7. Esan A, Wentowski C, Abdelwahed A, et al. The incidence of ventilator-associated tracheobronchitis and its relationship to ventilator-associated pneumonia. Am J Respir Crit Care Med 2010;181:A3246.

8. Craven DE, Lei Y, Ruthazer R, et al. Incidence and outcomes of ventilator-associated tracheobronchitis and pneumonia. Am J Med 2013;126:542–9.

9. Martin-Loeches I, Povoa P, Rodríguez A, et al. Incidence and prognosis of ventilator-associated tracheobronchitis (TAVeM): a multicentre, prospective, observational study. Lancet Respir Med 2015;3: 859–68.

10. Garner JS, Jarvis WR, Emori TG, et al. CDC definitions for nosocomial infections, 1988. Am J Infect Control 1988;16:128–40.

11. Nseir S, Favory R, Jozefowicz E, et al. Antimicrobial treatment for ventilator-associated tracheobronchitis: a randomized, controlled, multicenter study. Crit Care 2008;12:R62.

12. Chastre J, Fagon JY. Ventilator-associated pneumonia. Am J Respir Crit Care Med 2002;165: 867–903.

13. Tejerina E, Esteban A, Fernández-Segoviano P, et al. Accuracy of clinical definitions of ventilator-associated pneumonia: comparison with autopsy findings. J Crit Care 2010;25:62–8.

14. Chastre J, Luyt CE. Does this patient have VAP? Intensive Care Med 2016;42:1159–63.

15. Syrjälä H, Broas M, Suramo I, et al. High-resolution computed tomography for the diagnosis of community-acquired pneumonia. Clin Infect Dis 1998;27:358–63.

16. Esayag Y, Nikitin I, Bar-Ziv J, et al. Diagnostic value of chest radiographs in bedridden patients suspected of having pneumonia. Am J Med 2010;123: 88.e1-5.

17. Self WH, Courtney DM, McNaughton CD, et al. High discordance of chest x-ray and computed tomography for detection of pulmonary opacities in ED patients: implications for diagnosing pneumonia. Am J Emerg Med 2013;31:401–5.

18. Mongodi S, Via G, Girard M, et al. Lung ultrasound for early diagnosis of ventilator-associated pneumonia. Chest 2016;149:969–80.

19. Bourcier JE, Paquet J, Seinger M, et al. Performance comparison of lung ultrasound and chest x-ray for the diagnosis of pneumonia in the ED. Am J Emerg Med 2014;32:115–8.

20. Nseir S, Di Pompeo C, Pronnier P, et al. Nosocomial tracheobronchitis in mechanically ventilated patients: incidence, aetiology and outcome. Eur Respir J 2002;20:1483–9.

21. Nseir S, Povoa P, Salluh J, et al. Is there a continuum between ventilator-associated tracheobronchitis and ventilator-associated pneumonia? Intensive Care Med 2016;42:1190–2.

22. Martin-Loeches I, Coakley JD, Nseir S. Should we treat ventilator-associated tracheobronchitis with antibiotics? Semin Respir Crit Care Med 2017;38: 264–70.

23. Karvouniaris M, Makris D, Manoulakas E, et al. Ventilator-associated tracheobronchitis increases the length of intensive care unit stay. Infect Control Hosp Epidemiol 2013;34:800–8.

24. Heyland DK, Cook DJ, Griffith L, et al. The attribut-able morbidity and mortality of ventilator-associated pneumonia in the critically ill patient. Am J Respir Crit Care Med 1999;159:1249–56.

25. Safdar N, Dezfulian C, Collard HR, et al. Clinical and economic consequences of ventilator-associated pneumonia: a systematic review. Crit Care Med 2005;33(10):2184–93.

26. Nseir S, Di Pompeo C, Soubrier S, et al. Impact of ventilator-associated pneumonia on outcome in pa-tients with COPD. Chest 2005;128:1650–6.

27. Winer-Muram HT, Rubin SA, Ellis JV, et al. Pneu-monia and ARDS in patients receiving mechanical ventilation: diagnostic accuracy of chest radiog-raphy. Radiology 1993;188(2):479–85.

28. Wunderink RG. Radiologic diagnosis of ventilator-associated pneumonia. Chest 2000;117:S188.

29. Dudeck MA, Horan TC, Peterson KD, et al. National Healthcare Safety Network (NHSN) report, data summary for 2010, device-associated module. Am J Infect Control 2011;39:798–816.

30. Berton DC, Kalil AC, Teixeira PJ. Quantitative versus qualitative cultures of respiratory secretions for clin-ical outcomes in patients with ventilator-associated pneumonia. Cochrane Database Syst Rev 2014;(10):CD006482.

31. Bergmans DC, Bonten MJ, De Leeuw PW, et al. Reproducibility of quantitative cultures of endotra-cheal aspirates from mechanically ventilated pa-tients. J Clin Microbiol 1997;35:796–8.

32. Koenig SM, Truwit JD. Ventilator-associated pneu-monia: diagnosis, treatment, and prevention. Clin Microbiol Rev 2006;19:637–57.

33. Torres A, Ewig S, Lode H, et al, European HAP Work-ing Group. Defining, treating and preventing hospi-tal acquired pneumonia: European perspective. Intensive Care Med 2009;35:9–29.

34. Martin-Loeches I, Pobo A. What is new in ventilator-associated tracheobronchitis? Clin Pulm Med 2010;17:117–21.

35. Dallas J, Skrupky L, Abebe N, et al. Ventilator-associated tracheobronchitis in a mixed surgical and medical ICU population. Chest 2011;139:513–8.

36. Marquette CH, Copin MC, Wallet F, et al. Diagnostic tests for pneumonia in ventilated patients: prospec-tive evaluation of diagnostic accuracy using histol-ogy as a diagnostic gold standard. Am J Respir Crit Care Med 1995;151:1878–88.

37. Hashimoto S, Shime N. Evaluation of semi-quantitative scoring of Gram staining or semi-quantitative culture for the diagnosis of ventilator-associated pneumonia: a retrospective comparison with quantitative culture. J Intensive Care 2013;1:2.

38. Nseir S, Marquette CH. Diagnosis of hospital-acquired pneumonia: postmortem studies. Infect Dis Clin North Am 2003;17:707–16.

39. Nseir S, Lubret R. Ventilator-associated tracheo-bronchitis. Clin Pulm Med 2011;18:65–9.

40. Baselski V, Klutts JS. Point-counterpoint: quantitative cultures of bronchoscopically obtained specimens should be performed for optimal management of ventilator-associated pneumonia. J Clin Microbiol 2013;51:740–4.

41. Hotchkiss RS, Monneret G, Payen D. Immunosup-pression in sepsis: a novel understanding of the dis-order and a new therapeutic approach. Lancet Infect Dis 2013;13:260–8.

42. Luyt CE, Combes A, Trouillet JL, et al. Biomarkers to optimize antibiotic therapy for pneumonia due to multidrug-resistant pathogens. Clin Chest Med 2011;32:431–8.

43. Póvoa P, Martin-Loeches I, Ramirez P, et al. Biomarkers kinetics in the assessment of ventilator-associated pneumonia response to antibiotics-results from the BioVAP study. J Crit Care 2017;41:91–7.

44. Guo Y, Gao W, Yang H, et al. De-escalation of empiric antibiotics in patients with severe sepsis or septic shock: a meta-analysis. Heart Lung 2016;45:454–9.

45. Determann RM, Millo JL, Gibot S, et al. Serial changes in soluble triggering receptor expressed on myeloid cells in the lung during development of ventilator-associated pneumonia. Intensive Care Med 2005;31:1495–500.

46. Sierra R. C-reactive protein and procalcitonin as markers of infection, inflammatory response, and sepsis. Clin Pulm Med 2007;14:127–39.

47. Povoa P. Serum markers in community-acquired pneumonia and ventilator-associated pneumonia. Curr Opin Infect Dis 2008;21:157–62.

48. Martin-Loeches I, Bos LD, Povoa P, et al. Tumor necrosis factor receptor 1 (TNFRI) for ventilator-associated pneumonia diagnosis by cytokine multi-plex analysis. Intensive Care Med Exp 2015;3:26.

49. Ramirez P, Lopez-Ferraz C, Gordon M, et al. From starting mechanical ventilation to ventilator-associated pneumonia, choosing the right moment to start antibiotic treatment. Crit Care 2016;20:169.

50. Simon L, Gauvin F, Amre DK, et al. Serum procalci-tonin and C-reactive protein levels as markers of bacterial infection: a systematic review and meta-analysis. Clin Infect Dis 2004;39:206–17.

51. Póvoa P, Martin-Loeches I, Ramirez P, et al. Biomarker kinetics in the prediction of VAP diag-nosis: results from the BioVAP study. Ann Intensive Care 2016;6:32.

52. Nseir S, Cavestri B, Di Pompeo C, et al. Factors predicting bacterial involvement in severe acute ex-acerbations of chronic obstructive pulmonary dis-ease. Respiration 2008;76:253–60.

53. Suberviola B, Castellanos-Ortega A, Ballesteros MA, et al. Early identification of infectious complications

in lung transplant recipients using procalcitonin. Transpl Infect Dis 2012;14:461–7.

54. Grossman RF, Fein A. Evidence-based assessment of diagnostic tests for ventilator-associated pneumonia: executive summary. Chest 2000;117: 177S–81S.

55. Shorr AF, Sherner JH, Jackson WL, et al. Invasive approaches to the diagnosis of ventilator-associated pneumonia: a meta-analysis. Crit Care Med 2005;33:46–53.

56. Rea-Neto A, Youssef NC, Tuche F, et al. Diagnosis of ventilator-associated pneumonia: a systematic review of the literature. Crit Care 2008; 12:R56.

57. Lindholm CE, Oilman B, Snyder JV, et al. Cardiorespiratory effects of flexible fiberoptic bronchoscopy in critically Ill patients. Chest 1978;74:362–8.

58. Nayci A, Atis S, Duce MN, et al. Bronchoscopy is associated with decreased mesenteric arterial flow. Crit Care Med 2008;36:2517–22.

59. Miller RJ, Casal RF, Lazarus DR, et al. Flexible bronchoscopy. Clin Chest Med 2018;39(1):1–16.

60. Butler KL, Sinclair KE, Henderson VJ, et al. The chest radiograph in critically ill surgical patients is inaccurate in predicting ventilator-associated pneumonia. Am Surg 1999;65:805.

61. Graat ME, Choi G, Wolthuis EK, et al. The clinical value of daily routine chest radiographs in a mixed medical–surgical intensive care unit is low. Crit Care 2005;10:R11.

62. Wunderink RG, Woldenberg LS, Zeiss J, et al. The radiologic diagnosis of autopsy-proven ventilator-associated pneumonia. Chest 1992;101: 458–63.

63. Bouhemad B, Liu ZH, Arbelot C, et al. Ultrasound assessment of antibiotic-induced pulmonary reaeration in ventilator-associated pneumonia. Crit Care Med 2010;38:84–92.

64. Staub LJ, Biscaro RR, Maurici R. Accuracy and applications of lung ultrasound to diagnose ventilator-associated pneumonia: a systematic review. J Intensive Care Med 2017;33(8):447–55.

65. Wang G, Ji X, Xu Y, et al. Lung ultrasound: a promising tool to monitor ventilator-associated pneumonia in critically ill patients. Crit Care 2016;20: 320.

66. Taylor JO, Chulay JD, Landers CF, et al. Monitoring high-risk cardiac patients during transportation in hospital. Lancet 1970;296:1205–8.

67. Damm C, Vandelet P, Petit J, et al. Complications during the intrahospital transport in critically ill patients. Ann Fr Anesth Reanim 2005;24(1): 24–30.

68. Schwebel C, Clec'h C, Magne S, et al. Safety of intrahospital transport in ventilated critically ill patients: a multicenter cohort study. Crit Care Med 2013;41:1919–28.

69. Pugin J, Auckenthaler R, Mili N, et al. Diagnosis of ventilator-associated pneumonia by bacteriologic analysis of bronchoscopic and nonbronchoscopic "blind" bronchoalveolar lavage fluid. Am Rev Respir Dis 1991;143:1121–9.

70. Fartoukh M, Maître B, Honoré S, et al. Diagnosing pneumonia during mechanical ventilation: the clinical pulmonary infection score revisited. Am J Respir Crit Care Med 2003;168:173–9.

71. Luyt CE, Chastre J, Fagon JY, VAP Trial Group. Value of the clinical pulmonary infection score for the identification and management of ventilator-associated pneumonia. Intensive Care Med 2004;30:844–52.

72. Schurink CA, Van Nieuwenhoven CA, Jacobs JA, et al. Clinical pulmonary infection score for ventilator-associated pneumonia: accuracy and inter-observer variability. Intensive Care Med 2004; 30:217–24.

73. Croce MA, Swanson JM, Magnotti LJ, et al. The futility of the clinical pulmonary infection score in trauma patients. J Trauma 2006;60:523–8.

74. Pieracci FM, Rodil M, Haenel J, et al. Screening for ventilator-associated pneumonia in the surgical intensive care unit: a single-institution analysis of 1,013 lower respiratory tract cultures. Surg Infect (Larchmt) 2015;16:368–74.

75. Pham TN, Neff MJ, Simmons JM, et al. The clinical pulmonary infection score poorly predicts pneumonia in patients with burns. J Burn Care Res 2007;28:76–9.

76. Singh N, Rogers P, Atwood CW, et al. Short-course empiric antibiotic therapy for patients with pulmonary infiltrates in the intensive care unit: a proposed solution for indiscriminate antibiotic prescription. Am J Respir Crit Care Med 2000;162:505–11.

77. Grgurich PE, Hudcova J, Lei Y, et al. Diagnosis of ventilator-associated pneumonia: controversies and working toward a gold standard. Curr Opin Infect Dis 2013;26:140–50.

78. Kollef MH. Prevention of ventilator-associated pneumonia or ventilator-associated complications: a worthy, yet challenging, goal. Crit Care Med 2012; 40:271–7.

79. Rello J, Lisboa T, Koulenti D, et al. Determinants of prescription and choice of empirical therapy for hospital-acquired and ventilator-associated pneumonia. Eur Respir J 2011;37(6):1332–9.

80. Martin-Loeches I, Torres A, Rinaudo M, et al. Resistance patterns and outcomes in intensive care unit (ICU)-acquired pneumonia. Validation of European Centre for Disease Prevention and Control (ECDC) and the Centers for Disease Control and Prevention (CDC) classification of multidrug resistant organisms. J Infect 2015;70:213–22.

81. Zilahi G, McMahon MA, Povoa P, et al. Duration of antibiotic therapy in the intensive care unit. J Thorac Dis 2016;8:3774.

82. Wilke M, Grube R. Update on management options in the treatment of nosocomial and ventilator assisted pneumonia: review of actual guidelines and economic aspects of therapy. Infect Drug Resist 2014;7:1.

83. Available at: http://www.independent.co.uk/life-style/health-and-families/health-news/antibiotics-resistance-apocalypse-warning-chief-medical-officer-professor-dame-sally-davies-drugs-a7996806.html. Accessed March 5, 2018.

Management of Ventilator-Associated Pneumonia
Guidelines

Mark L. Metersky, MD[a],*, Andre C. Kalil, MD, MPH[b]

KEYWORDS

- Guideline • Hospital-acquired pneumonia • Ventilator-associated pneumonia
- Nosocomial pneumonia

KEY POINTS

- Although the guidelines for the diagnosis and treatment of hospital-acquired pneumonia (HAP) and ventilator associated pneumonia (VAP) recently released by the Infectious Diseases Society of America with the American Thoracic Society, and the European Respiratory Society have some noteworthy differences, they are more similar than different.
- Appropriate initial empiric antibiotic treatment of HAP and VAP is important for optimum patient outcomes. Both excessive antibiotic treatment and ineffective initial treatment have the potential to cause patient harm.
- There is considerable patient-level and hospital-level variation in the prevalence of resistant pathogens causing HAP and VAP. Empiric antibiotic regimens should be based on local antibiogram data and knowledge of patient-level factors that predict antibiotic-resistant pathogens.
- Most patients with HAP and VAP can be treated with a 7-day course of antibiotics.
- Procalcitonin measurement is not useful for determining if a patient with suspected VAP should receive antibiotics, but is useful in decreasing the length of antibiotic treatment in centers that do not routinely use short-course therapy.

INTRODUCTION

Ventilator-associated pneumonia (VAP) remains a common problem among patients who require invasive mechanical ventilation in acute care hospitals. Despite widespread implementation of care processes thought to decrease VAP rates, including head of bed elevation, sedation vacations, and daily assessment of readiness to wean, approximately 10% of patients ventilated for more than 2 days still develop VAP, a rate that has remained stable for more than a decade.[1]

The consequences of VAP are considerable. The attributable mortality is estimated at approximately 13%.[2] VAP also results in significant morbidity, evidenced by a markedly prolonged hospital length of stay[3] and increased ventilator days in patients[4] who develop VAP compared with those who do not, with associated increased costs estimated at $40,000.[3]

In 2005, the American Thoracic Society (ATS) and Infectious Diseases Society of America (IDSA) published guidelines for the prevention and management of VAP (and hospital-acquired

No authors report financial conflict of interest related to the subject of this article.
[a] Division of Pulmonary, Critical Care and Sleep Medicine, University of Connecticut School of Medicine, UConn Health, 263 Farmington Avenue, Farmington, CT 06030-1321, USA; [b] Department of Internal Medicine, Division of Infectious Diseases, University of Nebraska Medical Center, 985400 Nebraska Medical Center, Omaha, NE 68198, USA
* Corresponding author.
E-mail address: Metersky@uchc.edu

Clin Chest Med 39 (2018) 797–808
https://doi.org/10.1016/j.ccm.2018.08.002

pneumonia [HAP] and health care–associated pneumonia).[5] These guidelines were subsequently updated in 2016 by a panel convened jointly by the ATS and the IDSA.[6] The 2016 guideline did not address VAP prevention because a comprehensive VAP prevention guideline and subsequent update had been published shortly before.[7] Subsequently, in 2017, the European Respiratory Society (ERS) with involvement of the European Society of Intensive Care Medicine, the European Society of Clinical Microbiology and Infectious Diseases, and the Latin American Thoracic Association published their guidelines on the management of VAP.[8] Both guidelines used the Grading of Recommendations Assessment, Development and Evaluation (GRADE) methodology, which relies on framing specific clinical questions, systematic literature reviews, and a specified process for determining the direction and strength of recommendations that are based on the results of those systematic reviews.

This article summarizes the 2016 IDSA-ATS and 2017 ERS guideline recommendations, and in doing so highlights similarities and differences between the recommendations. We also comment on a few subsequent publications relevant to the recommendations we review.

DIAGNOSIS OF VENTILATOR-ASSOCIATED PNEUMONIA

The accurate diagnosis of VAP is difficult for numerous reasons, including the multitude of reasons why patients in the intensive care unit (ICU) can develop fever or elevated white blood cell count, difficulty in distinguishing between bacterial colonization of the airway and infection, and the limitations of portable chest imaging in the ICU. The IDSA/ATS guidelines suggest that blood cultures and respiratory cultures be obtained on all patients with suspected VAP, although they acknowledge that there is limited evidence to support either test.[6] The ERS guidelines also recommend respiratory tract cultures on all patients, but do not address blood cultures.[8] The rationale for blood cultures is that although bacteremic VAP is uncommon, the presence of bacteremia can provide definitive evidence of the infecting organism and consequently can improve the accuracy of using appropriate antibiotics. Also, if a pathogen not usually causing respiratory tract infection is isolated, it can point to a nonrespiratory source needing investigation.[9,10] Because of the high prevalence of multidrug resistant (MDR) pathogens causing VAP, there is no debate about the need to perform respiratory cultures to guide antibiotic therapy for VAP.

What has remained controversial since the publication of the 2005 ATS/IDSA guidelines[5] is the best way to obtain and process samples for respiratory culture. Two methods are most commonly used in clinical practice. One is the culture of suctioned endotracheal aspirates, in a semiquantitative fashion, which generates a report of bacterial growth as absent, or with one of three levels of growth (eg, no growth, small, moderate, large). The other method commonly used involves quantitative culturing of samples obtained in a manner that more preferentially samples the lower airways and alveoli (usually via protected bronchoalveolar lavage [BAL]), thereby minimizing collection of bacteria that may be colonizing the airways. Culture results are reported as colony-forming units (CFUs) per milliliter, with greater than 10^3 CFUs/mL considered as representing infection. The potential advantage of quantitative BAL culture is that it may decrease the frequency of false-positive diagnosis of VAP caused by airway colonization. The potential disadvantages include delays in antibiotic therapy while awaiting performance of the BAL, the potential for false-negative cultures in the setting of prior antibiotic therapy, and the cost and burden to the microbiology laboratory associated with quantitative cultures. The potential advantages of semiquantitative cultures of tracheal aspirates include the avoidance of the negative effects on gas exchange caused by BAL and the probable higher sensitivity in the setting of antibiotic treatment.

The 2005 ATS/IDSA guidelines described both methodologies and the competing rationales, but made no specific recommendation of one over the other.[5] The 2016 IDSA/ATS[6] and the 2017 ERS[8] guidelines both addressed this issue. A systematic review and meta-analysis of studies investigating outcomes of patients randomized to either invasive respiratory sampling with quantitative cultures versus noninvasive sampling and semiquantitative cultures demonstrated no improvement in patient outcomes including mortality, ventilator days or ICU days, or antibiotic changes.[11] Both guidelines concluded from the available data that invasive techniques with quantitative cultures are not likely to improve clinical outcomes, may decrease antibiotic exposure, may increase risk in the most severely ill patients, and that they increase laboratory cost. The ERS guidelines make the point that decreased antibiotic costs may mitigate the laboratory costs. Based on these findings, the IDSA/ATS guideline panel recommended not performing invasive modalities with quantitative cultures, whereas the ERS guideline recommended that one of the two modalities be used. In both guidelines, the recommendations were weak, indicating the limited and inconclusive evidence base. The IDSA/ATS panel recognized the degree of clinical equipoise associated with this issue, such that many institutions already performing invasive sampling and quantitative cultures are likely to continue to do so. The panel believed that if quantitative cultures were performed, the available evidence demonstrated that it was generally safe to discontinue antibiotics in patients with a quantitative culture below the accepted threshold.

It is noteworthy that despite using the same evidence base, and coming to a similar finding on the risks and benefits, the two guidelines panels arrived at different recommendations. This result demonstrates that despite the more structured methodology of the GRADE approach, when the magnitude of risks and benefits is unclear or is small, subjective expert opinion and experience can influence the ultimate recommendation.

BIOMARKERS FOR THE DIAGNOSIS OF VENTILATOR-ASSOCIATED PNEUMONIA

The IDSA/ATS guidelines also addressed the use of biomarkers to assist in the diagnosis of VAP.[6] Ideally, a recommendation to use one of these biomarkers would be based on evidence of improved outcomes with their use. However, there were no studies that reported patient outcomes related to the use of these biomarkers to diagnose the presence of VAP. Therefore, the recommendation was based solely on the performance characteristics of the test. Neither procalcitonin (PCT), C-reactive protein, nor soluble triggering receptor expressed on myeloid cells were found to have adequate sensitivity or specificity to inspire a recommendation for their use to assist in the diagnosis of VAP.

TREATMENT OF VENTILATOR-ASSOCIATED PNEUMONIA

Both the IDSA/ATS and ERS guidelines acknowledge the importance of appropriate initial antibiotic therapy,[6,8] because initial inappropriate therapy is associated with worsened patient outcomes.[12,13] Yet a major concern that has increased in magnitude is the danger posed by indiscriminant antibiotic usage, which results in increased resistance rates, *Clostridium difficile* colitis, and other antibiotic-associated side effects. Guidelines for VAP walk a tightrope trying to balance the risk of undertreatment versus the risks of overtreatment. It is an unfortunate reality that there are limited data that provide reliable estimates on the magnitude of morbidity and mortality associated with these competing risks. The IDSA/ATS guidelines accepted a somewhat arbitrary target of creating initial empiric antibiotic regimens that would provide appropriate therapy for 95% of patients. Even with triple antibiotics for all patients, it might not be possible to achieve 100% appropriate initial empiric therapy; there would be diminishing returns and increased antibiotic usage associated with attempting to achieve appropriate coverage rates greater than 95%.

The difficulty in crafting such regimens is that antibiotic resistance rates vary widely among ICUs in different hospitals and even among different ICUs in the same hospital. Furthermore, patient-related risk factors for MDR pathogens are not well understood; it remains difficult to predict at a patient level which case of VAP will be caused by resistant organisms.

Although there have been numerous randomized controlled trials (RCIs) of antibiotics for VAP, essentially all of them were for the purpose of obtaining regulatory approval of specific antibiotics and therefore were not always designed to answer the most clinically relevant questions. Consequently, most of these trials are limited in their ability to answer questions about initial empiric therapy for various reasons, including limiting enrollment of patients with risk factors for MDR pathogens, and allowing initial broader spectrum coverage for a period of time preceding enrollment or until culture results were obtained. For all of these reasons, recommendations for initial empiric antibiotic treatment of VAP must be considered as a "best effort," of knowledgeable and thoughtful guideline panelists, but based on an incomplete evidence base.

INITIAL EMPIRIC REGIMEN FOR "EARLY ONSET" VENTILATOR-ASSOCIATED PNEUMONIA

Several studies have suggested that patients with early onset VAP are less likely to develop VAP with MDR organisms, such as methicillin-resistant *Staphylococcus aureus* (MRSA) or *Pseudomonas aeruginosa*, than patients who develop VAP later in their hospital stay.[14–18] Importantly, early onset VAP should be defined as VAP occurring within 4 to 5 days of hospitalization, not within 4 to 5 days of the onset of mechanical ventilation. Hospitalized patients are at increased risk of infection with MDR pathogens even before being intubated. Based on these observations, the 2005 guidelines recommended that empiric therapy for early onset VAP need not include coverage for *P aeruginosa* or MRSA if the patient had no risk factors for infection with MDR pathogens.[5] The ERS guidelines specifically developed a recommendation for antibiotic treatment of early onset VAP,[8] whereas the IDSA/ATS guidelines considered late-onset VAP a risk for MDR pathogens.[6]

When one examines the rate of MDR pathogens as a cause of early onset VAP, there are considerable rates of MDR pathogens, including MRSA and potentially drug-resistant gram-negative bacilli, such as *Pseudomonas* (**Table 1**). Of course, many of these patients have risk factors for MDR pathogens independent of length of hospital stay. The important question, then, is whether a subpopulation of patients with early onset VAP can be identified who are at sufficiently low risk of MDR pathogens that narrow-spectrum antibiotic treatment can be safely used.

Patients with early onset VAP after traumatic or medical brain injury have been considered by some experts as especially likely to develop early onset VAP with community-type nonresistant organisms, given the significant risk for aspiration at the time of the brain injury. A study of 48 such patients by Ewig and colleagues[19] in 1999 found that at the time of ICU admission, no patients had MRSA in their tracheobronchial aspirate or protected specimen brush, at least 4 of 41 had gram-negative enterics, and at least four had *P aeruginosa*. Serial cultures demonstrated an increase rate of isolation of potentially MDR pathogens starting at around Day 5. A study published in 2010 found that among 45 patients with head

trauma who developed early onset VAP, one (2%) was caused by MRSA, four (9%) were caused by *P aeruginosa*, and nine (20%) were caused by gram-negative enterics. Although these percentages were generally lower than among the patients with late-onset VAP, they still represent a considerable risk for initial inappropriate antibiotic therapy if coverage for MDR pathogens was not used.[20]

In an observational study from a single ICU including 124 patients with nosocomial pneumonia (83% VAP), analysis identified certain factors associated with a lower risk of MDR pathogens. The absence of prior antimicrobial treatment, the presence of prior antimicrobial treatment with neurologic disturbances on ICU admission and early onset pneumonia, and the presence of prior antimicrobial treatment without neurologic disturbances but with aspiration on ICU admission were always associated with antimicrobial-susceptible pneumonia. The combination of these factors in a validation cohort of 26 patients allowed the validation of an algorithm that identified all patients with antimicrobial-susceptible nosocomial pneumonia.[21]

A prospective cohort study carried out to assess the rate of appropriateness of empirical antimicrobial therapy in 115 VAP patients showed that the mortality rate was significantly higher in the patients with inappropriate empirical therapy than in those with appropriate treatment (47% and 20%, respectively). A limited-spectrum therapy was used in 79 patients (69%) according to the criteria of early onset VAP (<5 days) without recent prior hospitalization or prior antibiotic treatment. Among these patients, there was a requirement for treatment escalation in 21 out of 79 patients (27%). The mortality rate was significantly higher in the patients in whom empirical therapy was inappropriate than in those in whom treatment was appropriate (47 vs 20%; $P = .04$).[12]

The ERS guidelines suggest using narrow-spectrum antibiotics (ertapenem, ceftriaxone, cefotaxime, moxifloxacin, or levofloxacin) in patients with suspected low risk of resistance and early onset HAP/VAP.[8] This was a weak recommendation, based on a very low quality of evidence. Patients defined as being at low risk were those without septic shock, with no other risk factors for MDR pathogens and those who are not in hospitals with a high background rate of resistant pathogens. However, the presence of other clinical conditions may make individuals unsuitable for this recommendation. A prevalence of resistant pathogens in the ICU caring for the patient in question of greater than 25% was considered a high background rate. It is not clear if patients with

Table 1 Frequency of potentially MDR pathogens in early onset nosocomial pneumonia versus late-onset pneumonia in studies published since 2010		
First Author, Year of Publication	Potential MDR Pathogens in Early Onset Nosocomial Pneumonia (%)	Potential MDR Pathogens in Late-Onset Nosocomial Pneumonia (%)
Ferrer et al,[14] 2010	26[a]	29[b]
Restrepo et al,[15] 2013	28	32
Martin-Loeches et al,[16] 2013	51[b]	60[b]
Arvanitis et al,[17] 2014	10	32
Khan et al,[18] 2016	32	41

[a] Includes only early onset nosocomial without risks for MDR pathogens.
[b] Includes early onset with risks for MDR pathogens.

septic shock were defined as higher risk because such patients are at higher risk of having MDR pathogens or because the danger to the patient resulting from inadequate initial therapy is greater. However, both issues are likely relevant.

The IDSA/ATS guidelines, in contrast, did not separate out early onset VAP for a less broad-spectrum initial empiric regimen.[6] The guideline panelists believed that there was not adequate data to safely use narrow-spectrum antibiotic therapy in this patient population. Rather, a hospital length of stay of 5 or more days was considered a risk factor for MDR pathogens. Patients with less than 5 days of hospitalization and no other risk factors for MDR pathogens were still suggested for MDR gram-negative coverage, but MRSA coverage could be omitted if there was a low prevalence of MRSA in the facility.

The available evidence suggests that there are some patients with early onset VAP who are at low risk of MDR pathogens. However, there is limited evidence to suggest that clinicians can accurately define such patients at this time, because a sizable proportion of these patients will be infected with potentially resistant gram negatives or MRSA. The ERS recommendation that either ertapenem, cefotaxime, or ceftriaxone alone (agents without activity against *Pseudomonas* or MRSA) can be used for early onset VAP in patients without other risk factors for MDR pathogens is arguably the most significant area of difference between the ERS and IDSA/ATS guidelines.

INITIAL EMPIRIC ANTIBIOTIC THERAPY FOR NON–EARLY ONSET VENTILATOR-ASSOCIATED PNEUMONIA

There are marked geographic variations in the prevalence of MRSA and MDR gram negatives, and what classes of antibiotics these gram negatives are susceptible to. This fact makes it imperative that the clinician be aware of antibiotic resistance patterns in their hospital, and if possible their ICU. Both the IDSA/ATS and the ERS guidelines stress the importance of knowledge of local antibiotic resistance patterns as being integral for the informed choice of empiric antibiotic for patients in a given ICU. The ERS stressed this in a "good practice," statement, whereas the IDSA/ATS performed a systematic review of the literature and provided a strong recommendation.

Both the IDSA/ATS and the ERS guidelines provide recommendations for initial empiric antibiotic regimens. However, the wording of the specific clinical question being addressed differs greatly

between the two guidelines. The ERS recommendation addresses the question of whether monotherapy can be used, or whether dual antibiotic coverage is always necessary.[8] Practically speaking, because essentially all patients whose VAP is not early onset require coverage for MDR gram-negative pathogens, for most patients, this is thought of as a question of whether MRSA coverage is required. Based on the risk for MDR pathogens and the patient's estimated risk of mortality, the ERS guidelines provided a suggested algorithm for initial empiric antibiotics in patients with HAP and VAP, although this algorithm was not directly linked to a formal recommendation (**Fig. 1**). Patients at low risk for mortality and low risk for MDR pathogens were recommended for monotherapy that would not cover MRSA, with some of the antibiotic choices potentially covering some isolates of nonfermenting gram negatives, such as *Pseudomonas*, and some not covering *Pseudomonas*.

The IDSA/ATS guidelines structured their question differently, addressing in a more general fashion the question of which antibiotics are recommended for the empiric treatment of VAP.[6] Gram-negative and gram-positive antibiotic coverage were addressed separately; the resulting regimen would be derived from the recommendations for gram-negative and gram-positive coverage relevant to the individual patient and the specific institution. IDSA/ATS an included coverage for MRSA and double coverage for MDR gram-negative bacilli for patients at high risk for MDR pathogens (**Table 2**). However, single gram-negative coverage was recommended in ICUs where the hospital or ICU antibiogram suggested that at least 90% of gram negatives would be sensitive to a single antibiotic. In such situations, certain antibiotics would allow monotherapy in settings where there were no risk factors for MRSA, as long as the antibiotic used was active against MSSA. Appropriate antibiotics in such situations could include piperacillin-tazobactam, cefepime, levofloxacin, or carbapenems depending on the local resistance patterns.

Both the IDSA/ATS and ERS guidelines recommend initial empiric coverage for *Pseudomonas* and MRSA in patients with risk factors for antibiotic resistance, including recent antibiotic exposure and treatment in an ICU with a high prevalence of MDR pathogens.

Recently, Ekren and colleagues[22] assessed the performance of the IDSA/ATS recommendations for initial empiric therapy in several ICUs in a single hospital. They found that guideline-concordant therapy resulted in initial appropriate empiric therapy for 97% of patients. In contrast, only 80% of

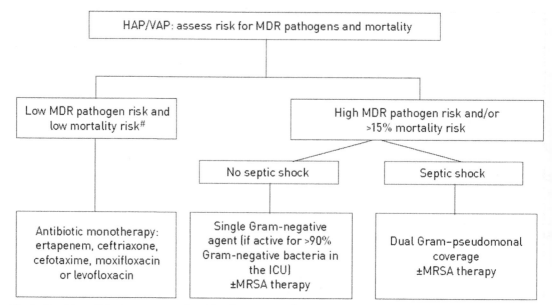

Fig. 1. Empiric antibiotic treatment algorithm for HAP/VAP. #Low risk for mortality is defined as a <15% chance of dying, a mortality rate that has been associated with better outcome using monotherapy than combination therapy when treating serious infection. (*From* Torres A, Niederman MS, Chastre J, et al. International ERS/ESICM/ESCMID/ALAT guidelines for the management of hospital-acquired pneumonia and ventilator-associated pneumonia: guidelines for the management of hospital-acquired pneumonia (HAP)/ventilator-associated pneumonia (VAP) of the European Respiratory Society (ERS), European Society of Intensive Care Medicine (ESICM), European Society of Clinical Microbiology and Infectious Diseases (ESCMID) and Asociación Latinoamericana del Tórax (ALAT). Eur Respir J 2017;50(3). [pii:1700582].)

patients with nonconcordant therapy receive appropriate empiric therapy (rate calculated based on numbers reported in the research letter). This high appropriate therapy rate associated with guideline-concordant therapy might have come at a cost of antibiotic overuse; 60% of patients receiving guideline-concordant therapy received what was defined as overtreatment. However, the authors did not describe how they defined overtreatment; for example, it is unclear if double gram-negative coverage was defined as overtreatment if only one of the antibiotics would have covered the gram-negative pathogen ultimately isolated. Also, if antibiotic de-escalation and short-course treatment were appropriately performed as recommended in both guidelines, the initial empiric coverage should not have led to significant antibiotic overtreatment. The authors also noted that 25% of patients would have been adequately covered with community-acquired pneumonia-type antibiotics. It would have been interesting to know if these patients had characteristics that could have allowed then to be reliably identified. For example, were they mostly early onset? Despite the limitations represented by a single-center study and the unanswered questions, this study represents an interesting preliminary evaluation of a few aspects of the IDSA/ATS guidelines. It is hoped that further studies can help identify factors that would allow progress toward the "Holy Grail" of less broad-spectrum antibiotic coverage combined with a high rate of initial appropriate coverage. Unfortunately, we suspect that no single guideline will be able to achieve this goal, because of the marked variations in antibiotic resistance rates from ICU to ICU, hospital to hospital, and region to region. Ideally, hospitals will review their antibiograms in specific subpopulations, such as early onset VAP, to adapt antibiotic decisions to their local situation.

LENGTH OF ANTIBIOTIC THERAPY

The 2005 ATS/IDSA guidelines recommended 7 to 8 days of antibiotic therapy for most VAP patients who respond well to therapy, with the exception of patients infected by nonfermenting gram-negative bacilli (NF-GNB), including *Pseudomonas* spp, *Acinetobacter* spp, and *Stenotrophomonas maltophilia*.[5] This was based on a large multicenter trial demonstrating overall similar outcomes with the shorter course treatment, compared with a 15-day course of antibiotics.[23] However, the investigators noted a higher rate of recurrent VAP in the

Table 2
Suggested empiric treatment options for clinically suspected ventilator-associated pneumonia in units where empiric methicillin-resistant *Staphylococcus aureus* coverage and double antipseudomonal/gram-negative coverage are appropriate

A. Gram-Positive Antibiotics with MRSA Activity	B. Gram-Negative Antibiotics with Antipseudomonal Activity: β-Lactam-Based Agents	C. Gram-Negative Antibiotics with Antipseudomonal Activity: Non-β-Lactam-Based Agents

Glycopeptides[a]
  Vancomycin, 15 mg/kg IV q 8–12 h (consider a loading dose of 25–30 mg/kg × 1 for severe illness)
	Antipseudomonal penicillins[b]
	  Piperacillin-tazobactam, 4.5 g IV q 6 h[b]
		Fluoroquinolones
		  Ciprofloxacin, 400 mg IV q 8 h
		  Levofloxacin, 750 mg IV q 24 h

OR	OR	OR

Oxazolidinones
  Linezolid, 600 mg IV q 12 h
	Cephalosporins[b]
	  Cefepime, 2 g IV q 8 h
	  Ceftazidime, 2 g IV q 8 h
		Aminoglycosides[a,c]
		  Amikacin, 15–20 mg/kg IV q 24 h
		  Gentamicin, 5–7 mg/kg IV q 24 h
		  Tobramycin, 5–7 mg/kg IV q 24 h

	OR
	Carbapenems[b,d]
	  Imipenem, 500 mg IV q 6 h[a]
	  Meropenem, 1 g IV q 8 h
		OR
		Polymyxins[a,e]
		  Colistin, 5 mg/kg IV × 1 (loading dose) followed by 2.5 mg × (1.5 × CrCl + 30) IV daily, divided q 12 h (maintenance dose)
		Polymyxin B, 2.5–3.0 mg/kg/d divided in 2 daily IV doses

	OR Monobactams[f] Aztreonam, 2 g IV q 8 h	

Abbreviations: CrCl, creatinine clearance; IV, Intravenous.

Choose one gram-positive option from column A, one gram-negative option from column B, and one gram-negative option from column C. Note that the initial doses suggested in this table may need to be modified for patients with hepatic or renal dysfunction.

[a] Drug levels and adjustment of doses and/or intervals required.

[b] Extended infusions may be appropriate. Please see the section on pharmacokinetic/pharmacodynamic optimization of antibiotic therapy.

[c] On meta-analysis, aminoglycoside regimens were associated with lower clinical response rates with no differences in mortality.

[d] The dose may need to be lowered in patients weighing less than 70 kg to prevent seizures.

[e] Polymyxins should be reserved for settings where there is a high prevalence of multidrug resistance and local expertise in using this medication. Dosing is based on colistin-base activity; for example, 1 million IU of colistin is equivalent to about 30 mg of colistin-base activity, which corresponds to about 80 mg of the prodrug colistimethate. Polymyxin B (1 mg = 10,000 units).

[f] In the absence of other options, it is acceptable to use aztreonam as an adjunctive agent with another β-lactam-based agent because it has different targets within the bacterial cell wall.

From Kalil AC, Metersky ML, Klompas M, et al. Management of adults with hospital-acquired and ventilator-associated pneumonia: 2016 clinical practice guidelines by the infectious diseases society of America and the American Thoracic Society. Clin Infect Dis 2016;63:e64; with permission.

patients with NF-GNB who received short-course therapy. This finding was likely caused by the way in which the end point of recurrent VAP was calculated (at 28 days after the beginning of treatment). This meant that the short-course group had 21 days during which they were at risk for recurrence, whereas the longer course group had only 14 days at risk. When the recurrence rate was calculated per day at risk, there was no significant difference in recurrent VAP rate. Furthermore, the short course NF-GNB VAP patients had similar mortality, clinical cure, and ventilator days to patients receiving long-course therapy, suggesting that at least some of the recurrences may have been colonization, without clinical significance. The IDSA/ATS guideline panel further performed a systematic review with data provided by the authors of previous trials: the data analysis separated VAP caused by nonfermenting gram-negative rods, mostly *Pseudomonas* spp, *Acinetobacter* spp, and *Stenotrophomonas* spp, and found no significant differences between long and short courses for the following outcomes: mortality, clinical cure, pneumonia recurrence, and ventilation days. Two systematic reviews have concluded that short-course therapy (7–8 days) results in similar outcomes compared with longer course therapy (10–15 days).[24,25] Based on these data, the IDSA/ATS and the ERS guidelines recommended 7 to 8 days of therapy for most patients.[6,8] Although the ERS guideline does not exclude patients infected with NF-GNB from the recommendation for short-course therapy, they note that short-course therapy "may not be possible" for such patients and that therapy should be individualized. Of course, this is true for all patients; no matter what the infecting organism, if a patient is still febrile and producing copious amounts of purulent sputum on Day 5, a course of therapy greater than 7 days is likely appropriate. Furthermore, the ERS guidelines note that patients who received initially inappropriate therapy, might not be candidates for short-course therapy (perhaps the way to approach this issue is to consider the days of appropriate therapy when determining the length of therapy). The ERS guidelines also recommend that short-course therapy not be considered for patients with lung abscess or necrotizing pneumonia, although evidence is not provided to support this statement.[8] That being said, patients with lung abscess or necrotizing pneumonia are more likely to have prolonged symptomatology and/or slower clinical recovery, so they would likely fall within the IDSA/ATS recommendation to provide longer therapy based on individual patient response.

INHALED ANTIBIOTICS

The theoretic advantage of using inhaled antibiotics in VAP is the ability to deliver high concentrations of antibiotic directly to the airways. This might be especially relevant for such antibiotics as aminoglycosides, which penetrate poorly into the alveolar lining fluid when given intravenously. Several studies have evaluated the role of adjunctive inhaled antibiotics combined with intravenous antibiotics in patients with VAP. Most recruited patients were infected with organisms sensitive to only aminoglycosides or polymyxins (colistin or polymyxin B). A meta-analysis of these studies

performed by the IDSA/ATS guidelines panelists demonstrated improved outcomes in patients who received adjunctive inhaled antibiotics.[6] The evidence was considered low quality because most were observational, unblinded studies, therefore subject to bias. Nonetheless, given the limited treatment options for these pathogens and lack of significant toxicity of adjunctive inhaled antibiotics in these studies, the IDSA/ATS guidelines suggested adjunctive inhaled antibiotics, but only for patients infected with MDR pathogens sensitive to only aminoglycosides or polymyxins. Fortunately, this remains a rare occurrence in the United States.

Recent studies of adjunctive inhaled amikacin[26] and amikacin-fosfamycin[27] with standard of care intravenous antibiotics failed to show benefit of adding inhaled antibiotics. However, the studies were not limited to pneumonia due to extremely drug resistant pathogens. At this point, evidence seems to be accumulating that adjunctive inhaled antibiotics should not be routinely used for VAP, but there is limited evidence suggesting that there may be benefit in the setting of pathogens that are only sensitive to aminoglycosides or polymyxins.

PHARMACOKINETIC/PHARMACODYNAMIC OPTIMIZED ANTIBIOTIC DOSING

A wealth of evidence in animal models has demonstrated that some antibiotics are more effective in killing bacteria when given in a manner not consistent with the parameters recommended by the manufacturers. For example, β-lactam antibiotics kill bacteria in a time-dependent fashion, such that killing is more effective the longer the serum antibiotic concentration remains higher than minimum inhibitory concentration. This finding suggests that continuous or prolonged infusion would be more effective than the traditional episodic bolus dosing. In contrast, such antibiotics as fluoroquinolones and aminoglycosides exhibit concentration-dependent killing, meaning that the higher the concentration achieved, the more effective the killing. This evidence, in addition to evidence suggesting lower toxicity with once-daily aminoglycoside dosing, has led to widespread adoption of this practice. The IDSA/ATS guideline panelists performed a systematic review of patient outcomes in patients who received pharmacokinetic/pharmacodynamic (PK/PD) optimized antibiotic dosing.[6] For the purposes of this recommendation, all antibiotics were considered in a single analysis, but most of the included studies were of prolonged infusion of β-lactam antibiotics. Two studies investigated serum concentration monitoring compared with manufacturer recommended dosing (eg, for vancomycin). Meta-analyses demonstrated a significant improvement in patient outcomes, including mortality, ICU length of stay, and clinical cure, associated with the use of PK/PD optimized dosing versus standard dosing. Based on these results, the IDSA/ATS guidelines gave a weak recommendation in favor of PK/PD optimized dosing. In doing so, the panel acknowledged the limitations of the data, because the amount of evidence for any specific antibiotic was limited. The Agency for Healthcare Research and Quality convened a panel to address this same question, and published their results in 2014.[28] In contrast to the IDSA/ATS recommendations, the Agency for Healthcare Research and Quality panel found insufficient evidence to either recommend or discourage PK/PD optimized dosing for VAP. The disparity between the findings of the two panels is likely because the Agency for Healthcare Research and Quality panel considered each antibiotic individually and excluded all observational studies, markedly limiting the amount of available evidence. Subsequent to the publication of the IDSA/ATS guidelines, a meta-analysis of RCTs investigating continuous infusion of β-lactams in severe sepsis was published. Approximately 55% of the patients had a pulmonary source of the sepsis. A significant improvement in mortality was noted; 19.6% versus 26.3% (relative risk, 0.74; 95% confidence interval, 0.56–1.00; $P = .045$).[29] A subsequent RCT in patients with severe sepsis also demonstrated improved clinical cure rates associated with continuous infusion of β-lactams.[30] Last, a newly updated systematic review and meta-analysis by a different research group also showed significant sepsis mortality reduction with prolonged antibiotic infusion compared with short-duration infusion.[31]

PROCALCITONIN FOR SHORTENING THE COURSE OF VENTILATOR-ASSOCIATED PNEUMONIA THERAPY

Three randomized trials,[32–34] including one published only in abstract form,[34] have assessed whether serial measurement of PCT can allow clinicians to safely shorten the length of antibiotic treatment of patients with VAP. Pooled analysis of these three trials demonstrated that the use of serial PCT measurement, when combined with clinical criteria, resulted in decreased antibiotic exposure (9.1 vs 12.1 days; $P<.00001$) with no difference in mortality. Other outcomes, such as ICU days and hospital length of stay, were assessed in some of these studies and also were not significantly different between groups. Based on these

results, the IDSA/ATS guidelines gave a weak recommendation in favor of using serial PCT in combination with clinical criteria to shorten antibiotic exposure to patients with VAP.[6] However, the guideline noted that there is no evidence that doing so could decrease antibiotic exposure to less than 7 days, so this strategy is not likely to be of benefit in settings where clinicians accept the recommendation for 7 days as the standard length of antibiotic treatment of VAP. Subsequent to the publication of the IDSA/IDSA guidelines, a large multicenter RCT of ICU patients with suspected bacterial infection of any type demonstrated a significant decrease in antibiotic days with the use of serial PCT measurement.[35] In this study, the median length of antibiotic treatment in the PCT group was 5 days, whereas the standard of care treated group received antibiotics for a median of 7 days. Furthermore, the PCT-guided patients had a significantly higher survival (hazard ratio, 1.26; 95% confidence interval, 1.07–1.49). However, the applicability of this study to VAP is unclear. Although 65% of the patients included in the study had a suspected pulmonary source of infection, only about 49% of the patients had a hospital-acquired infection. A recent patient-level data meta-analysis by Schuetz and colleagues[36] also showed a significant mortality reduction and a significant decrease in antibiotic treatment duration specifically for acute respiratory infections from 8.1 days to 5.7 days.

The IDSA/ATS recommendation[6] differs somewhat from that made in the ERS guidelines, although the interpretation of the available literature and the intent of the two recommendations seem to be similar.[8] The European panel, similarly noting that an intended antibiotic course of 7 to 8 days was unlikely to be shortened by the use of PCT, recommended against routine PCT testing for this purpose when the anticipated length of antibiotic treatment was 7 to 8 days. However, they noted that in certain patient populations, a routine 7- to 8-day course of antibiotics might be unlikely. These include patients who had initially inappropriate antibiotic therapy, those with severe immunocompromise (neutropenia or stem cell transplant), patients with highly antibiotic-resistant pathogens (*P aeruginosa*, carbapenem-resistant *Acinetobacter* spp, carbapenem-resistant *Enterobacteriaceae*), and those being treated with second-line antibiotic therapy (eg, colistin, tigecycline). A good practice statement in the European guidelines suggested that the use of PCT in these settings, with the aim of decreasing the length of antibiotic therapy, represents good clinical practice. Of note, the use of PCT has not been studied specifically

---

Box 1
Recommendations from the 2016 IDSA/ATS HAP/VAP guidelines not discussed in this review

Recommendation against use of the clinical pulmonary infection score to assist with the decision of whether to start antibiotics in patients with suspected VAP

Recommendation against routine antibiotic treatment of ventilator-associated tracheobronchitis

Recommendations for initial empiric antibiotic regimens for HAP

Pathogen-specific therapy

    Recommendation for use of either vancomycin or linezolid for treatment of HAP/VAP caused by MRSA

    Recommendation against aminoglycoside monotherapy for treatment of *Pseudomonas* HAP/VAP

    Recommendation for combination therapy for *Pseudomonas* HAP/VAP for patients in septic shock or high risk of death at the time antibiotic susceptibility results become known

    No specific antibiotic class recommended for the treatment of extended-spectrum β-lactamase-producing gram-negative bacilli

    Recommendation for either ampicillin/sulbactam or a carbapenem for susceptible *Acinetobacter* species and against tigecycline

Recommendation in favor of antibiotic de-escalation

Recommendation against use of the clinical pulmonary infection score to assist with the decision of how long to continue antibiotics for VAP

---

in any of these situations, either in original studies or as secondary/subgroup analyses of previously published studies.

OTHER RECOMMENDATIONS FOR HOSPITAL-ACQUIRED PNEUMONIA AND VENTILATOR-ASSOCIATED PNEUMONIA

Both the IDSA/ATS and the ERS guidelines included additional recommendations that are

---

Box 2
Recommendations from the 2017 European Respiratory Society Guidelines not discussed in this review

Recommendation against the routine use of biomarkers in patients being treated for nosocomial pneumonia to predict clinical response or likelihood of adverse outcomes

Recommendation against routine use of antibiotics for more than 3 days in patients with low probability of hospital-acquired pneumonia and no clinical deterioration within 3 days of symptom onset

Recommendation for the use of selective oral decontamination with nonabsorbable antibiotics to prevent VAP, in settings with low use of antibiotics (ICU with <1000 daily doses per patient days) and less than 5% prevalence of antibiotic-resistant bacteria

No recommendation on use of selective oral decontamination with chlorhexidine caused by unclear balance between potential reduction of pneumonia and increase in mortality

---

not discussed in this review. They are briefly listed in **Box 1** (IDSA/ATS guidelines) and **Box 2** (ERS guidelines).

SUMMARY

During the past 2 years, two guidelines for the diagnosis and treatment of patients with HAP and VAP were released. Although these guidelines have some notable differences in their recommendations, they share more similarities than differences. A common theme among both guidelines is that high-quality evidence is lacking for many of the most commonly encountered diagnostic and treatment decisions. It is hoped that the publication of these guidelines will serve to define the areas of greatest need for clinical and basic research in HAP/VAP.

REFERENCES

1. Metersky ML, Wang Y, Klompas M, et al. Trend in ventilator-associated pneumonia rates between 2005 and 2013. JAMA 2016;316:2427–9.
2. Melsen WG, Rovers MM, Groenwold RH, et al. Attributable mortality of ventilator-associated pneumonia: a meta-analysis of individual patient data from randomised prevention studies. Lancet Infect Dis 2013;13:665–71.
3. Kollef MH, Hamilton CW, Ernst FR. Economic impact of ventilator-associated pneumonia in a large matched cohort. Infect Control Hosp Epidemiol 2012;33:250–6.

4. Muscedere JG, Day A, Heyland DK. Mortality, attributable mortality, and clinical events as end points for clinical trials of ventilator-associated pneumonia and hospital-acquired pneumonia. Clin Infect Dis 2010; 51(Suppl 1):S120–5.

5. American Thoracic Society; Infectious Diseases Society of America. Guidelines for the management of adults with hospital-acquired, ventilator-associated, and healthcare-associated pneumonia. Am J Respir Crit Care Med 2005;171:388–416.

6. Kalil AC, Metersky ML, Klompas M, et al. Management of adults with hospital-acquired and ventilator-associated pneumonia: 2016 clinical practice guidelines by the infectious diseases society of America and the American Thoracic society. Clin Infect Dis 2016;63:e61–111.

7. Klompas M, Branson R, Eichenwald EC, et al. Strategies to prevent ventilator-associated pneumonia in acute care hospitals: 2014 update. Infect Control Hosp Epidemiol 2014;35(Suppl 2):S133–54.

8. Torres A, Niederman MS, Chastre J, et al. International ERS/ESICM/ESCMID/ALAT guidelines for the management of hospital-acquired pneumonia and ventilator-associated pneumonia: guidelines for the management of hospital-acquired pneumonia (HAP)/ventilator-associated pneumonia (VAP) of the European Respiratory Society (ERS), European Society of Intensive Care Medicine (ESICM), European Society of Clinical Microbiology and Infectious Diseases (ESCMID) and Asociacion Latinoamericana del Tórax (ALAT). Eur Respir J 2017;50 [pii:1700582].

9. Kunac A, Sifri ZC, Mohr AM, et al. Bacteremia and ventilator-associated pneumonia: a marker for contemporaneous extra-pulmonic infection. Surg Infect (Larchmt) 2014;15:77–83.

10. Luna CM, Videla A, Mattera J, et al. Blood cultures have limited value in predicting severity of illness and as a diagnostic tool in ventilator-associated pneumonia. Chest 1999;116(4):1075–84.

11. Berton DC, Kalil AC, Teixeira PJ. Quantitative versus qualitative cultures of respiratory secretions for clinical outcomes in patients with ventilator-associated pneumonia. Cochrane Database Syst Rev 2014;(10):CD006482.

12. Leone M, Garcin F, Bouvenot J, et al. Ventilator-associated pneumonia: breaking the vicious circle of antibiotic overuse. Crit Care Med 2007;35:379–85 [quizz: 386].

13. Luna CM, Vujacich P, Niederman MS, et al. Impact of BAL data on the therapy and outcome of ventilator-associated pneumonia. Chest 1997;111: 676–85.

14. Ferrer M, Liapikou A, Valencia M, et al. Validation of the American Thoracic Society-Infectious Diseases Society of America guidelines for hospital-acquired pneumonia in the intensive care unit. Clin Infect Dis 2010;50:945–52.

15. Restrepo MI, Peterson J, Fernandez JF, et al. Comparison of the bacterial etiology of early-onset and late-onset ventilator-associated pneumonia in subjects enrolled in 2 large clinical studies. Respir Care 2013;58:1220–5.

16. Martin-Loeches I, Deja M, Koulenti D, et al. Potentially resistant microorganisms in intubated patients with hospital-acquired pneumonia: the interaction of ecology, shock and risk factors. Intensive Care Med 2013;39:672–81.

17. Arvanitis M, Anagnostou T, Kourkoumpetis TK, et al. The impact of antimicrobial resistance and aging in VAP outcomes: experience from a large tertiary care center. PLoS One 2014;9:e89984.

18. Khan R, Al-Dorzi HM, Tamim HM, et al. The impact of onset time on the isolated pathogens and outcomes in ventilator associated pneumonia. J Infect Public Health 2016;9:161–71.

19. Ewig S, Torres A, El-Ebiary M, et al. Bacterial colonization patterns in mechanically ventilated patients with traumatic and medical head injury. Incidence, risk factors, and association with ventilator-associated pneumonia. Am J Respir Crit Care Med 1999;159:188–98.

20. Lepelletier D, Roquilly A, Demeure dit latte D, et al. Retrospective analysis of the risk factors and pathogens associated with early-onset ventilator-associated pneumonia in surgical-ICU head-trauma patients. J Neurosurg Anesthesiol 2010;22:32–7.

21. Leroy O, Jaffre S, D'Escrivan T, et al. Hospital-acquired pneumonia: risk factors for antimicrobial-resistant causative pathogens in critically ill patients. Chest 2003;123:2034–42.

22. Ekren PK, Ranzani OT, Ceccato A, et al. Evaluation of the 2016 Infectious Diseases Society of America/American Thoracic Society guideline criteria for risk of multidrug-resistant pathogens in patients with hospital-acquired and ventilator-associated pneumonia in the ICU. Am J Respir Crit Care Med 2018;197:826–30.

23. Chastre J, Wolff M, Fagon JY, et al. Comparison of 8 vs 15 days of antibiotic therapy for ventilator-associated pneumonia in adults: a randomized trial. JAMA 2003;290:2588–98.

24. Pugh R, Grant C, Cooke RP, et al. Short-course versus prolonged-course antibiotic therapy for hospital-acquired pneumonia in critically ill adults. Cochrane Database Syst Rev 2015;(8):CD007577.

25. Dimopoulos G, Poulakou G, Pneumatikos IA, et al. Short- vs long-duration antibiotic regimens for ventilator-associated pneumonia: a systematic review and meta-analysis. Chest 2013;144:1759–67.

26. Phase III study with Amikacin Inhale in intubated and mechanically ventilated patients with gram-negative pneumonia does not meet primary endpoint of superiority. 2017. https://www.prnewswire.com/news-releases/phase-iii-study-with-amikacin-inhale-in-intubated-and-mechanically-ventilated-patients-with-gram-negative-

pneumonia-does-not-meet-primary-endpoint-of-superiority-300561095.html. Accessed April 10, 2018.

27. Kollef MH, Ricard JD, Roux D, et al. A randomized trial of the Amikacin Fosfomycin inhalation system for the adjunctive therapy of gram-negative ventilator-associated pneumonia: IASIS trial. Chest 2017;151:1239–46.

28. Lux LJ, Posey RE, Daniels LS, et al. Pharmacokinetic/pharmacodynamic measures for guiding antibiotic treatment for hospital-acquired pneumonia. Rockville (MD): Agency for Healthcare Research and Quality; 2014.

29. Abdul-Aziz MH, Dulhunty JM, Bellomo R, et al. Continuous beta-lactam infusion in critically ill patients: the clinical evidence. Ann Intensive Care 2012;2:37.

30. Abdul-Aziz MH, Sulaiman H, Mat-Nor MB, et al. Beta-Lactam Infusion in Severe Sepsis (BLISS): a prospective, two-centre, open-labelled randomised controlled trial of continuous versus intermittent beta-lactam infusion in critically ill patients with severe sepsis. Intensive Care Med 2016;42: 1535–45.

31. Vardakas KZ, Voulgaris GL, Maliaros A, et al. Prolonged versus short-term intravenous infusion of antipseudomonal beta-lactams for patients with sepsis: a systematic review and meta-analysis of randomised trials. Lancet Infect Dis 2018;18: 108–20.

32. Stolz D, Smyrnios N, Eggimann P, et al. Procalcitonin for reduced antibiotic exposure in ventilator-associated pneumonia: a randomised study. Eur Respir J 2009;34:1364–75.

33. Bouadma L, Luyt CE, Tubach F, et al. Use of procalcitonin to reduce patients' exposure to antibiotics in intensive care units (PRORATA trial): a multicentre randomised controlled trial. Lancet 2010;375: 463–74.

34. Pontet J, Paciel D, Olivera W, et al. Procalcitonin (PCT) guided antibiotic treatment in ventilator associated pneumonia (VAP). Multi-centre, clinical prospective, randomized-controlled study. Am J Respir Crit Care Med 2007;175:A212.

35. de Jong E, van Oers JA, Beishuizen A, et al. Efficacy and safety of procalcitonin guidance in reducing the duration of antibiotic treatment in critically ill patients: a randomised, controlled, open-label trial. Lancet Infect Dis 2016;16:819–27.

36. Schuetz P, Wirz Y, Sager R, et al. Effect of procalcitonin-guided antibiotic treatment on mortality in acute respiratory infections: a patient level meta-analysis. Lancet Infect Dis 2018;18: 95–107.

Is Zero Ventilator-Associated Pneumonia Achievable?
Practical Approaches to Ventilator-Associated Pneumonia Prevention

Cristina Vazquez Guillamet, MD[a,b], Marin H. Kollef, MD[c],*

KEYWORDS

- Ventilator-associated pneumonia • Prevention bundle • Antimicrobial resistance • Chlorhexidine
- Selective digestive decontamination

KEY POINTS

- Ventilator-associated pneumonia (VAP) rates remain high across the world, including North America. These rates are predicated on long durations of mechanical ventilation and increasing rates of antimicrobial resistance.
- VAP prevention is a worthwhile goal, and designing an efficient bundle is a core measure for both governmental agencies and hospitals alike.
- Some previously recommended prevention measures have been questioned by recent data.

INTRODUCTION

Ventilator-associated pneumonia (VAP) accounts for approximately half of all nosocomial pneumonia cases and remains the most common infection in patients requiring mechanical ventilation (**Table 1**).[1] It is associated with additive mortality, prolonged length of stay both in the intensive care unit (ICU) and the hospital, greater antimicrobial use, and significant health care costs.[2,3] Therefore, the prevention of VAP has become a cornerstone quality improvement program for most governing bodies and ICUs.[4] Despite recent advances in microbiologic diagnostics and ICU-specific therapies, such as new antibiotics, the epidemiology and definition of VAP are still debated, rendering efforts aimed at VAP prevention and outcome data interpretation to be inconclusive.

The initial Centers for Disease Control and Prevention (CDC) VAP definition relied heavily on radiographic criteria for establishing this diagnosis. This infection was shown to add unwanted subjectivity to the already subjective nature of symptoms and physical signs interpretation within the VAP criteria.[5,6] Data reported to the CDC over the past 2 decades suggested a dramatic decrease in VAP rates in US hospitals, with some

Disclosures: Dr M.H. Kollef's efforts were supported by the Barnes-Jewish Hospital Foundation. Dr C. Vazquez Guillamet has no conflicts of interest to report.
[a] Division of Pulmonary, Critical Care, and Sleep Medicine, University of New Mexico School of Medicine, 2425 Camino de Salud, Albuquerque, NM 87106, USA; [b] Division of Infectious Diseases, University of New Mexico School of Medicine, 2425 Camino de Salud, Albuquerque, NM 87106, USA; [c] Division of Pulmonary and Critical Care Medicine, Washington University School of Medicine, 4523 Clayton Avenue, Campus Box 8052, St Louis, MO 63110, USA
* Corresponding author.
E-mail address: kollefm@wustl.edu

Clin Chest Med 39 (2018) 809–822
https://doi.org/10.1016/j.ccm.2018.08.004
0272-5231/18/© 2018 Elsevier Inc. All rights reserved.

chestmed.theclinics.com

Table 1
Recommendations for prevention of ventilator-associated pneumonia and applicable patient populations

Mechanism	Recommendation	Level of Support	Patient Population	Cons/Observations
Decrease duration/avoid mechanical ventilation	Consider NIPPV in certain types of respiratory failure, preintubation, or as weaning modalities	RCT[90,91]	COPD, certain types of hypoxemic respiratory failure	Delaying intubation when clinically indicated may jeopardize patient's stability
Decrease colonization with resistant pathogens	Optimal hand hygiene practices	Observational studies	All patients	Very low compliance rates[40,92]
Decrease colonization with resistant pathogens	Gown/glove isolation for patients with resistant bacteria	Observational studies	All patients	Universal gown/glove precautions only decreased MRSA acquisition rates as a secondary outcome[93]
Reduce duration of mechanical ventilation	Spontaneous breathing trials	RCT[28,34]	All patients	Low compliance rates
Reduce duration of mechanical ventilation	Spontaneous awakening trials	RCT[30,32]	All patients	None
Reduce duration of mechanical ventilation	Early mobilization	RCT[38,39]	All stable patients	Larger resources needed
Reduce aspiration	Head of bed elevation to 30°–45°	RCT[23,27–29]	All stable patients	None
Reduce aspiration	Avoid unnecessary suctioning and ventilatory circuit changes	RCT[42]	All patients	Safe practice, decreased costs when tubes changed only as needed
Decrease aspiration, reduce bacterial load to the airways	Orogastric tubes	Observational studies[61]	All patients	Lower rates of nosocomial sinusitis
Decrease oral bacterial load	Administer chlorhexidine-based oral care	RCT[76–78]	Postsurgical patients with short intubation	Recent trials showed increased mortality in medical intubated patients[28,80,81]
Decrease oral bacterial load	Administer topical oral antibiotics (SOD)	RTC[80]	ICUs with low antimicrobial resistance rates and low antibiotic utilization[a]	Unclear long-term impact on antimicrobial resistance in ICUs with moderate-, high-resistance rates

Goal	Intervention	Evidence	Population	Comments
Decrease oral and gastric bacterial load	Selective digestive decontamination	RCT[63-65]	Unclear	Unclear long-term impact on antimicrobial resistance in ICUs with moderate-, high-resistance rates
Decrease bacterial load in the airways	Subglottic drainage	RCT[43-45]	All patients	New data questioning benefit
Decrease bacterial load in the airways	Silver impregnated endotracheal tubes	RCT[57]	All patients especially at high risk for VAP	May not be cost-effective
Reduce bacterial load/improve dysbiosis	Probiotics	RCT[82]	All patients	Low-quality RCT
Reduce airway bacterial load	Inhaled antibiotics	Small RCT[87,88]	Patients colonized with or at high risk for MDR microbes	Studies combined parenteral and inhaled antibiotics
Reduce skin bacterial colonization	Perform chlorhexidine skin baths	RCT[94]	ICUs with high resistance rates, patients colonized with MRSA	Theoretic benefit, studies showed reduction in CLABSI and MRSA but not in VAP
Reduce gastric bacterial load	Avoid inappropriate use of proton-pump inhibitors	Observational studies[28,95]	Septic patients	Possible increased hospital-acquired pneumonia rates without lowering the gastrointestinal bleeding rates

Abbreviations: CLABSI, central line-associated blood stream infection; COPD, chronic obstructive pulmonary disease; MDR, multidrug resistant; NIPPV, noninvasive positive pressure ventilation; RCT, randomized controlled trial.

^a Less than 5% and daily antibiotic doses less than 1000 per 1000 d of admission.

hospitals achieving an impressive and unthinkable rate of zero episodes.[7,8] However, clinical data showed a different pattern, with VAP still being diagnosed by ICU clinicians and treated with antibiotics.[9,10] Although US rates were plummeting, VAP rates remained consistently higher (approximately 3- to 5-fold greater) in Western Europe and middle-income countries across 4 continents.[8–10] To balance this discrepancy between the rates of VAP reported by US hospitals and the rest of the world, as well as between hospital surveillance data and clinician diagnosed VAP, attempts were made at redefining VAP as part of the ventilator-associated events (VAEs) criteria.[11] The main changes from the old definition were excluding the radiographic criteria and adding a significant change in oxygenation that followed a period of 48 hours of clinical stability. VAEs, along with infection-related ventilator-associated complications (IVACs) and the possible and probable VAP criteria, have been proposed by the CDC as a methodology for improving the evaluation of medical care quality rendered in the ICU setting. Unfortunately, these new definitions do not seem to correlate well with the clinical understanding and incidence of VAP. It is reasonable to think that not all VAEs are VAPs, but it also appears that not all VAPs are VAEs, which leads to underestimating current rates of VAP.[12,13]

The diagnostic uncertainty and confusion around the diagnosis of VAP represent the first layer of complexity in VAP prevention. How do we define and assess VAP prevention in the context of fluctuating VAP definitions? Despite previous overly optimistic reports, newer data suggest that VAP is still prevalent in US ICUs at constant and predictable rates. When Medicare reviewers analyzed randomly selected postsurgical and medical patients admitted with acute myocardial infarction and congestive heart failure between 2006 and 2010, they discovered a constant VAP rate of approximately 10 cases per 100 ventilated patients.[14] In addition, ventilated hospital-acquired pneumonia (HAP) has been shown to be even more prevalent than VAP with a rising incidence, adding a significant burden to patients' risk of mortality and prolonged hospital stays.[15,16]

The second layer of complexity in understanding VAP prevention stems from the inherent limitations of before-after time series studies that examined the impact of prevention bundles on VAP rates. Randomized controlled double-blinded trials are ideally suited to minimize the subjectivity and inherent observer bias in assessing patient outcomes. Lack of subjectivity is not the case with before-after studies whereby observers' biases are likely to be prevalent. Also,

with frequent implementation and reinforcement, a cultural shift, similar to the acceptance of rapid response team initiatives, may have occurred, resulting in the routine acceptance of VAP prevention interventions. Health care providers have seemingly become more aware of the importance of preventing VAP as well as implementing prevention strategies that may or may not be part of the bundle components, potentially biasing any assessment of the true occurrence of VAP and the impact of VAP on patient outcomes. The contextual effect whereby multiple levels of variability (hospital population, type of ICU, patient characteristics) contribute to the outcome of interest may also weigh significantly on the interpretation of VAP prevention studies, especially those using before-after study designs.

Because VAP definitions are in flux, determining the benefits of VAP prevention may need to focus on other objective outcomes besides incidence rates. However, VAP attributable mortality is also difficult to discern with various studies citing a varying impact of attributable mortality from VAP ranging between 0% and 50%.[17,18] Mechanical ventilation-free days, length of stay, and antibiotic utilization may serve as more accurate and objective outcomes of interest to gauge the success of VAP prevention programs. Given the difficulties in adequately assessing the impact of VAP prevention strategies on patient outcomes, it is important to question whether it is really possible to achieve zero rates for this infection. Zero rates seems highly unlikely; nevertheless hospitals should attempt to reduce their VAP rates to the lowest degree possible in order to improve patient outcomes and reduce the use of antimicrobial agents. This review focuses on reviewing the practical evidence-based approaches for the prevention of VAP.

POTENTIAL STRATEGIES IN VENTILATOR-ASSOCIATED PNEUMONIA PREVENTION

VAP represents a heterogeneous disease affecting both medical and surgical ICU patients with different predisposing conditions thus resulting in variable incidence rates. The microbiology of VAP and resultant antibacterial treatment are dependent on host factors but also the duration of ventilation, hospital length of stay before pneumonia onset, and the spectrum of antibiotic-resistant microbes present within the hospital. The cost of VAP prevention strategies is also a relevant issue whereby more expensive prevention strategies or devices should be reserved for patients at the highest risk for developing VAP or for ICUs demonstrating a higher prevalence of infection attributed to antibiotic-resistant pathogens. The most useful and cost-effective strategies should generally be applied to at-risk patients in the ICU according to the availability of such resources at the local hospital level. Therefore, a multilevel approach may be more beneficial in thinking about how VAP prevention programs should be implemented in various patient populations, although such an approach could limit acceptance by health care providers.[19]

Many elements considered to have a significant impact on reducing the incidence of VAP have been investigated either solely or as part of a ventilator bundle. The most robust prevention bundles attempt to account for the dual pathogenesis of VAP, colonization with pathogenic bacteria, and aspiration of contaminated secretions, when designing the individual component elements included within the prevention bundle. However, the duration of mechanical ventilation is one of the most important determinants for the occurrence of VAP. Thus, preventing the need for intubation and mechanical ventilation in the first place and shortening the duration of mechanical ventilation should be key components of all prevention bundles. It has also been established that hospitalized patients become colonized with nosocomial microbes as early as 48 hours after admission, especially in the ICU setting. The implication of this is that clinicians should have a keen understanding of the predominant antibiotic-resistant microbes present within their hospitals when designing prevention strategies. Moreover, numerous host factors have been described increasing the likelihood of VAP attributed to antibiotic-resistant bacteria, including immune suppression, previous hospitalizations and antibiotic courses, and admission from nursing homes or long-term acute care facilities, where infection control practices may not be as rigorous as in acute care hospitals. These antibiotic-resistant infections are the VAPs that are most likely to impact patient outcomes due to the administration of ineffective antibiotic therapy and thus the ones that should be targeted for prevention.

Aspiration of contaminated oropharyngeal secretions or stomach contents refluxing into the oropharynx and then into the airways plays a paramount role in VAP pathogenesis and likely represents one of the most preventable factors that should be factored into the design of VAP prevention strategies. Radiolabeling studies clearly described passage of contaminated gastric contents into the airways via the pharynx in supine mechanically ventilated patients.[20] Similarly, other studies have shown the frequent occurrence of bacterial-laden oral secretions being aspirated into the bronchial tree as a potential starting point

for the VAP process.[21,22] Therefore, the most likely successful strategy for the prevention of VAP should be one that emphasizes shorter durations of mechanical ventilation, prevention of colonization of the aerodigestive tract with pathogenic bacteria, and prevention of the subsequent aspiration of bacterial contaminated secretions.

PRACTICAL APPROACHES TO VENTILATOR-ASSOCIATED PNEUMONIA PREVENTION

In designing a prevention bundle, clinicians must first consider the sine qua non elements that have been proven to impact VAP rates and ideally other objective outcomes. Easy application and cost-effectiveness may be desirable attributes, but additional considerations should include the potential for future changes in either patient population or predominant bacterial pathogens. Secondary elements can then be added to the baseline prevention bundle depending on the hospital's resources while also avoiding overburdening the health care teams. Sometimes less may be more effective as indiscriminate use of multiple interventions not tied to improved outcomes may lead to unnecessary workload increases and decreased compliance with the bundle elements.

CORE MEASURES

Some prevention measures have strong evidence to support their routine use, whereas others have been proven to be associated with decreased transmission and propagation of resistant microbes. Intuitively, all measures that shorten the duration of intubation and decrease the transmission of resistant microbes should positively impact rates of complications associated with mechanical ventilation, including VAP. Although many interventions have been tested as part of a prevention bundle, making it difficult to ascertain the relative weight or importance of the individual element, potential bundle elements are presented with the best supporting evidence.

Head of Bed Elevation to 30° to 45°

Bed elevation is probably one of the oldest and simplest prevention measures used after gastroesophageal reflux was shown to worsen in supine positioned patients.[20] However, one can also argue that semirecumbent positioning favors gravitational pulling of oropharyngeal secretions into the airways, making aspiration around endotracheal tube cuffs more likely.

A trial in 86 patients showed that semirecumbent positioning reduced the rates of clinically suspected and microbiologically proven nosocomial pneumonia by 4-fold.[23] Subsequent studies showed poor compliance with head of bed elevation,[24] but easy solutions like visual cues and small bedside devices are now available to improve compliance.[25,26] A Cochrane literature review based on small and potentially biased studies found an overall benefit in reducing VAP rates when patients were positioned at 30° to 60° versus 0° to 10°, but there was no significant difference in the occurrence of microbiologically confirmed episodes of VAP.[27]

While trying to discern the relative contribution of individual VAP bundle components, Klompas and colleagues[28] found that head of bed elevation was associated with relatively high rates of compliance (>85%) and faster times to extubation, but it did not significantly impact rates of possible VAP, IVACs, or VAEs.

Trying to counteract the gravitational disadvantage of the semirecumbent positioning, a large multicenter trial randomized patients to semirecumbent positioning versus the lateral Trendelenburg position.[29] Overall, the VAP incidence was very low in this trial at 0.5%, and even though there were fewer microbiologically confirmed cases of VAP in the lateral Trendelenburg group, none of the primary or secondary outcomes reached statistical significance. Moreover, greater numbers of adverse events were reported with the lateral Trendelenburg positioning, including vomiting, intracranial hemorrhage, and brachial plexus injury, making this an unacceptable component of any prevention bundle.

To date, the authors think that head of bed elevation to 30° to 45° provides the safest positioning for the prevention of VAP in hemodynamically stable patients. The availability of endotracheal tubes with subglottic suctioning also mitigates the gravitational pull of oropharyngeal secretions that might occur in the semirecumbent position. The simplicity and minimal risk of semirecumbent positioning, as well as its ability to facilitate patient mobility and weaning from mechanical ventilation compared with supine positioning, makes it a core element within prevention bundles.

Decrease Sedation: Daily Awakening Trials

In general, daily awakening trials have been associated with shortening the duration of mechanical ventilation by 2 to 4 days.[30] Reduced duration of mechanical ventilation has been extrapolated to result in decreased risk for VAP and has become part of the Society for Healthcare Epidemiology of America (SHEA) guidelines for VAP prevention. Kress and colleagues[30] randomized patients to daily sedation interruptions until awake, resulting

in shorter duration of mechanical ventilation (4.9 vs 7.3 days, $P = .004$) and shorter stays in the ICU. Analgesia alone without accompanying sedation may also provide the same benefit of shorter durations of mechanical ventilation based on a Danish study,[31] although both the control and the intervention groups had longer durations of mechanical ventilation compared with patients in the study by Kress and colleagues. When coupled with daily spontaneous breathing trials, the use of sedation interruption was associated with a larger number of ventilator-free days (14.7 vs 11.6, $P = .02$) and faster discharge from the ICU and the hospital as demonstrated in a multicenter trial of 336 patients.[32] Daily interruption in sedation was one of the strongest measures associated with higher likelihood of extubation, shorter hospital stay, and even lower ventilator mortality in the study by Klompas and colleagues[28] analyzing the association between individual bundle components and outcomes. A multicenter trial in 16 Canadian hospitals that relied on benzodiazepines as the main sedatives found no difference in duration of intubation between a nursing-driven protocol targeting light sedation and daily interruptions in sedation.[33] However, the total daily doses and boluses used in the interruption group were also higher than those used in the comparator group and those reported in previous studies. Taken together, the evidence in support of minimizing sedation to achieve more timely liberation from mechanical ventilation should be seen as a fundamental element of any ventilator or VAP bundle.

Spontaneous Breathing Trials

Many studies have described the positive impact of readiness assessment and spontaneous breathing trials in shortening the duration of mechanical ventilation, reducing ICU length of stay and costs associated with ICU hospitalization.[34] Subsequently, these interventions became protocolized, making their applicability more facile.[35,36] Heterogenous meta-analyses grouping randomized and quasi-randomized trials obtained the same results.[37] At the present time, daily sedation interruption and spontaneous breathing trials are performed synchronously. Unfortunately, daily breathing trials have been shown to have among the lowest compliance rates[28] compared with other prevention bundle elements and have primarily been associated with the prevention of VAEs but without a significant impact on possible VAP rates (odds ratio [OR] 0.7, 95% confidence interval [CI] 0.4-1.6, $P = .5$). Nevertheless, given the strong evidence linking VAP to more prolonged episodes of mechanical ventilation, the authors favor using spontaneous breathing trials as part of all ventilator bundles and VAP prevention bundles.

Early Mobilization

Along the same lines, physical therapy and early mobilization have been proven to be safe, even in high-risk patients, including those with acute respiratory distress syndrome, continuous renal replacement therapy, vasopressor requiring shock, and body mass indexes greater than 30, to shorten the length of mechanical ventilation.[38] When applied to patients already benefiting from daily sedation interruptions, the benefit of early mobilization resulted in further shortening of mechanical ventilation duration (ventilator-free days 23.5 vs 21.1, $P = .05$).[39] Therefore, early mobilization should be included in VAP prevention bundles along with daily spontaneous breathing and awakening trials.

Hand Hygiene

Hand hygiene with either soap or alcohol-based solutions has been repeatedly linked to decreased transmission of nosocomial pathogens and the occurrence of nosocomial infections. In a quasi-experimental study with interrupted time series analysis, a simple ventilator bundle that consisted only of hand hygiene, oral care with chlorhexidine, and health care provider education decreased VAP rates by 59%.[40] Nevertheless, hand hygiene remains the measure with the lowest compliance rates across prevention bundle components even as low as 10% to 15%.[41] The use of protective gloves and gowns when necessary for contact with individuals infected or colonized with highly resistant bacteria can also decrease the rate of transmission of multidrug-resistant pathogens.

Ventilator Circuit Manipulation

Maintenance of the ventilator circuit without needless disconnections and manipulation is safe and may decrease entry of bacteria into the trachea even though no impact on VAP rates has been noted.[42] Avoiding unnecessary suctioning may also protect against unneeded contamination of the bronchial tree with pathogenic bacteria.

ADDITIONAL ADJUNCTIVE PREVENTION MEASURES
Subglottic Drainage/Suctioning, Cuff Pressure Monitoring, and Endotracheal Tube Cuff Design

Subglottic drainage refers to specially designed endotracheal tubes that allow suctioning of contaminated oropharyngeal secretions that accumulate above the endotracheal tube cuff. By decreasing the quantity of these secretions and therefore the bacterial load that trickles in the lower airway, VAP may presumably be avoided. Many studies, including meta-analyses examining subglottic drainage, have shown a reduction in early-onset VAP rates by approximately 50%.[43–45] Randomized controlled trials have varied in terms of pneumonia definitions, expected durations of mechanical ventilation cutoffs, and suctioning techniques (continuous vs intermittent). The earliest meta-analysis by Dezfulian and colleagues[43] included 5 randomized trials and demonstrated shorter mechanical ventilation and also ICU length of stay with the use of subglottic drainage. A subsequent meta-analysis by Muscedere and colleagues[44] included 2442 patients from 13 trials and partially replicated the findings by Dezfulian and colleagues; however, the analyses for duration of mechanical ventilation and length of stay were biased by significant study heterogeneity. The most recent meta-analysis by Caroff and colleagues[45] included 4 newer trials but did not find the same benefit in terms of shorter durations of mechanical ventilation and overall length of stay. The findings within that meta-analysis were reinforced after excluding a Chinese study thought to be an outlier[46] that had contributed approximately 20% weight to the previous meta-analysis.

Ideally, endotracheal tube cuff pressures should be maintained at 25 to 30 cm H_2O to allow for optimal closure within the trachea, thus avoiding aspiration around the cuff while also minimizing the occurrence of tracheal ischemia. Small, single-center studies have looked at intermittent versus continuous cuff pressure monitoring (pneumatic or electronic devices) with conflicting results in terms of reducing aspiration, tracheal secretion bacterial loads, and incidence of VAP.[47–49] A larger study is underway to determine the role of continuous pneumatic cuff pressure monitoring in severe trauma patients and its impact on outcome.[50] However, a recent trial of 2 different manual cuff monitoring practices found that more frequent cuff pressure monitoring was not associated with any identifiable clinical outcome benefit, including VAP.[51]

It has also been postulated that various tube shapes (eg, tapered cuff) or materials (polyurethane) may help to hold the secretions above the cuff and avert microaspiration. Initial animal and small human studies showed contradictory results. Two randomized controlled trials also failed to find a benefit when using tapered cuffs or polyurethane tubes.[52,53] In the most recent trial, 326 patients were enrolled across 10 French ICUs looking at the advantage of tapered cuffs on microaspiration of gastric contents.[54] Microaspiration was measured using pepsin and salivary amylase levels in the tracheal aspirates, although a previous study found tracheal salivary amylase to only moderately correlate with microaspiration events (AUROC 0.56)[55] All outcomes including microaspiration and pneumonia rates were similar, but tracheo-bronchial bacterial colonization was less in the tapered cuff group.[54] Six randomized trials were included in the most recent meta-analysis that again failed to reveal a reduction in VAP rates in critically ill and postoperative patients receiving tapered endotracheal tube cuffs.[56]

A relative risk reduction of 36% for microbiologically confirmed VAP was observed in a large randomized trial using silver-coated endotracheal tubes to prevent VAP.[57] However, it is unclear whether the routine use of these coated tubes is cost-effective given their high cost and the relatively low incidence of VAP in many ICUs.[58,59]

Gastric Distention/Selective Gastric Decontamination

Clinically, gastric overdistention augments gastro-esophageal reflux and can contribute to microaspiration and macroaspiration events. Nasogastric or orogastric tubes are routinely inserted in mechanically ventilated patients for both enteral nutrition administration and also decompression of the stomach. However, routine monitoring of gastric residual volumes is not currently recommended based on a large randomized trial, and orogastric tubes are preferred to reduce the occurrence of nosocomial sinusitis.[60,61]

Selective digestive decontamination (SDD) has been a promising strategy in European countries with low incidences of resistant microbes, and it is now a core recommendation in the French guidelines on VAP prevention.[62] SDD is associated with not only decreasing VAP rates but also decreasing mortality and other objective outcomes.[63–65] In a large, cluster randomized, cross-over Dutch study including close to 6000 ICU patients, SDD was compared with selective oral decontamination (SOD) and regular care.[64] The initial study was retracted and revised after it was discovered that the control and intervention periods were misclassified for one of the 16 participating ICUs. SOD included colistin, tobramycin, and amphotericin paste, whereas these agents were also administered via a nasogastric tube for the patients in the SDD arm. A third-generation cephalosporin was also given for the initial 4 days intravenously for patients in the SDD group. The results favored SDD in terms of mortality, ICU length of stay, bacteremia, and candidemia rates but also reduced rectal carriage of resistant microbes. However, there was an increase in the isolation of aminoglycoside-resistant gram-negative bacteria among patients in the SDD group. When examining the patient population from one of the participating ICUs, it was noted that the VAP rates were approximately half in the SDD group compared with SOD.[66] However, the main concern regarding the routine use of SDD and SOD is the long-term detrimental effect of these agents on antimicrobial resistance. Use of third-generation cephalosporins may increase the rates of methicillin-resistant *Staphylococcus aureus* (MRSA), extended-spectrum β-lactamase *Enterobacteriaceae*, and *Pseudomonas aeruginosa*, which usually arise after previous exposure to antibiotics.

No increased resistance to aminoglycosides or colistin was noted among sites using SDD and SOD in prior studies[67,68]; in fact, decreased colonization with antibiotic-resistant strains and lower overall rates of resistance to third-generation cephalosporins was described during some of the larger SDD trials.[69,70] Although a transient increase in the rate of susceptible *S aureus* and *Enterococcus fecalis* were reported at the initiation of SDD, these effects reportedly dissolved after 5 years of SDD utilization.[71] Oostdijk and colleagues[72] looked at the ecological effects of SDD and SOD in all ICU patients, not only the ones who had received SDD or SOD. Both rectal and respiratory colonization with ceftazidime-resistant strains more than doubled after the end of the SDD period after initially declining during the SDD period (from 5% to 15%, $P = .05$ for the trend of ceftazidime resistance in respiratory samples). Other interesting findings came from a recent Dutch study that followed mechanically ventilated patients receiving SDD between 2011 and 2015.[73] The investigators found that rectal colonization with gram-negative bacteria correlated with ICU-acquired infections, more than half being respiratory tract infections. The congruence between the rectal colonizing species and respiratory species was low at 35%, questioning the role of gastrointestinal bacteria in producing VAP. More importantly, it remains to be seen which patient populations would benefit the most from the use of SDD and SOD especially in countries with higher rates of patient colonization with antimicrobial-resistant bacteria.

Considering all these aspects from the available clinical trials, and the potential impact on bacterial resistance from escalating the routine use of SDD and SOD, the authors agree with the European guidelines on VAP prevention recommending SOD but not SDD in ICUs with low antimicrobial resistance rates less than 5% and low antibiotic consumption (<1000 daily doses per 1000 admission days).[74]

Oral Care/Selective Oral Decontamination

Because aspiration of oropharyngeal secretions seems to be the principal mechanism for the development of VAP, a plethora of modalities trying to curb the oral bacterial load have been tested. These modalities have ranged from brushing teeth with toothpaste to the oral application of antiseptics (chlorhexidine and povidone iodine) and topical antibiotics such as SOD.

Based on 4 studies, tooth brushing did not reduce the incidence of VAP or other objective outcomes.[75] Antiseptics were thought to be ideal tools in oral care, and initial randomized trials in cardiac surgery patients showed a benefit in reducing VAP rates and at times mortality.[76] In subsequent meta-analyses, it seemed the benefit was not so striking for povidone iodine as it was for chlorhexidine and that the main achievement was lower VAP rates without significant impact on mortality or duration of ventilation and ICU stays.[77–79] More recent studies have questioned chlorhexidine's positive role. When isolating the impact on mortality using a network meta-analysis methodology, British investigators found chlorhexidine to augment the risk of dying in a general ICU population[80] (OR 1.25, 95% CI 1.05–1.5). However, in the same study, SDD was the most beneficial in terms of improving outcomes with OR 0.73 (0.64–0.84), whereas SOD had OR of 0.85 (0.74–0.97). In a detailed meta-analysis, Klompas and colleagues[81] found that the benefit of VAP reduction with chlorhexidine of approximately 27% was mainly derived from studies in cardiac surgery patients. For noncardiac patients, the OR crossed 1 (OR 0.78, 95% CI 0.6-1.02), and the investigators also discovered that chlorhexidine may increase the risk of dying in these patients, although this finding did not reach statistical significance (relative risk 1.13, 0.99–1.29). The same group found a stronger association between chlorhexidine use and ventilator mortality when analyzing the bundle components separately (hazard ratio 1.6, 95% CI 1.2-2.3, $P = .06$).[28] Taking into account these findings, the European Respiratory Society guidelines favored SOD but did not make any recommendation on chlorhexidine use for VAP prevention.[74]

Probiotics

Use of probiotics has been associated with improved VAP rates but without significant changes in mortality, duration of mechanical ventilation, and length of stay.[82] A feasibility pilot trial in Canada and the United States returned supporting findings so the results of a large randomized trail looking at the impact of *Lactobacillus rhamnosus* on VAP will further the topic.[83]

BUNDLE COMPLIANCE

Just recommending a list of bundled measures will never suffice. Health care providers need to be engaged and be active participants in the quality improvement process. A sustained effort is expected along with auditing, feedback, and continuous education. In general, the higher the compliance rates with the proposed bundles, the better the outcomes, although some studies recorded improved VAP rates even with compliance less than 30%.[41] Studies have also shown that a higher level of understanding of VAP among health care providers helps to improve compliance rates.[84] The highest reductions in VAP rates have been achieved with sequential introduction of mandatory measures, but it can take up to 1 to 2 years for the full benefit to be seen.[85] Compliance rates vary across bundle components,[41,84] but it remains unclear which bundle elements should be focused on given the significant interactions between these elements in the available studies. It is expected that compliance with bundle elements will wane over time in the absence of constant reinforcement and that there is a threshold effect beyond which VAP incidence cannot be lowered any further even in the presence of well-constructed and managed prevention programs.[86]

Because VAP represents the consequence of prolonged mechanical ventilation and also the bacterial load that gains access to the lower respiratory tract, the future holds promise in introducing new approaches to counteract these mechanisms. There is hope that inhaled antibiotics could be delivered in high concentrations to the airways, thereby reducing the presence of resistant microbes and decreasing the risk of VAP and the need for systemic antibiotics.[87,88] Studies so far have used inhaled and systemic antibiotics concomitantly for treatment of respiratory infections without long-term follow-up. Lessons extrapolated from the neutropenic fever literature suggest that the use of nonabsorbable antibiotics may not fully prevent serious infections, and thus, the need for preventive systemic antibiotics in patients at high risk seems reasonable for future investigation.

Immune therapies like monoclonal antibodies and targeted vaccines may also gain a niche in the prevention and treatment of VAP[89] as they have shown promise as adjunctive therapies for pneumonia.

COST-EFFECTIVENESS

With a myriad of available interventions, cost-effectiveness becomes relevant. Unfortunately cost-effectiveness is a very dynamic process, and the medical costs change for interventions that have been accepted over long periods of time. Branch-Elliman and colleagues[58] tried to identify the most cost-effective strategy for VAP prevention from both hospital and societal perspectives. From the hospital standpoint, the Institute for Healthcare Improvement VAP prevention bundle, subglottic suctioning, and probiotics were found to be preferred. The preferred methods from the societal perspective included oral care with chlorhexidine and SDD. Cost-effectiveness goals could also differ between various types of ICUs and types of patients, and they should also consider the impact on longer-term outcomes, including the emergence of antimicrobial resistance.

SUMMARY

In an era dominated by antimicrobial resistance that defines nosocomial pneumonia, especially VAP, it is unlikely that our vulnerable, immunocompromised patients requiring prolonged hospitalizations for new surgeries or cancer treatments will not be at risk for developing VAP. Better defining VAP in an honest manner is needed so the impact of VAP on patient outcomes and the impact of prevention bundles on VAP incidence can truly be appreciated. If VAP remains a subjective, elusive diagnosis, the focus should be on objective improvements like ventilator-free days, length of stay, and antibiotic use. Prevention bundles should generally be as simple as possible, made up of evidence-based interventions, but also taking into account variables that determine long-term compliance rates and workload burden. In the future, new mathematical models may be able to identify which prevention strategies would perform best in hospitals with high rates versus low rates of bacterial resistance, or surgical versus medical ICUs, therefore creating a more ICU personalized efficient bundle.

REFERENCES

1. Vincent JL, Bihari DJ, Suter PM, et al. The prevalence of nosocomial infection in intensive care units in Europe. Results of the European Prevalence of Infection in Intensive Care (EPIC) study. EPIC International Advisory Committee. JAMA 1995;274:639–44.
2. Melsen WG, Rovers MM, Groenwold RHH, et al. Attributable mortality of ventilator-associated pneumonia: a meta-analysis of individual patient data from randomised prevention studies. Lancet Infect Dis 2013;13:665–71.
3. Kollef MH, Hamilton CW, Ernst FR. Economic impact of ventilator-associated pneumonia in a large matched cohort. Infect Control Hosp Epidemiol 2012;33:250–6.
4. Klompas M, Branson R, Eichenwald EC, et al. Strategies to prevent ventilator-associated pneumonia in acute care hospitals: 2014 update. Infect Control Hosp Epidemiol 2014;35:915–36.
5. Wunderink RG, Woldenberg LS, Zeiss J, et al. The radiologic diagnosis of autopsy-proven ventilator-associated pneumonia. Chest 1992;101:458–63.
6. Klompas M. Interobserver variability in ventilator-associated pneumonia surveillance. Am J Infect Control 2010;38:237–9.
7. Dudeck MA, Weiner LM, Allen-Bridson K, et al. National Healthcare Safety Network (NHSN) report, data summary for 2012, device-associated module. Am J Infect Control 2013;41:1148–66.
8. Rosenthal VD, Al-Abdely HM, El-Kholy AA, et al. International nosocomial infection control consortium report, data summary of 50 countries for 2010-2015: device-associated module. Am J Infect Control 2016;44:1495–504.
9. Kollef MH, Chastre J, Fagon J-Y, et al. Global prospective epidemiologic and surveillance study of ventilator-associated pneumonia due to Pseudomonas aeruginosa. Crit Care Med 2014;42:2178–87.
10. Skrupky LP, McConnell K, Dallas J, et al. A comparison of ventilator-associated pneumonia rates as identified according to the National Healthcare Safety Network and American College of Chest Physicians criteria. Crit Care Med 2012;40:281–4.
11. Magill SS, Klompas M, Balk R, et al. Developing a new, national approach to surveillance for ventilator-associated events: executive summary. Clin Infect Dis 2013;57:1742–6.
12. Kobayashi H, Uchino S, Takinami M, et al. The impact of ventilator-associated events in critically ill subjects with prolonged mechanical ventilation. Respir Care 2017;62:1379–86.
13. Fan Y, Gao F, Wu Y, et al. Does ventilator-associated event surveillance detect ventilator-associated pneumonia in intensive care units? A systematic review and meta-analysis. Crit Care 2016;20:338.
14. Metersky ML, Wang Y, Klompas M, et al. Trend in ventilator-associated pneumonia rates between 2005 and 2013. JAMA 2016;316:2427–9.
15. Esperatti M, Ferrer M, Theessen A, et al. Nosocomial pneumonia in the intensive care unit acquired by mechanically ventilated versus nonventilated patients. Am J Respir Crit Care Med 2010;182:1533–9.
16. Giuliano KK, Baker D, Quinn B. The epidemiology of nonventilator hospital-acquired pneumonia in the United States. Am J Infect Control 2018;46(3):322–7.

17. Bekaert M, Timsit J-F, Vansteelandt S, et al. Attributable mortality of ventilator-associated pneumonia: a reappraisal using causal analysis. Am J Respir Crit Care Med 2011;184:1133–9.

18. Nguile-Makao M, Zahar J-R, Français A, et al. Attributable mortality of ventilator-associated pneumonia: respective impact of main characteristics at ICU admission and VAP onset using conditional logistic regression and multi-state models. Intensive Care Med 2010;36:781–9.

19. Kollef MH. Ventilator-associated pneumonia prevention. Is it worth it? Am J Respir Crit Care Med 2015; 192:5–7.

20. Torres A, Serra-Batlles J, Ros E, et al. Pulmonary aspiration of gastric contents in patients receiving mechanical ventilation: the effect of body position. Ann Intern Med 1992;116:540–3.

21. Garrouste-Orgeas M, Chevret S, Arlet G, et al. Oropharyngeal or gastric colonization and nosocomial pneumonia in adult intensive care unit patients. A prospective study based on genomic DNA analysis. Am J Respir Crit Care Med 1997;156:1647–55.

22. Bonten MJ, Gaillard CA, van Tiel FH, et al. The stomach is not a source for colonization of the upper respiratory tract and pneumonia in ICU patients. Chest 1994;105:878–84.

23. Drakulovic MB, Torres A, Bauer TT, et al. Supine body position as a risk factor for nosocomial pneumonia in mechanically ventilated patients: a randomised trial. Lancet 1999;354:1851–8.

24. van Nieuwenhoven CA, Vandenbroucke-Grauls C, van Tiel FH, et al. Feasibility and effects of the semirecumbent position to prevent ventilator-associated pneumonia: a randomized study. Crit Care Med 2006;34:396–402.

25. Williams Z, Chan R, Kelly E. A simple device to increase rates of compliance in maintaining 30-degree head-of-bed elevation in ventilated patients. Crit Care Med 2008;36:1155–7.

26. Wolken RF, Woodruff RJ, Smith J, et al. Observational study of head of bed elevation adherence using a continuous monitoring system in a medical intensive care unit. Respir Care 2012;57: 537–43.

27. Wang L, Li X, Yang Z, et al. Semi-recumbent position versus supine position for the prevention of ventilator-associated pneumonia in adults requiring mechanical ventilation. Cochrane Database Syst Rev 2016;(1):CD009946.

28. Klompas M, Li L, Kleinman K, et al. Associations between ventilator bundle components and outcomes. JAMA Intern Med 2016;176:1277–83.

29. Li Bassi G, Panigada M, Ranzani OT, et al. Randomized, multicenter trial of lateral Trendelenburg versus semirecumbent body position for the prevention of ventilator-associated pneumonia. Intensive Care Med 2017;43:1572–84.

30. Kress JP, Pohlman AS, O'Connor MF, et al. Daily interruption of sedative infusions in critically ill patients undergoing mechanical ventilation. N Engl J Med 2000;342:1471–7.

31. Strøm T, Martinussen T, Toft P. A protocol of no sedation for critically ill patients receiving mechanical ventilation: a randomised trial. Lancet 2010;375: 475–80.

32. Girard TD, Kress JP, Fuchs BD, et al. Efficacy and safety of a paired sedation and ventilator weaning protocol for mechanically ventilated patients in intensive care (Awakening and Breathing Controlled trial): a randomised controlled trial. Lancet 2008; 371:126–34.

33. Mehta S, Burry L, Cook D, et al. Daily sedation interruption in mechanically ventilated critically ill patients cared for with a sedation protocol: a randomized controlled trial. JAMA 2012;308: 1985–92.

34. Ely EW, Baker AM, Dunagan DP, et al. Effect on the duration of mechanical ventilation of identifying patients capable of breathing spontaneously. N Engl J Med 1996;335:1864–9.

35. Kollef MH, Shapiro SD, Silver P, et al. A randomized, controlled trial of protocol-directed versus physician-directed weaning from mechanical ventilation. Crit Care Med 1997;25:567–74.

36. Lellouche F, Mancebo J, Jolliet P, et al. A multicenter randomized trial of computer-driven protocolized weaning from mechanical ventilation. Am J Respir Crit Care Med 2006;174:894–900.

37. Blackwood B, Burns KEA, Cardwell CR, et al. Protocolized versus non-protocolized weaning for reducing the duration of mechanical ventilation in critically ill adult patients. Cochrane Database Syst Rev 2014;(11):CD006904.

38. Pohlman MC, Schweickert WD, Pohlman AS, et al. Feasibility of physical and occupational therapy beginning from initiation of mechanical ventilation. Crit Care Med 2010;38:2089–94.

39. Schweickert WD, Pohlman MC, Pohlman AS, et al. Early physical and occupational therapy in mechanically ventilated, critically ill patients: a randomised controlled trial. Lancet 2009;373: 1874–82.

40. Su K-C, Kou YR, Lin F-C, et al. A simplified prevention bundle with dual hand hygiene audit reduces early-onset ventilator-associated pneumonia in cardiovascular surgery units: an interrupted time-series analysis. PLoS One 2017;12:e0182252.

41. Rello J, Afonso E, Lisboa T, et al. A care bundle approach for prevention of ventilator-associated pneumonia. Clin Microbiol Infect 2013;19:363–9.

42. Kollef MH, Shapiro SD, Fraser VJ, et al. Mechanical ventilation with or without 7-day circuit changes. A randomized controlled trial. Ann Intern Med 1995; 123:168–74.

43. Dezfulian C, Shojania K, Collard HR, et al. Subglottic secretion drainage for preventing ventilator-associated pneumonia: a meta-analysis. Am J Med 2005;118:11–8.

44. Muscedere J, Rewa O, McKechnie K, et al. Subglottic secretion drainage for the prevention of ventilator-associated pneumonia: a systematic review and meta-analysis. Crit Care Med 2011;39:1985–91.

45. Caroff DA, Li L, Muscedere J, et al. Subglottic secretion drainage and objective outcomes: a systematic review and meta-analysis. Crit Care Med 2016;44:830–40.

46. Zheng R-Q, Lin H, Shao J, et al. A clinical study of subglottic secretion drainage for prevention of ventilation associated pneumonia. Zhongguo Wei Zhong Bing Ji Jiu Yi Xue 2008;20:338–40 [in Chinese].

47. Sole ML, Penoyer DA, Su X, et al. Assessment of endotracheal cuff pressure by continuous monitoring: a pilot study. Am J Crit Care 2009;18:133–43.

48. Nseir S, Lorente L, Ferrer M, et al. Continuous control of tracheal cuff pressure for VAP prevention: a collaborative meta-analysis of individual participant data. Ann Intensive Care 2015;5:43.

49. Nseir S, Zerimech F, Fournier C, et al. Continuous control of tracheal cuff pressure and microaspiration of gastric contents in critically ill patients. Am J Respir Crit Care Med 2011;184:1041–7.

50. Marjanovic N, Frasca D, Asehnoune K, et al. Multicentre randomised controlled trial to investigate the usefulness of continuous pneumatic regulation of tracheal cuff pressure for reducing ventilator-associated pneumonia in mechanically ventilated severe trauma patients: the AGATE study protocol. BMJ Open 2017;7:e017003.

51. Letvin A, Kremer P, Silver PC, et al. Frequent versus infrequent monitoring of endotracheal tube cuff pressures. Respir Care 2018;63(5):495–501.

52. Monsel A, Lu Q, Le Corre M, et al. Tapered-cuff endotracheal tube does not prevent early postoperative pneumonia compared with spherical-cuff endotracheal tube after major vascular surgery: a randomized controlled trial. Anesthesiology 2016;124:1041–52.

53. Philippart F, Gaudry S, Quinquis L, et al. Randomized intubation with polyurethane or conical cuffs to prevent pneumonia in ventilated patients. Am J Respir Crit Care Med 2015;191:637–45.

54. Jaillette E, Brunin G, Girault C, et al. Impact of tracheal cuff shape on microaspiration of gastric contents in intubated critically ill patients: study protocol for a randomized controlled trial. Trials 2015;16:429.

55. Dewavrin F, Zerimech F, Boyer A, et al. Accuracy of alpha amylase in diagnosing microaspiration in intubated critically-ill patients. PLoS One 2014;9:e90851.

56. Maertens B, Blot K, Blot S. Prevention of ventilator-associated and early postoperative pneumonia through tapered endotracheal tube cuffs: a systematic review and meta-analysis of randomized controlled trials. Crit Care Med 2018;46:316–23.

57. Kollef MH, Afessa B, Anzueto A, et al. Silver-coated endotracheal tubes and incidence of ventilator-associated pneumonia: the NASCENT randomized trial. JAMA 2008;300:805–13.

58. Branch-Elliman W, Wright SB, Howell MD. Determining the ideal strategy for ventilator-associated pneumonia prevention. Cost-benefit analysis. Am J Respir Crit Care Med 2015;192:57–63.

59. Shorr AF, Zilberberg MD, Kollef M. Cost-effectiveness analysis of a silver-coated endotracheal tube to reduce the incidence of ventilator-associated pneumonia. Infect Control Hosp Epidemiol 2009;30:759–63.

60. Reignier J, Mercier E, Le Gouge A, et al. Effect of not monitoring residual gastric volume on risk of ventilator-associated pneumonia in adults receiving mechanical ventilation and early enteral feeding: a randomized controlled trial. JAMA 2013;309:249–56.

61. George DL, Falk PS, Umberto Meduri G, et al. Nosocomial sinusitis in patients in the medical intensive care unit: a prospective epidemiological study. Clin Infect Dis 1998;27:463–70.

62. Leone M, Bouadma L, Bouhemad B, et al. Hospital-acquired pneumonia in ICU. Anaesth Crit Care Pain Med 2018;37:83–98.

63. de Smet AM, Kluytmans JA, Cooper BS, et al. Decontamination of the digestive tract and oropharynx in ICU patients. N Engl J Med 2009;360:20–31.

64. Oostdijk EAN, Kesecioglu J, Schultz MJ, et al. Notice of retraction and replacement: Oostdijk et al. Effects of decontamination of the oropharynx and intestinal tract on antibiotic resistance in ICUs: a randomized clinical trial. JAMA. 2014;312(14):1429-1437. JAMA 2017;317:1583–4.

65. Roquilly A, Marret E, Abraham E, et al. Pneumonia prevention to decrease mortality in intensive care unit: a systematic review and meta-analysis. Clin Infect Dis 2015;60:64–75.

66. Bos LD, Stips C, Schouten LR, et al. Selective decontamination of the digestive tract halves the prevalence of ventilator-associated pneumonia compared to selective oral decontamination. Intensive Care Med 2017;43:1535–7.

67. Daneman N, Sarwar S, Fowler RA, et al, SuDDICU Canadian Study Group. Effect of selective decontamination on antimicrobial resistance in intensive care units: a systematic review and meta-analysis. Lancet Infect Dis 2013;13:328–41.

68. Wittekamp BHJ, Oostdijk EAN, de Smet AMGA, et al. Colistin and tobramycin resistance during

long- term use of selective decontamination strategies in the intensive care unit: a post hoc analysis. Crit Care 2015;19:113.

69. de Smet AM, Kluytmans JA, Blok HE, et al. Selective digestive tract decontamination and selective oropharyngeal decontamination and antibiotic resistance in patients in intensive-care units: an open-label, clustered group-randomised, crossover study. Lancet Infect Dis 2011;11:372–80.

70. Houben AJM, Oostdijk E a N, van der Voort PHJ, et al. Selective decontamination of the oropharynx and the digestive tract, and antimicrobial resistance: a 4 year ecological study in 38 intensive care units in The Netherlands. J Antimicrob Chemother 2014;69: 797–804.

71. van der Bij AK, Frentz D, Bonten MJM, ISIS-AR Study Group. Gram-positive cocci in Dutch ICUs with and without selective decontamination of the oropharyngeal and digestive tract: a retrospective database analysis. J Antimicrob Chemother 2016; 71:816–20.

72. Oostdijk EAN, de Smet AMGA, Blok HEM, et al. Ecological effects of selective decontamination on resistant gram-negative bacterial colonization. Am J Respir Crit Care Med 2010;181:452–7.

73. Frencken JF, Wittekamp BHJ, Plantinga NL, et al. Associations between enteral colonization with gram-negative bacteria and intensive care unit-acquired infections and colonization of the respiratory tract. Clin Infect Dis 2018;66:497–503.

74. Torres A, Niederman MS, Chastre J, et al. International ERS/ESICM/ESCMID/ALAT guidelines for the management of hospital-acquired pneumonia and ventilator-associated pneumonia: guidelines for the management of hospital-acquired pneumonia (HAP)/ventilator-associated pneumonia (VAP) of the European Respiratory Society (ERS), European Society of Intensive Care Medicine (ESICM), European Society of Clinical Microbiology and Infectious Diseases (ESCMID) and Asociación Latinoamericana del Tórax (ALAT). Eur Respir J 2017;50(3) [pii: 1700582].

75. Gu W-J, Gong Y-Z, Pan L, et al. Impact of oral care with versus without toothbrushing on the prevention of ventilator-associated pneumonia: a systematic review and meta-analysis of randomized controlled trials. Crit Care 2012;16:R190.

76. DeRiso AJ, Ladowski JS, Dillon TA, et al. Chlorhexidine gluconate 0.12% oral rinse reduces the incidence of total nosocomial respiratory infection and nonprophylactic systemic antibiotic use in patients undergoing heart surgery. Chest 1996;109: 1556–61.

77. Labeau SO, Van de Vyver K, Brusselaers N, et al. Prevention of ventilator-associated pneumonia with oral antiseptics: a systematic review and meta-analysis. Lancet Infect Dis 2011;11:845–54.

78. Chan EY, Ruest A, Meade MO, et al. Oral decontamination for prevention of pneumonia in mechanically ventilated adults: systematic review and meta-analysis. BMJ 2007;334:889.

79. Hua F, Xie H, Worthington HV, et al. Oral hygiene care for critically ill patients to prevent ventilator-associated pneumonia. Cochrane Database Syst Rev 2016;10:CD008367.

80. Price R, MacLennan G, Glen J, SuDDICU Collaboration. Selective digestive or oropharyngeal decontamination and topical oropharyngeal chlorhexidine for prevention of death in general intensive care: systematic review and network meta-analysis. BMJ 2014;348:g2197.

81. Klompas M, Speck K, Howell MD, et al. Reappraisal of routine oral care with chlorhexidine gluconate for patients receiving mechanical ventilation: systematic review and meta-analysis. JAMA Intern Med 2014;174:751–61.

82. Bo L, Li J, Tao T, et al. Probiotics for preventing ventilator-associated pneumonia. Cochrane Database Syst Rev 2014;(10):CD009066.

83. Cook DJ, Johnstone J, Marshall JC, et al. Probiotics: prevention of severe pneumonia and endotracheal colonization trial-PROSPECT: a pilot trial. Trials 2016;17:377.

84. Darawad MW, Sa'aleek MA, Shawashi T. Evidence-based guidelines for prevention of ventilator-associated pneumonia: evaluation of intensive care unit nurses' adherence. Am J Infect Control 2018; 46(6):711–3.

85. Bouadma L, Mourvillier B, Deiler V, et al. A multifaceted program to prevent ventilator associated pneumonia: impact on compliance with preventive measures. Crit Care Med 2010;38: 789–96.

86. Rosenthal VD, Rodrigues C, Álvarez-Moreno C, et al. Effectiveness of a multidimensional approach for prevention of ventilator-associated pneumonia in adult intensive care units from 14 developing countries of four continents: findings of the International Nosocomial Infection Control Consortium. Crit Care Med 2012;40:3121–8.

87. Palmer LB, Smaldone GC. Reduction of bacterial resistance with inhaled antibiotics in the intensive care unit. Am J Respir Crit Care Med 2014;189: 1225–33.

88. Falagas ME, Siempos II, Bliziotis IA, et al. Administration of antibiotics via the respiratory tract for the prevention of ICU-acquired pneumonia: a meta-analysis of comparative trials. Crit Care 2006;10: R123.

89. Que Y-A, Lazar H, Wolff M, et al. Assessment of panobacumab as adjunctive immunotherapy for the treatment of nosocomial Pseudomonas aeruginosa pneumonia. Eur J Clin Microbiol Infect Dis 2014; 33:1861–7.

90. Girou E, Brun-Buisson C, Taillé S, et al. Secular trends in nosocomial infections and mortality associated with noninvasive ventilation in patients with exacerbation of COPD and pulmonary edema. JAMA 2003;290:2985–91.

91. Burns KEA, Meade MO, Premji A, et al. Noninvasive positive-pressure ventilation as a weaning strategy for intubated adults with respiratory failure. Cochrane Database Syst Rev 2013;(12):CD004127.

92. Allegranzi B, Pittet D. Role of hand hygiene in healthcare-associated infection prevention. J Hosp Infect 2009;73:305–15.

93. Harris AD, Pineles L, Belton B, et al. Universal glove and gown use and acquisition of antibiotic-resistant bacteria in the ICU: a randomized trial. JAMA 2013; 310:1571–80.

94. Frost SA, Alogso M-C, Metcalfe L, et al. Chlorhexidine bathing and health care-associated infections among adult intensive care patients: a systematic review and meta-analysis. Crit Care 2016;20:379.

95. Sasabuchi Y, Matsui H, Lefor AK, et al. Risks and benefits of stress ulcer prophylaxis for patients with severe sepsis. Crit Care Med 2016;44:e464–9.

Aerosol Therapy for Pneumonia in the Intensive Care Unit

Charles-Edouard Luyt, MD, PhD[a], Guillaume Hékimian, MD[a],
Nicolas Bréchot, MD, PhD[a], Jean Chastre, MD[a,b,*]

KEYWORDS

- Ventilator-associated pneumonia • Aerosol • Amikacin • Colistin

KEY POINTS

- Aerosol antibiotic administration may allow achieving very high drug concentrations at the infection site in the lung, with low systemic absorption.
- However, optimal deposition in the tracheobronchial tree and alveolar compartment requires specific devices, drug formulations and ventilator settings, with close clinical monitoring.
- To date, antibiotic aerosolization in adults with pneumonia can only be recommended when the infection is caused by extensively resistant pathogens only susceptible to antibiotics with limited efficacy and high toxicity when given by the IV route (ie, aminoglycosides and colistin).

INTRODUCTION

Hospital-acquired pneumonia (HAP), including ventilator-associated pneumonia (VAP), is still a common intensive care unit (ICU) infection, with a high attributable morbidity and mortality. With current standard-of-care therapy, clinical success rates are often less than 60%, related to the many challenges that encompass antibiotic therapy in critically ill patients, including alterations in pharmacokinetics (PK) and pharmacodynamics (PD), relative low penetration of most antibiotics into the lung tissue, and the frequency of difficult-to-treat or highly resistant pathogens in that setting.[1]

Aerosol antibiotic administration offers the theoretic advantages of achieving high drug concentrations at the infection site, considerably more than the minimal inhibitory concentration (MIC) of most causative microorganisms, and low systemic absorption, thereby avoiding toxicity, particularly the renal toxicity of aminoglycosides or colistin. The poor development of this potentially advantageous technique in patients on mechanical ventilation (MV) is caused partly by high amounts of the particles dispersed by conventional nebulizers depositing in the ventilatory circuits and the tracheobronchial tree during MV, therefore not reaching the distal lung, and hence less drug is available in the alveolar compartment. Current nonstandardized clinical practice, the difficulties of implementing optimal nebulization technique, and lack of robust clinical data

Conflicts of Interest: J. Chastre and C.-E. Luyt have received honoraria from Bayer HealthCare for having participated in advisory boards on nebulized amikacin, and are investigators of Inhale 2, a phase 3 study on nebulized amikacin using the PDDS Clinical device in patients with gram-negative pneumonia, sponsored by Bayer HealthCare.
a Service de Réanimation Médicale, Institut de Cardiologie, Groupe Hospitalier Pitié–Salpêtrière, Assistance Publique–Hôpitaux de Paris, 47-83 Boulevard de l'Hôpital, Paris Cedex 13 75651, France; b Sorbonne Universités, UPMC Université Paris 06, INSERM, UMRS_1166-ICAN Institute of Cardiometabolism and Nutrition, Paris, France
* Corresponding author. Service de Réanimation Médicale, Institut de Cardiologie, Groupe Hospitalier Pitié–Salpêtrière, Assistance Publique–Hôpitaux de Paris, 47-83 Boulevard de l'Hôpital, Paris Cedex 13 75651, France.
E-mail address: jean.chastre@aphp.fr

Clin Chest Med 39 (2018) 823–836
https://doi.org/10.1016/j.ccm.2018.08.005
0272-5231/18/© 2018 Elsevier Inc. All rights reserved.

considerably limit widespread adoption. However, with the recent development of new nebulizers,[2–6] antibiotic aerosolization in patients with pneumonia has renewed interest.[7–9] This article focuses on patients with VAP.

RATIONALE FOR THE USE OF INHALED ANTIBIOTICS IN MECHANICALLY VENTILATED PATIENTS

Effective antimicrobial therapy requires adequate drug concentrations at the target site of infection, which is often not possible when using conventional intravenous (IV) therapy in ICU patients requiring MV because of the poor lung tissue penetration of many antimicrobial agents and the unpredictable modifications observed in their pharmacokinetics.[10–14] For many drugs, significant increases in the volume of distribution and/or variability in clearance are observed in the most severe ICU patients. When standard doses are used, such pharmacokinetic changes can result in subtherapeutic plasma concentrations, treatment failure, and the development of antibiotic resistance. Thus, even when the microorganism is susceptible to currently available antibiotics, the outcome is frequently suboptimal with a high rate of failure and/or relapse. This suboptimal outcome is particularly problematic when the microorganism responsible for infection has an MIC very close to the breakpoint defining the potential efficacy of these antibiotics, as is more and more frequently encountered nowadays in many countries. To treat these strains, raising the dose of systemic antibiotics and/or modifying the modalities of administration (ie, using continuous infusion) are the only options, but it can be responsible for an increased toxicity and lead to acute renal failure and/or neurologic complications.[15]

Inhalation therapy has the capability of directly targeting the airways, creating increased and more sustained local concentrations and thereby increasing the therapeutic index, improving efficacy, and minimizing toxicities. Although never shown, the microflora of the gut is probably less altered with nebulized antibiotics than with systemic antibiotics, which might also decrease the emergence and dissemination of resistant strains, including *Clostridium difficile*.

However, many clinicians do not fully appreciate the complexities associated with inhaled therapy, in part because of misconceptions based on inadequate techniques performed in the past, including instilling antibiotic solutions through the endotracheal tube and using existing parenteral formulations for inhalation.[16]

HOW TO OPTIMIZE LUNG DELIVERY OF ANTIBIOTICS DURING AEROSOLIZATION

One of the main limitations of nebulization is that a part of the nebulized drug is trapped in the ventilator circuit and the upper airways by impaction.[17] This impaction of aerosol droplets is driven by the size of particles but also by the turbulences generated in the gas flow. Several factors can influence nebulization efficiency: the generator, the size of the particles (which are largely dependent of the generator), the ventilator settings and circuit, the drug (dose, formulation), and the patients themselves. Although the patients are an unchangeable factor, other factors can be modified to increase the nebulization efficiency (**Fig. 1**).[18]

The Aerosol Generator

There are 3 types of nebulizers: jet, ultrasonic, and vibrating-mesh or plate nebulizers.[3,7] **Table 1** shows the potential advantages and drawbacks of the 3 types of nebulizers.

The generation of aerosol with jet nebulizers uses air or oxygen under high pressure. The gas may come either from a wall system (the generated flow is continuous, during the inspiratory and expiratory phases), or from the ventilator (the device is connected to the ventilator and the driving pressure is provided by the ventilator itself, delivering an intermittent flow during the inspiratory phase). With this kind of nebulizer, drug delivery into the lungs might be highly variable from one generator to another, depending on the brand, the pressure of the driving gas, and the position of the device on the ventilatory circuit.[19] This variability is decreased with newer generations of ventilators, marketed with built-in nebulizers that have been tested to generate efficient aerosols during intermittent operation.[3] The efficiency of jet nebulizers is increased when the connection with the inspiratory limb is at a distance from the endotracheal tube, compared with its connection between the Y piece and the endotracheal tube.[7,20,21]

Ultrasonic nebulizers use the vibration of a piezoelectric crystal to produce the aerosol. The aerosol particle size is inversely proportional to the piezoelectric crystal vibration frequency, and drug output is directly proportional to the amplitude of crystal vibration.[2] The main advantages of this technique are the short time of nebulization and the high flow of nebulization.[2,22] However, the use of these devices may increase the temperature of the solution by 10°C to 15°C after a few minutes of ultrasonic nebulization, which can lead to antibiotic denaturation and inactivation.[2,23] Moreover, the drug solution becomes

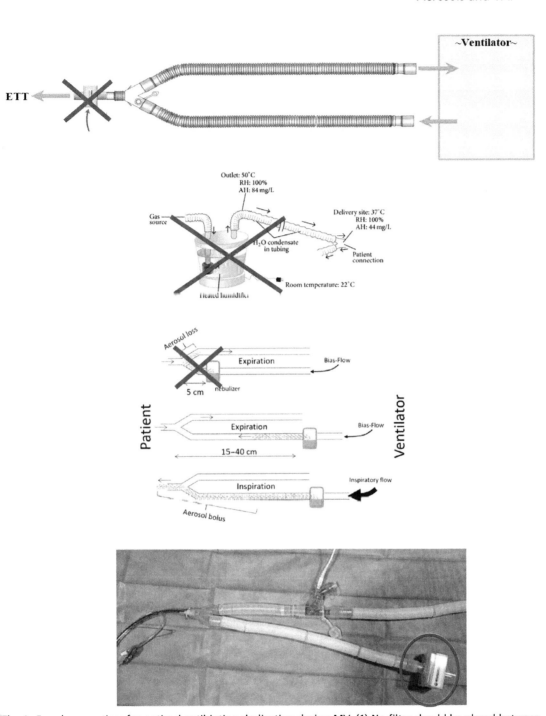

Fig. 1. Four key practices for optimal antibiotic nebulization during MV. (1) No filter should be placed between the nebulizer and the endotracheal prosthesis. (2) If a heated humidifier was used for humidifying and warming the inspiratory gases delivered by the mechanical ventilator, it should be switched off during aerosolization. (3) At best, vibrating-mesh nebulizers have to be placed on the inspiratory limb of the ventilator, 10 to 40 cm from the Y piece. To decrease impaction, the Y piece should have no acute or right angles, and should be connected directly to the endotracheal tube. (4) A filter (*red circle*) should be placed on the expiratory limb of the circuit to avoid antibiotic nebulization in the environment. This filter has to be replaced after each nebulization.

Table 1
Comparison of jet, ultrasonic, and vibrating-mesh nebulizers

	Advantages	Drawbacks
Jet nebulizer	Low cost Unique use Can be breath synchronized	Variable size of particles Long duration of nebulization Lower efficiency High performance variability High residual volume of drug Potential interference with the tidal volume delivered by the ventilator
Ultrasonic nebulizer	High efficiency High speed of drug delivery Easy to use Low residual volume of drug	High cost Increase in the solution temperature, which can degrade heat-sensitive drugs Hygiene concern No breath synchronization
Vibrating-mesh nebulizer	Small particle size, precisely calibrated Very high efficiency Easy to use Low residual volume of drug	High cost No breath synchronization Low efficacy with viscous solutions

more concentrated during operation. Whether or not increase in temperature and concentration of the drug can lead to antibiotic inactivation remains to be determined for each molecule to be used.

Although they are more efficient than jet nebulizers,[22,24] they are not widely used, mostly because of their cost and potential drawbacks.

Vibrating-mesh nebulizers are a newer generation of nebulizers. The nebulizer/reservoir unit comprises the aerosol generator and a drug reservoir. The aerosol is generated by the vibration of a plate with uniform holes. This vibration creates a rapid pumping of liquid droplets through the holes, thereby producing the aerosol. The size of the droplets depends directly on the diameter of the tapered holes, and can vary from 1 to 5 μm. The nebulizer/reservoir unit is connected to the ventilator circuit through a T-piece adapter placed on the inspiratory limb of the circuit. Unlike ultrasonic nebulizers, the temperature of the solution does not change during operation of the vibrating-mesh nebulizers, and drugs can be nebulized with minimal risk of denaturation. The vibrating-mesh nebulizers have many advantages compared with jet nebulizers, as indicated in **Table 1**, but they are costly.[7]

Size of the Particles

During MV, part of the aerosol is trapped in the ventilator circuit and the endotracheal tube.[21] Large droplets (>3 μm) are more likely to affect the circuit, whereas smaller particles (<0.5 μm) diffuse and are more likely to be expelled during expiration.[21,25,26]

Consequently, the optimal size of the generated particles to achieve the best alveolar deposition is between 1 and 3 μm. The size of the particles depends on the aerosol generator and its settings: on jet nebulizers, droplet size decreases when gas flow increases, whereas droplet size increases with increase in the ratio of liquid to gas flow. On ultrasonic nebulizers, aerosol particle size is inversely proportional to the piezoelectric crystal vibration frequency, and drug output is directly proportional to the amplitude of crystal vibration. On vibrating-mesh nebulizers, droplet size is homogeneous and can be precisely calibrated.[7,19,25,26]

Ventilator Settings

Ventilator settings are of importance for improving lung deposition. Indeed, any turbulence in inspiratory flow may cause an increase in impaction and deposition of droplets that leads to decreased lung drug deposition. Air turbulence can be decreased by optimizing ventilator settings: the best ventilator mode is volume-controlled mode (compared with pressure-controlled mode) with a constant inspiratory flow.[27] The tidal volume is also important, because a high tidal volume is associated with a better lung deposition. Experts recommend a Vt of 8 mL/kg,[28,29] with a long inspiratory time (which can be obtained by increasing the I/E ratio).[30,31] A low inspiratory flow achieves better lung deposition than a high flow. Consequently, the authors recommend setting the inspiratory flow at 40 L/min[28,31,32] whenever possible, because it can be poorly supported by the patient, and requesting increasing sedation.

Ventilator Circuit

Aerosol impaction on the respiratory circuit and the tracheal tube is a limitation of nebulization. Impaction (and thus aerosol lung deposition) is modified by the position of the nebulizer. Heated humidity decreases the amount of delivered drug by increasing the size of the droplets.[4,19,33] When using a heat/moisture exchanger, this has to be repositioned at the end of the expiratory circuit during nebulization (to avoid contamination of the environment by the product) and replaced at the end of the session (to avoid obstruction of the filter and thus of the expiratory circuit).[4,19] When using a heated humidifier, it should be switched off during nebulization, or the amount of drug should be increased.[4,19]

It has recently been shown, in an experimental study, that jet nebulizers provide the highest efficiency when placed proximal to the ventilator.[33] For ultrasonic nebulizers, the distal or proximal placement in the ventilator circuit had no impact on its efficiency.[24] However, in a recent experimental study on a dual-chamber test lung using an ultrasonic nebulizer, the investigators compared the deposition of albuterol according to its position.[33] The highest lung deposition was obtained when the nebulizer was placed 15 to 40 cm from the Y piece in the inspiratory limb. Other positions of the nebulizer on the circuit (between the Y piece and the endotracheal tube, on the inspiratory limb of the circuit at 15 cm from the ventilator) were associated with less efficiency. Heated/humidified and nonhumidified conditions did not change the deposition of albuterol.[33]

Few data are available for vibrating-mesh nebulizers. Experts recommend the placement of the device in the inspiratory limb of the circuit, 15 to 40 cm from the Y piece (see **Fig. 1**). In an experimental study, Ari and colleagues[33] showed that, during simulated adult MV, placement of a vibrating-mesh nebulizer in the inspiratory limb 15 cm from the Y piece provided the best deposition, compared with other places, which has recently been confirmed in another in vitro study.[31]

A new system not currently marketed, the Amikacin Inhale vibrating-mesh nebulizer, was recently developed by Aerogen/Bayer in an on-ventilator configuration for intubated and mechanically ventilated patients and in a handheld configuration for patients who are not intubated. The latter allows patients to continue treatment if extubated during the course of therapy. Several design features of Amikacin Inhale offer improvements compared with other aerosol generators for mechanically ventilated patients: it generates particles with a consistent mean size of 2.9 to 3.3 μm, suitable for deposition throughout the lower airway; it is synchronized with the ventilator in order to deliver nebulization during the first 75% of the patient's inspiratory cycle; it does not request modifying the ventilatory setting; it does not require patient sedation or changes in the inspiratory to expiratory cycle ratio or other ventilator changes needed to improve deposition with generic devices; and it has a high in vitro delivery efficiency of ~50%, which is unaffected by circuit humidification.[8,9,28]

AEROSOLIZATION DRAWBACKS

Although antibiotic nebulization seems attractive, it has several drawbacks and some questions have not yet been resolved.

Adverse Effects of Antibiotic Nebulization

In addition to the effects of the systematically absorbed antibiotic (ie, renal toxicity for aminoglycosides and polymyxins), most adverse events result from the direct toxicity on airways and lung parenchyma (mucosal irritation). Cough and a disagreeable taste, which are minor and transient, are frequently reported.[34] Bronchospasm is a more severe, but less common, side effect that has been described in patients receiving nebulized antibiotic, especially when the IV formulation was used. Bronchospasm during aerosolization imposes the immediate withdrawal of the aerosol and β-agonist nebulization.[28,34–36] In case of bronchospasm occurring during antibiotic nebulization, reintroduction of the same drug by the same route should be avoided. One of the most dreadful complications of antibiotic nebulization is the obstruction of the expiratory filter, which can lead to cardiac arrest and death, as reported by Lu and colleagues.[37] This complication can be avoided by a systematic change of the expiratory filter after each aerosol.

Parenchymal Lung Penetration

In healthy humans, nebulized antibiotic penetration into lung tissues is good.[38] However, in patients with alveolar consolidations, it is less certain. Most studies evaluating aerosolized antibiotics in patients with VAP found high antibiotic levels in tracheal aspirates,[34,39] but high sputum antibiotic levels do not necessarily mean high levels at the infection site (ie, in the lung parenchyma). In piglets with experimental pneumonia, Goldstein and colleagues[40] found that amikacin penetration into the lung was less in consolidated areas than in well-aerated alveoli, but greater than with IV administration. In humans, Luyt and colleagues[35,36] found that administering aerosolized amikacin to patients with gram-negative VAP achieved very high aminoglycoside concentrations in epithelial lining fluids (ELFs) and VAP-affected lung zones while maintaining safe serum drug concentrations. Those ELF concentrations were always greater than the antibiotic's MIC for gram-negative microorganisms usually responsible for VAP.

Emergence of Resistant Strains

Two studies looked for the emergence of resistant strains in proximal airways' respiratory secretions among chronically ill patients who received an adjunctive inhaled antibiotic.[41,42] Aerosolized antibiotics successfully eradicated existing multidrug-resistant (MDR) microorganisms and reduced the pressure from systemic agents for new respiratory resistance. However, no prolonged surveillance of patients included in these studies was performed, raising some doubt about the true efficacy of such a strategy, because the on-going use of antibiotics at subtherapeutic levels outside the respiratory tract, particularly at the level of the digestive tract, may lead to selection of antibiotic-resistant organisms.[43] Thus, as for all prevention and/or therapeutic strategies based on the use of antimicrobial agents, antibiotic nebulization must be managed prudently, particularly concerning treatment duration, which should be kept as short as possible.[44,45]

Prolonged Duration of Aerosolization

Another limitation of antibiotic aerosolization is the long aerosolization time required in some situations, which could lead to the prolongation of MV and ICU stay. Indeed, to be more efficient, antibiotic aerosolization must be accompanied by specific ventilator settings (discussed earlier). However, decreasing the inspiratory flow may increase patient discomfort. For many patients, physicians need to increase or start sedation to maintain patients who are perfectly adapted to their ventilators, which might lead to MV prolongation. As an example, in their study comparing aerosol therapy with the IV route for *Pseudomonas aeruginosa* VAP, Lu and colleagues[37] found that duration of MV and ICU stay after randomization were longer (although not statistically significant) in patients receiving aerosols, probably in part because of the need for an increased sedation level.

Cost

Most of the devices, especially the latest generations of vibrating-mesh nebulizer, are expensive.

Moreover, to be nebulized, a special antibiotic formulation must be prepared, which can also be costly. In addition, most companies developed antibiotic formulations to be administered via a specific device, thereby further increasing the cost of delivery by nebulization.[34]

Legal Concerns

Inhaled drug formulation considerations are extremely important when considering administering inhaled antimicrobial therapy to a patient with a bacterial pneumonia. Only drugs prepared and manufactured specifically for inhalation should be used. They should be pyrogen free; isotonic; sterile; pH balanced to the airway epithelium (pH 6); and dispensed in unit-dose, single-use containers. Importantly, preservatives and sulfites should be avoided if possible, because they have been specifically associated with adverse effects when inhaled.

Most antibiotics have only been approved for IV use and not for direct delivery to the lungs. A special formulation for nebulization exists in France for colistin and tobramycin, but the use of other antibiotics is off label.[28,34] The situation is the same in most European countries and the United States, and it may have legal issues. It should also be noted that there is very limited information regarding the doses that should be used when aerosolizing antibiotics (discussed later).

EXPERIMENTAL DATA SUPPORTING THE USE OF ANTIBIOTIC AEROSOLIZATION

Several studies in animal models of VAP have shown that antibiotic aerosolization led to higher antibiotic concentration into the lung than IV infusion. From a pharmacodynamic point of view, aminoglycosides and colistin are concentration-dependent antibiotics with a postantibiotic effect. They are particularly suitable for nebulization because high lung concentrations can be expected and only 1 to 3 daily administrations are required. Time-dependent antibiotics, like β-lactams or glycopeptides, require that drug concentrations be maintained at more than the MIC throughout the dosing interval. Continuous or closely repeated administration is hence required, which could limit the clinical feasibility of nebulized delivery of such drugs.

In healthy piglets, Goldstein and colleagues[46] compared amikacin lung tissue concentrations after nebulization with those after IV administration. The lung concentrations of amikacin were more than 10-fold higher after nebulization than the lung concentrations after IV administration, and were homogeneously distributed throughout the lung parenchyma. These concentrations were far in excess of the MIC of most gram-negative strains responsible for VAP. These data were confirmed in piglets with experimental pneumonia caused by *Escherichia coli*: the amikacin lung concentration was 3-fold to 30-fold higher after nebulization than after IV administration.[40] In the lungs of piglets having received nebulized amikacin, amikacin concentrations were lower in the infected (consolidated) segments of the lungs than in the nonconsolidated, noninfected parts of the lungs, but even in the infected parenchyma it was higher than the concentration achieved with IV amikacin. Moreover, bactericidal efficacy seemed better after nebulization than after IV administration, the lung bacterial burden being significantly lower in the lungs of animals receiving aerosolized amikacin than in the lungs of animals receiving IV amikacin.[10]

Recently, the same team evaluated lung deposition of colistin administered intravenously or via a vibrating-mesh nebulizer in piglets. Colistin was not detected in lung tissue following IV infusion, whereas it was detected in the lung parenchyma of animals receiving nebulized colistin, with peak lung tissue concentrations greater in lung segments with mild pneumonia than in lung segments with severe pneumonia.[47] Accordingly, bacterial burden in the lungs of aerosol-treated animals was lower than in the lung of IV-treated animals.[47]

In humans, lung penetration of aerosolized antibiotics (at least for aminoglycosides and colistin) seems better than when using the IV route: in 1993, Le Conte and colleagues[48] found that a single nebulization of tobramycin in healthy subjects led to high lung parenchymal concentrations with low serum level. These results were recently confirmed by Niederman and colleagues[49] in a pharmacokinetic study of nebulized amikacin using the breath-synchronized vibrating-mesh nebulizer developed by Aerogen/Bayer in ventilated patients with microbiologically confirmed gram-negative pneumonia. Two other pharmacokinetic studies using bronchoalveolar lavage for assessing amikacin penetration into the alveolar ELF found high amikacin concentrations from infected alveolar spaces, whereas serum amikacin concentration remained low, less than the toxicity level, in patients with or without acute renal failure.[35,36]

There are no recommended doses for colistin or aminoglycoside nebulization. In patients with VAP or ventilator-associated tracheobronchitis (VAT) who were administered 1 million international units (MIU, ie, 80 mg) of colistimethate sodium (CMS), the precursor of colistin, via a vibrating-mesh nebulizer every 8 hours, peak ELF concentrations were high but then decreased to less than the

sensitivity breakpoint at 4 hours, thus indicating that this dose may not be optimal for treating.[50] Steady-state plasma concentrations of colistin, indirectly reflecting alveolar deposition, were significantly higher in studies evaluating high doses of nebulized CMS (4–5 MIU/8 h)[46,47] compared with 2 MIU/8 h.[51] In the largest retrospective study published to date, the investigators gave 300 mg of tobramycin twice daily or 1000 mg of amikacin twice daily.[52] Palmer and colleagues[41] administered 80 mg of gentamicin every 8 hours in patients with ventilator-associated tracheobronchitis. In the most recent studies that used a breath-synchronized vibrating-mesh nebulizer, 400 mg of amikacin twice daily allowed high tracheal and ELF levels.[35,36] Using nebulizers to administer aminoglycosides allows reducing the dose of aminoglycosides compared with IV doses,[11,60] but the exact amount of aminoglycosides to be nebulized remains to be determined and depends on the device used.

Taken together, these results suggest that nebulization of antibiotics can effectively deliver antibiotics in higher concentrations to the lungs of patients with pneumonia than the IV route.

ANTIBIOTIC AEROSOLIZATION: FOR WHOM AND WITH WHAT EFFICACY?

Aerosolized antibiotics can be used either as an adjunctive therapy to standard IV antibiotics, instead of IV antibiotics, or in patients with pneumonia caused by extensively drug-resistant (XDR) pathogens for which no IV therapy is readily available.

Aerosolization as an Adjunctive Treatment to Active Intravenous Antibiotics

In this setting, aerosol antibiotic administration is associated with IV antibiotics active against the pathogen responsible for pneumonia, with the aim of increasing efficiency, accelerating clinical and bacteriologic cure, and improving outcome. However, practically all studies performed to date showed no improvement in clinically relevant outcomes when comparing aerosolized antibiotics with aerosolized placebo.

In a randomized, placebo-controlled, double-blind study, Rattanaumpawan and colleagues[53] evaluated patients with gram-negative VAP having received either nebulized colistin (n = 51) or nebulized placebo (n = 49) in addition to IV antibiotics. Clinical outcomes including clinical cure, mortality, and VAP-attributed mortality were similar in the two groups, whereas microbiological cure rate was higher in patients receiving nebulized colistin than in those receiving placebo. Complications were similar in the two groups.[53] Using a breath-synchronized vibrating-mesh nebulizer, the PDDS Clinical, Niederman and colleagues[49] randomized 69 mechanically ventilated patients with gram-negative VAP to receive 7 to 14 days of aerosolized amikacin 400 mg twice a day (n = 21), amikacin 400 mg once daily and placebo 12 hours later (n = 26), or placebo twice a day (n = 22) (33) in addition to IV antimicrobials. Aerosolized amikacin was well tolerated, without any severe adverse event, and patients who received amikacin twice daily required significantly less antibiotic than patients receiving nebulized placebo (mean number of systemic antibiotics per patient per day at the end of treatment, 0.9 vs 1.9, respectively; $P = .02$), perhaps because their disease improved more rapidly, but no other benefit could be shown.

Results of 2 large, double-blind, placebo-controlled, randomized trials were recently made available. In the first, the investigators compared standard of care in each arm plus 300 mg amikacin/120 mg fosfomycin or placebo (saline), delivered by aerosol twice daily for 10 days via an efficient mesh-vibrating nebulizer, the PARI eFlow.[54] A total of 143 patients with gram-negative bacterial VAP were studied. Comparison of Clinical Pulmonary Infection Score change from baseline between treatment groups was not different, as well as the secondary hierarchical end point of no mortality and clinical cure at day 14. Patients randomized in the amikacin/fosfomycin nebulized group had significantly fewer positive tracheal cultures within the 7 days following randomization, but the relevance of such an end point is doubtful because of the presence of high antibiotic concentrations in respiratory secretions obtained from patients having received aerosolized antibiotics, which could have rendered falsely negative culture results.[54]

The second study, not yet published, was the Bayer Inhaled study, a multicenter, randomized, placebo-controlled, double-blind trial that investigated the clinical efficacy and safety of adjunctive nebulized amikacin compared with standard care and nebulized placebo for the treatment of gram-negative pneumonia in adult ICU ventilated patients (phase III study program with Amikacin Inhale in addition to standard of care in intubated and mechanically ventilated patients with gram-negative pneumonia does not meet primary end point of superiority. News release: Friday, November 24, 2017. http://press.bayer.com/baynews/baynews.nsf/id/Phase-III-study-program-Amikacin-Inhale-addition-standard-intubated-mechanically-ventilated-patients). The primary outcome measure was survival at day 30.

Secondary outcome measures included pneumonia-related mortality to day 30, early clinical response up to day 10, number of days on MV, and number of ICU days up to day 30. Seven-hundred and twenty-five eligible patients were randomized into 2 arms. Patients in the first arm received 400 mg of a specially formulated Amikacin Inhalation Solution every 12 hours for 10 days administered using the Synchronized Inhalation System, a mesh-vibrating nebulizer synchronized with inspiration. Patients in the comparator arm received aerosolized placebo every 12 hours for 10 days, also administered using the Synchronized Inhalation System. Both groups received standard-of-care IV antibiotics following American Thoracic Society (ATS) guidelines or local guidelines. The primary end point (overall mortality at day 28), as well as secondary end points, were similar in both treatment arms, and therefore the study failed to show he superiority of adjunctive aerosolized amikacin versus standard of care.

Based on these results and data obtained from previous trials, the use of aerosolized antibiotics as an adjunctive treatment to IV antibiotics active against the pathogen responsible for pneumonia cannot be recommended.[55–60]

Aerosolized Antibiotics Used Alone, Instead of Intravenous Antibiotics

Nebulization of antibiotics offers the possibility of delivering very high lung tissue concentrations of antibiotics in normal and infected lungs with rapid bacterial killing, as documented in experimental studies.[40] As such, it can provide similar efficiency in terms of clinical cure of VAP caused by susceptible microorganisms, while not using potentially toxic IV antibiotics. The feasibility and clinical utility of such a strategy was assessed in a randomized controlled trial that included 40 patients with VAP caused by *P aeruginosa*.[37] Twenty patients infected with susceptible or intermediate strains received nebulized ceftazidime and amikacin. Seventeen patients infected with susceptible strains received IV ceftazidime by continuous administration and amikacin. In 3 patients infected with intermediate strains, amikacin was replaced by ciprofloxacin. After 8 days of antibiotic administration, aerosol and IV groups were similar in terms of successful treatment (70% vs 55%), treatment failure (15% vs 30%), and superinfection with other microorganisms (15% vs 15%). Acquisition of per-treatment antibiotic-resistant strains was observed exclusively in the IV group. However, patients allocated to the aerosol arm required prolonged aerosolization over a total of 8 to 9 h/d and increased sedation, which might have contributed to MV prolongation. Indeed, although not significant, the median duration of MV after randomization was longer in the aerosol arm than in the IV arm (14 vs 8 days, P = nonsignificant).[37] Patients with positive blood cultures (10% of patients with VAP[61]) are not eligible to such a strategy. Therefore, whether such a strategy can be recommended in patients with VAP is highly doubtful.

Aside from investigating curative nebulized antibiotics to treat patients with VAT and/or VAP, some investigators have also tested nebulized colistin, ceftazidime, or aminoglycosides for prophylaxis in intubated patients. Two small studies obtained positive results with such a preemptive inhaled therapy in terms of VAP incidence, with no significant change in the bacterial antibiotic sensitivity pattern.[60,62] Further studies are required to assess this benefit as well as the risk of antibiotic resistance selection pressure.

Patients with Pneumonia Caused by Extensively Drug-Resistant Pathogens

Adjunctive aerosolization of still-active antibiotics (namely colistin and aminoglycosides) seems a logical step in patients with pneumonia caused by XDR pathogens only susceptible to these drugs. Because of their systemic toxicity, it is difficult to use them intravenously at an optimized PK/PD dosing, and thus, aerosolization seems to be the best way to achieve the high drug concentrations that are required at the site of infection for maximal bacterial killing while avoiding nephrotoxicity.

Czosnowski and colleagues[52] evaluated 49 patients who received aerosolized antibiotics for the treatment of a total of 60 episodes of VAP caused by P aeruginosa and/or Acinetobacter baumannii. Investigators used nebulized tobramycin, amikacin, and colistimethate in 44, 9, and 9 episodes, respectively. Systemic antibiotics were used in all except 1 patient. The main outcome measure was clinical success, which was achieved in 36 (73%) of the 49 first episodes of VAP, 8 (73%) of 11 subsequent episodes, 17 (85%) of 20 episodes that were failing IV monotherapy, and 30 (79%) of 38 episodes with MDR P aeruginosa or A baumannii. Microbiologic success was achieved in 29 (71%) of 41 evaluable episodes.[52] **Table 2** shows other important studies having reported patients treated with nebulized colistin. Most patients were treated with a combination of IV antibiotics in addition to nebulized colistin. In one of the most recent studies reported, the investigators compared 122 patients with P aeruginosa VAP caused by sensitive strains

treated with IV antibiotics with 43 patients with P aeruginosa VAP caused by MDR strains that received nebulized colistin either alone (n = 28, 65%) or in combination with a 3-day IV aminoglycoside therapy (n = 15, 35%) (36). VAP cure, VAP recurrence, and mortality were similar in patients infected with sensitive-strain P aeruginosa VAP and in patients infected with MDR strains.[63] None of these studies reported the emergence of colistin-resistant pathogens or renal toxicity caused by colistin nebulization.[63–67] The effect of aerosolized colistin as adjunctive treatment on the outcomes of microbiologically documented VAP caused by colistin-only susceptible gram-negative bacteria was also assessed by Tumbarello and colleagues[68] in a retrospective, 1:1 matched case-control study that included 208 patients. Compared with the IV-only colistin cohort, patients who received a combination of IV and aerosolized colistin had a higher clinical cure rate (69% vs 55%, P = .03) and required fewer days of MV after VAP onset (8 days vs 12 days, P = .001). In the 166 patients with posttreatment cultures, eradication of the causative organism was also more common in the aerosolized-IV colistin group (63% vs 50%, P = .08). No between-cohort differences were observed in all-cause ICU mortality or rates of acute kidney injury during colistin therapy.

Three meta-analyses were recently performed, with mixed results.[69–71] Valachis and colleagues[71] evaluated the efficacy and safety of aerosolized colistin as adjunctive therapy with IV antimicrobials or as monotherapy in the treatment of VAP: 16 studies were included in their meta-analysis for a total of 690 patients. A significant improvement in clinical response (odds ratio, 1.57; P = .006), microbiological eradication (odds ratio, 1.61; P = .01), and infection-related mortality (odds ratio, 0.58; P = .04) was observed with the addition of aerosolized colistin to IV treatment, whereas overall mortality was not affected (odds ratio, 0.74; P = .06), nor was nephrotoxicity (odds ratio, 1.18; P = .45). Similar results were found by Liu and colleagues[70] in an analysis of 9 studies having compared a combination of IV plus nebulized polymyxin versus IV polymyxin alone in a total of 672 patients: the combination of IV plus nebulized colistin was associated with higher rates of clinical cure or improvement and pathogen eradication and lower all-cause mortality. However, in the meta-analysis done by Zampieri and colleagues,[69] which included 6 randomized controlled trials for a total of 812 patients, nebulized antibiotics were not associated with microbiological cure (relative risk (RR) = 1.24; 95% confidence interval [CI], 0.95–1.62), mortality

Table 2
Main studies having evaluated nebulized colistin for the treatment of ventilator-associated pneumonia

Author	Study Design	Number of Patients	Control Group	Pathogens	Pathogen Eradication (%)	Clinical Cure (%)	Time of Evaluation	Mortality (%)
Kwa et al,[66] 2005	Retrospective cohort	21	None	P aeruginosa, A baumannii	86	57	NR	47
Berlana et al,[67] 2005	Retrospective cohort	70	None	P aeruginosa, A baumannii	92	NR	NR	18
Michalopoulos et al,[65] 2008	Prospective cohort	80	None	P aeruginosa, A baumannii, Klebsiella pneumoniae	83	83	End of antimicrobial treatment	25
Lin et al,[74] 2010	Retrospective cohort	45	None	A baumannii	38	58	NR	42
Athanassa et al,[75] 2011	Retrospective cohort	12	None	A baumannii, P aeruginosa, K pneumoniae	67	75	NR	25
Kofteridis et al,[76] 2010	Retrospective matched cohort study	43 patients receiving IV + AS colistin	43 patients receiving IV colistin alone	A baumannii, P aeruginosa, K pneumoniae	45 IV + AS, 50 IV alone	50 IV + AS, 32.5 IV alone	10–13 d	23 IV + AS, 42 IV alone
Lu et al,[63] 2012	Prospective cohort	43	122 patients with susceptible strains	P aeruginosa, A baumannii	69	67	14 d	16
Doshi et al,[77] 2013	Retrospective cohort study	44 patients receiving IV + AS colistin	51 patients receiving IV colistin	A baumannii, P aeruginosa, K pneumoniae	54.5 IV + AS, 39.2 IV alone	44.4 IV + AS, 40.7 IV alone	NR	36.4 IV + AS, 52.9 IV alone
Tumbarello et al,[68] 2013	Retrospective matched cohort study	104 patients receiving IV + AS colistin	104 patients receiving IV colistin alone	A baumannii, P aeruginosa, K pneumoniae	63.4 IV + AS, 50 IV alone	69.2 IV + AS, 54.8 IV alone	End of antimicrobial treatment	43 IV + AS, 46 IV alone
Abdellatif et al,[78] 2016	Randomized controlled study	73 patients receiving nebulized colistin (13 had monotherapy)	76 patients receiving IV colistin (12 had monotherapy)	A baumannii, P aeruginosa, Enterobacteriaceae	67.1 AS 72.3 IV colistin	NR	End of antimicrobial treatment (14 d)	27.4 AS group 23.7 IV group

RR = 0.90; CI 95%, 0.76–1.08), duration of MV standardized mean difference = −0.10 days; 95% CI, −1.22 to 1.00), ICU length of stay (standardized mean difference = 0.14 days; 95% CI, −0.46 to 0.73), or renal toxicity (RR = 1.05; 95% CI, 0.70–1.57).

SUMMARY AND PERSPECTIVES

To date, based on data reviewed earlier, antibiotic aerosolization in adults with pneumonia can only be recommended in patients with HAP/VAP caused by extensively resistant pathogens only susceptible to antibiotics with limited efficacy and high toxicity when given by the IV route (ie, aminoglycosides and colistin). Clinicians should also be aware that administration of aerosol to patients needs specific devices, drug formulations, and ventilator settings, and also close monitoring. These recommendations are consistent with existing guidelines, including those recently published by the ATS and the Infectious Diseases Society of America (IDSA).[72] In the latter, experts only recommend adjunctive inhaled antibiotic therapy for patients who are most likely to benefit; specifically, those who have VAP caused by bacteria that are only susceptible to the classes of antibiotics for which evidence of efficacy by the IV alone route is the most limited (ie, aminoglycosides or colistin; weak recommendation, very low-quality evidence). However, experts from ATS-IDSA also believe that it is reasonable to consider adjunctive inhaled antibiotic therapy as a treatment of last resort for patients who are not responding to IV antibiotics alone, whether or not the infecting organism is MDR.

Careful design of future large randomized trials to turn the favorable PK/PD profile of nebulized antibiotics into improved clinical outcomes and reduced toxicity in patients with VAP is needed, with a focus on patients who can benefit the most from such a strategy (ie, those infected with very-difficult-to-treat pathogens, as indicated earlier). Defining populations at high risk of toxicity (mainly patients with acute kidney injury) may also be a worthwhile challenge. At the other end of the severity spectrum, in patients colonized by difficult-to-treat bacteria and at high risk of developing pneumonia but who do not yet show parenchymal infection, the benefits of an exclusively nebulized therapeutic strategy may warrant further evaluation.[42,73]

A paradigm change may occur in the future with the development of inhaled antiinfective nanoparticles, antibodies, or phage therapy, but administering aerosolized antibiotics alone to patients with VAP is premature at present and should be reserved for the specific patients for whom no other therapy is available.

REFERENCES

1. Weiss E, Essaied W, Adrie C, et al. Treatment of severe hospital-acquired and ventilator-associated pneumonia: a systematic review of inclusion and judgment criteria used in randomized controlled trials. Crit Care 2017;21(1):162.
2. Dhand R. Aerosol delivery during mechanical ventilation: from basic techniques to new devices. J Aerosol Med Pulm Drug Deliv 2008;21(1):45–60.
3. Dhand R, Guntur VP. How best to deliver aerosol medications to mechanically ventilated patients. Clin Chest Med 2008;29(2):277–96, vi.
4. Dhand R, Mercier E. Effective inhaled drug administration to mechanically ventilated patients. Expert Opin Drug Deliv 2007;4(1):47–61.
5. Waldrep JC, Berlinski A, Dhand R. Comparative analysis of methods to measure aerosols generated by a vibrating mesh nebulizer. J Aerosol Med 2007; 20(3):310–9.
6. Waldrep JC, Dhand R. Advanced nebulizer designs employing vibrating mesh/aperture plate technologies for aerosol generation. Curr Drug Deliv 2008; 5(2):114–9.
7. Luyt C-E, Combes A, Nieszkowska A, et al. Aerosolized antibiotics to treat ventilator-associated pneumonia. Curr Opin Infect Dis 2009;22(2):154–8.
8. Bassetti M, Luyt C-E, Nicolau DP, et al. Characteristics of an ideal nebulized antibiotic for the treatment of pneumonia in the intubated patient. Ann Intensive Care 2016;6(1):35.
9. Nicolau DP, Dimopoulos G, Welte T, et al. Can we improve clinical outcomes in patients with pneumonia treated with antibiotics in the intensive care unit? Expert Rev Respir Med 2016;10(8):907–18.
10. Rodvold KA, George JM, Yoo L. Penetration of antiinfective agents into pulmonary epithelial lining fluid: focus on antibacterial agents. Clin Pharmacokinet 2011;50(10):637–64.
11. Panidis D, Markantonis SL, Boutzouka E, et al. Penetration of gentamicin into the alveolar lining fluid of critically ill patients with ventilator-associated pneumonia. Chest 2005;128(2):545–52.
12. Lodise TP, Sorgel F, Melnick D, et al. Penetration of meropenem into epithelial lining fluid of patients with ventilator-associated pneumonia. Antimicrob Agents Chemother 2011;55(4):1606–10.
13. Sime FB, Roberts MS, Peake SL, et al. Does betalactam pharmacokinetic variability in critically ill patients justify therapeutic drug monitoring? a systematic review. Ann Intensive Care 2012;2(1):35.
14. Roberts JA, Abdul-Aziz MH, Lipman J, et al. Individualised antibiotic dosing for patients who are

critically ill: challenges and potential solutions. Lancet Infect Dis 2014;14(6):498–509.

15. Schliamser SE, Cars O, Norrby SR. Neurotoxicity of beta-lactam antibiotics: predisposing factors and pathogenesis. J Antimicrob Chemother 1991;27(4): 405–25.

16. Solé-Lleonart C, Rouby J-J, Chastre J, et al. Intratracheal administration of antimicrobial agents in mechanically ventilated adults: an international survey on delivery practices and safety. Respir Care 2016;61(8):1008–14.

17. Wenzler E, Fraidenburg DR, Scardina T, et al. Inhaled antibiotics for gram-negative respiratory infections. Clin Microbiol Rev 2016;29(3):581–632.

18. Dhanani J, Fraser JF, Chan H-K, et al. Fundamentals of aerosol therapy in critical care. Crit Care 2016; 20(1):269.

19. Miller DD, Amin MM, Palmer LB, et al. Aerosol delivery and modern mechanical ventilation: in vitro/in vivo evaluation. Am J Respir Crit Care Med 2003;168(10):1205–9.

20. O'Riordan TG, Greco MJ, Perry RJ, et al. Nebulizer function during mechanical ventilation. Am Rev Respir Dis 1992;145(5):1117–22.

21. O'Riordan TG, Palmer LB, Smaldone GC. Aerosol deposition in mechanically ventilated patients. Optimizing nebulizer delivery. Am J Respir Crit Care Med 1994;149(1):214–9.

22. Harvey CJ, O'Doherty MJ, Page CJ, et al. Comparison of jet and ultrasonic nebulizer pulmonary aerosol deposition during mechanical ventilation. Eur Respir J 1997;10(4):905–9.

23. Steckel H, Eskandar F. Factors affecting aerosol performance during nebulization with jet and ultrasonic nebulizers. Eur J Pharm Sci 2003;19(5):443–55.

24. O'Doherty MJ, Thomas SH, Page CJ, et al. Delivery of a nebulized aerosol to a lung model during mechanical ventilation. Effect of ventilator settings and nebulizer type, position, and volume of fill. Am Rev Respir Dis 1992;146(2):383–8.

25. Newman SP. How well do in vitro particle size measurements predict drug delivery in vivo? J Aerosol Med 1998;11(Suppl 1):S97–104.

26. Newman SP, Chan H-K. In vitro/in vivo comparisons in pulmonary drug delivery. J Aerosol Med Pulm Drug Deliv 2008;21(1):77–84.

27. Hess DR, Dillman C, Kacmarek RM. In vitro evaluation of aerosol bronchodilator delivery during mechanical ventilation: pressure-control vs. volume control ventilation. Intensive Care Med 2003;29(7): 1145–50.

28. Luyt C-E, Bréchot N, Combes A, et al. Delivering antibiotics to the lungs of patients with ventilator-associated pneumonia: an update. Expert Rev Anti Infect Ther 2013;11(5):511–21.

29. Rouby J-J, Bouhemad B, Monsel A, et al. Aerosolized antibiotics for ventilator-associated pneumonia: lessons from experimental studies. Anesthesiology 2012;117(6):1364–80.

30. Fink JB, Dhand R, Grychowski J, et al. Reconciling in vitro and in vivo measurements of aerosol delivery from a metered-dose inhaler during mechanical ventilation and defining efficiency-enhancing factors. Am J Respir Crit Care Med 1999;159(1): 63–8.

31. Dugernier J, Wittebole X, Roeseler J, et al. Influence of inspiratory flow pattern and nebulizer position on aerosol delivery with a vibrating-mesh nebulizer during invasive mechanical ventilation: an in vitro analysis. J Aerosol Med Pulm Drug Deliv 2015;28(3): 229–36.

32. Dolovich MA. Influence of inspiratory flow rate, particle size, and airway caliber on aerosolized drug delivery to the lung. Respir Care 2000;45(6): 597–608.

33. Ari A, Areabi H, Fink JB. Evaluation of aerosol generator devices at 3 locations in humidified and non-humidified circuits during adult mechanical ventilation. Respir Care 2010;55(7):837–44.

34. Dhand R. The role of aerosolized antimicrobials in the treatment of ventilator-associated pneumonia. Respir Care 2007;52(7):866–84.

35. Luyt C-E, Clavel M, Guntupalli K, et al. Pharmacokinetics and lung delivery of PDDS-aerosolized amikacin (NKTR-061) in intubated and mechanically ventilated patients with nosocomial pneumonia. Crit Care 2009;13(6):R200.

36. Luyt C-E, Eldon MA, Stass H, et al. Pharmacokinetics and tolerability of amikacin administered as BAY41-6551 aerosol in mechanically ventilated patients with gram-negative pneumonia and acute renal failure. J Aerosol Med Pulm Drug Deliv 2011; 24(4):183–90.

37. Lu Q, Yang J, Liu Z, et al. Nebulized ceftazidime and amikacin in ventilator-associated pneumonia caused by Pseudomonas aeruginosa. Am J Respir Crit Care Med 2011;184(1):106–15.

38. Michalopoulos A, Papadakis E. Inhaled anti-infective agents: emphasis on colistin. Infection 2010;38(2): 81–8.

39. Palmer LB, Smaldone GC, Simon SR, et al. Aerosolized antibiotics in mechanically ventilated patients: delivery and response. Crit Care Med 1998;26(1): 31–9.

40. Goldstein I, Wallet F, Nicolas-Robin A, et al. Lung deposition and efficiency of nebulized amikacin during Escherichia coli pneumonia in ventilated piglets. Am J Respir Crit Care Med 2002;166(10):1375–81.

41. Palmer LB, Smaldone GC, Chen JJ, et al. Aerosolized antibiotics and ventilator-associated tracheobronchitis in the intensive care unit. Crit Care Med 2008;36(7):2008–13.

42. Palmer LB, Smaldone GC. Reduction of bacterial resistance with inhaled antibiotics in the intensive

care unit. Am J Respir Crit Care Med 2014;189(10): 1225–33.

43. Feeley TW, Du Moulin GC, Hedley-Whyte J, et al. Aerosol polymyxin and pneumonia in seriously ill patients. N Engl J Med 1975;293(10):471–5.

44. Chastre J, Wolff M, Fagon J-Y, et al. Comparison of 8 vs 15 days of antibiotic therapy for ventilator-associated pneumonia in adults: a randomized trial. JAMA 2003;290(19):2588–98.

45. Luyt C-E, Bréchot N, Trouillet J-L, et al. Antibiotic stewardship in the intensive care unit. Crit Care 2014;18(5):480.

46. Goldstein I, Wallet F, Robert J, et al. Lung tissue concentrations of nebulized amikacin during mechanical ventilation in piglets with healthy lungs. Am J Respir Crit Care Med 2002;165(2):171–5.

47. Lu Q, Girardi C, Zhang M, et al. Nebulized and intravenous colistin in experimental pneumonia caused by *Pseudomonas aeruginosa*. Intensive Care Med 2010;36(7):1147–55.

48. Le Conte P, Potel G, Peltier P, et al. Lung distribution and pharmacokinetics of aerosolized tobramycin. Am Rev Respir Dis 1993;147(5):1279–82.

49. Niederman MS, Chastre J, Corkery K, et al. BAY41-6551 achieves bactericidal tracheal aspirate amikacin concentrations in mechanically ventilated patients with Gram-negative pneumonia. Intensive Care Med 2012;38(2):263–71.

50. Athanassa ZE, Markantonis SL, Fousteri M-ZF, et al. Pharmacokinetics of inhaled colistimethate sodium (CMS) in mechanically ventilated critically ill patients. Intensive Care Med 2012;38(11): 1779–86.

51. Boisson M, Jacobs M, Grégoire N, et al. Comparison of intrapulmonary and systemic pharmacokinetics of colistin methanesulfonate (CMS) and colistin after aerosol delivery and intravenous administration of CMS in critically ill patients. Antimicrob Agents Chemother 2014;58(12):7331–9.

52. Czosnowski QA, Wood GC, Magnotti LJ, et al. Adjunctive aerosolized antibiotics for treatment of ventilator-associated pneumonia. Pharmacotherapy 2009;29(9):1054–60.

53. Rattanaumpawan P, Lorsutthitham J, Ungprasert P, et al. Randomized controlled trial of nebulized colistimethate sodium as adjunctive therapy of ventilator-associated pneumonia caused by Gram-negative bacteria. J Antimicrob Chemother 2010; 65(12):2645–9.

54. Kollef MH, Ricard J-D, Roux D, et al. A randomized trial of the amikacin fosfomycin inhalation system for the adjunctive therapy of gram-negative ventilator-associated pneumonia: IASIS trial. Chest 2017; 151(6):1239–46.

55. Solé-Lleonart C, Rouby J-J, Blot S, et al. Nebulization of antiinfective agents in invasively mechanically

ventilated adults: a systematic review and meta-analysis. Anesthesiology 2017;126(5):890–908.

56. Rello J, Solé-Lleonart C, Rouby J-J, et al. Use of nebulized antimicrobials for the treatment of respiratory infections in invasively mechanically ventilated adults: a position paper from the European Society of Clinical Microbiology and Infectious Diseases. Clin Microbiol Infect 2017;23(9):629–39.

57. Russell CJ, Shiroishi MS, Siantz E, et al. The use of inhaled antibiotic therapy in the treatment of ventilator-associated pneumonia and tracheobronchitis: a systematic review. BMC Pulm Med 2016; 16:40.

58. Wood GC, Boucher BA, Croce MA, et al. Aerosolized ceftazidime for prevention of ventilator-associated pneumonia and drug effects on the proinflammatory response in critically ill trauma patients. Pharmacotherapy 2002;22(8):972–82.

59. Poulakou G, Siakallis G, Isiodras S, et al. Nebulized antibiotics in mechanically ventilated patients: roadmap and challenges. Expert Rev Anti Infect Ther 2017;15(3):211–29.

60. Florescu DF, Qiu F, McCartan MA, et al. What is the efficacy and safety of colistin for the treatment of ventilator-associated pneumonia? A systematic review and meta-regression. Clin Infect Dis 2012; 54(5):670–80.

61. Chastre J, Fagon J-Y. Ventilator-associated pneumonia. Am J Respir Crit Care Med 2002;165(7): 867–903.

62. Karvouniaris M, Makris D, Zygoulis P, et al. Nebulised colistin for ventilator-associated pneumonia prevention. Eur Respir J 2015;46(6):1732–9.

63. Lu Q, Luo R, Bodin L, et al. Efficacy of high-dose nebulized colistin in ventilator-associated pneumonia caused by multidrug-resistant Pseudomonas aeruginosa and *Acinetobacter baumannii*. Anesthesiology 2012;117(6):1335–47.

64. Falagas ME, Agrafiotis M, Athanassa Z, et al. Administration of antibiotics via the respiratory tract as monotherapy for pneumonia. Expert Rev Anti Infect Ther 2008;6(4):447–52.

65. Michalopoulos A, Fotakis D, Virtzili S, et al. Aerosolized colistin as adjunctive treatment of ventilator-associated pneumonia due to multidrug-resistant Gram-negative bacteria: a prospective study. Respir Med 2008;102(3):407–12.

66. Kwa ALH, Loh C, Low JGH, et al. Nebulized colistin in the treatment of pneumonia due to multidrug-resistant *Acinetobacter baumannii* and *Pseudomonas aeruginosa*. Clin Infect Dis 2005;41(5):754–7.

67. Berlana D, Llop JM, Fort E, et al. Use of colistin in the treatment of multiple-drug-resistant gram-negative infections. Am J Health Syst Pharm 2005;62(1): 39–47.

68. Tumbarello M, De Pascale G, Trecarichi EM, et al. Effect of aerosolized colistin as adjunctive treatment

on the outcomes of microbiologically documented ventilator-associated pneumonia caused by colistin-only susceptible gram-negative bacteria. Chest 2013;144(6):1768–75.

69. Zampieri FG, Nassar AP, Gusmao-Flores D, et al. Nebulized antibiotics for ventilator-associated pneumonia: a systematic review and meta-analysis. Crit Care 2015;19:150.

70. Liu D, Zhang J, Liu H-X, et al. Intravenous combined with aerosolised polymyxin versus intravenous polymyxin alone in the treatment of pneumonia caused by multidrug-resistant pathogens: a systematic review and meta-analysis. Int J Antimicrob Agents 2015;46(6):603–9.

71. Valachis A, Samonis G, Kofteridis DP. The role of aerosolized colistin in the treatment of ventilator-associated pneumonia: a systematic review and metaanalysis. Crit Care Med 2015;43(3): 527–33.

72. Kalil AC, Metersky ML, Klompas M, et al. Management of adults with hospital-acquired and ventilator-associated pneumonia: 2016 clinical practice guidelines by the Infectious Diseases Society of America and the American Thoracic Society. Clin Infect Dis 2016;63(5):e61–111.

73. Nseir S, Martin-Loeches I, Makris D, et al. Impact of appropriate antimicrobial treatment on transition from ventilator-associated tracheobronchitis to ventilator-associated pneumonia. Crit Care 2014; 18(3):R129.

74. Lin C-C, Liu T-C, Kuo C-F, et al. Aerosolized colistin for the treatment of multidrug-resistant *Acinetobacter baumannii* pneumonia: experience in a tertiary care hospital in northern Taiwan. J Microbiol Immunol Infect 2010;43(4):323–31.

75. Athanassa ZE, Myrianthefs PM, Boutzouka EG, et al. Monotherapy with inhaled colistin for the treatment of patients with ventilator-associated tracheobronchitis due to polymyxin-only-susceptible Gram-negative bacteria. J Hosp Infect 2011;78(4):335–6.

76. Kofteridis DP, Alexopoulou C, Valachis A, et al. Aerosolized plus intravenous colistin versus intravenous colistin alone for the treatment of ventilator-associated pneumonia: a matched case-control study. Clin Infect Dis 2010;51(11):1238–44.

77. Doshi NM, Cook CH, Mount KL, et al. Adjunctive aerosolized colistin for multi-drug resistant gram-negative pneumonia in the critically ill: a retrospective study. BMC Anesthesiol 2013;13(1):45.

78. Abdellatif S, Trifi A, Daly F, et al. Efficacy and toxicity of aerosolised colistin in ventilator-associated pneumonia: a prospective, randomised trial. Ann Intensive Care 2016;6(1):26.

Optimizing Antibiotic Administration for Pneumonia

Ana Motos, MSc[a,b], James M. Kidd, PharmD[a],
David P. Nicolau, PharmD, FCCP, FIDSA[a,c],*

KEYWORDS

- Pharmacokinetics • Pharmacodynamics • Hospital-acquired bacterial pneumonia
- Community-acquired bacterial pneumonia • Ventilator-acquired bacterial pneumonia
- Critical illness

KEY POINTS

- In the multidrug-resistance era, dosing decisions should be driven by pharmacokinetic and pharmacodynamic principles, maximizing microbiological response as minimizing toxicity and emergence of resistance.
- Pharmacokinetics/pharmacodynamics studies are a central part of preclinical/clinical antibiotic development programs; however, labeled dosing recommendations are frequently not specific to the treatment of pneumonia.
- Aerosolized antibiotics could deliver an effective drug concentration directly to the respiratory system and rapidly achieve eradication, while reducing drug resistance and systemic antibiotics exposure.
- The combination of antibiotics and its potential synergy have been investigated, revealing the need to confirm that in vitro data are consistent with clinical outcomes.
- Despite the evidence supporting the clinical significance of therapeutic drug monitoring, a lack of consistency among hospitals drives the need for standardized guidelines.

INTRODUCTION

Pneumonia is the third most common cause of death worldwide[1] and remains responsible for approximately 50% of all episodes of sepsis and septic shock.[2] Both community-acquired bacterial pneumonia (CABP) and hospital-acquired bacterial pneumonia (HABP) are associated with increased morbidity, mortality, hospital length of stay, and health care costs.[3–6] Furthermore, patients with ventilator-acquired bacterial pneumonia (VABP) have longer mean hospital and intensive care unit (ICU) stays, more mechanical ventilation days, and higher mortality than ICU non-VABP patients.[7] In 2013, pneumonia was among the 10 most economically charged diseases to the US health care systems, with an aggregate cost of approximately $9.5 billion.[8]

Despite advances in antimicrobial therapy and improvement in the clinical management of pneumonia, treatment failure rates for HABP and CABP

Disclosure Statement: A. Motos and J. M. Kidd have nothing to disclose. D.P. Nicolau is a consultant, is involved with speaker bureau, or has received research funding from Achaogen, Bayer, Cepheid, Merck, Melinta, Pfizer, and Shionogi.
[a] Center for Anti-Infective Research and Development, Hartford Hospital, 80 Seymour Street, Hartford, CT 06102, USA; [b] Division of Animal Experimentation, Department of Pulmonary and Critical Care, Hospital Clinic, 170 Villarroel Street, Barcelona 08036, Spain; [c] Division of Infectious Diseases, Hartford Hospital, 80 Seymour Street, Hartford, CT 06102, USA
* Corresponding author. Center for Anti-Infective Research and Development, Hartford Hospital, 80 Seymour Street, Hartford, CT 06102.
E-mail address: david.nicolau@hhchealth.org

Clin Chest Med 39 (2018) 837–852
https://doi.org/10.1016/j.ccm.2018.08.006
0272-5231/18/© 2018 Elsevier Inc. All rights reserved.

remain high at 30.0% to 62.0%[9] and 2.4% to 31.0%,[10] respectively. Although many factors contribute to treatment failures, several of these factors concern the provision of antibacterial therapy. Foremost, an antibiotic must be selected to which the suspected causative organism is susceptible. However, the emergence of multidrug resistant (MDR) or extensive-drug resistant (XDR) pathogens[11] makes this a challenge, both in ensuring adequate likelihood of efficacy and in preventing the inappropriate use of broad-spectrum antibacterials. Indeed, drug resistance is particularly important, given that the ESKAPE pathogens (*Enterococcus faecium*, *Staphylococcus aureus*, *Klebsiella pneumoniae*, *Acinetobacter baumannii*, *Pseudomonas aeruginosa*, and *Enterobacter* species) represent more than 80%[12] of HABP. In addition to selecting the right drug, the right dose must be used. Many antibacterials lack labeled indications for the treatment of pneumonia. Labeled doses for other indications may yield insufficient concentrations in lung tissues or fail to account for variation among patients, such as those with critical illness, obesity, augmented renal clearance, or those receiving organ replacement therapies, such as hemodialysis or extracorporeal membrane oxygenation.

Optimal antibacterial treatment, which includes the correct selection of 1 or more antibiotics, dosing, route of administration, and appropriate duration of therapy, significantly improves outcomes of patients with pneumonia.[13] Certainly, the ideal approach should maximize the likelihood of a satisfactory microbiological response as well as minimize the exposure-related toxicity and the emergence and spread of bacterial resistance.[14] In this context, intelligent dosing decisions should be driven by the principles of pharmacokinetics (PK) and pharmacodynamics (PD).

Although a significant portion of PK/PD studies are performed to identify optimal doses for use in clinical trials, these methods can also be used in a patient-specific fashion to guide dosing. The latest Infectious Diseases Society of America/American Thoracic Society (IDSA/ATS) guidelines for the treatment of HABP/VABP weakly recommend PK/PD-driven dosing strategies.[15] Although the downsides of this approach are scant, involving cost and personnel burden, limited clinical evidence exists supporting the practice, garnering the weak recommendation. Under these circumstances, the extent to which patient-specific adjustment of antibacterial regimens based on PK/PD data should be used and its potential impact on major outcomes are still under debate.

In the era of multidrug resistance, the optimization of antibiotic efficacy is a priority. Although several promising new antibiotics are in development,[16–18] some may lack the clear guidance of a labeled indication, and others will be routinely used in poorly studied subpopulations. For patient-specific treatment decisions, an understanding of PK/PD is indispensable. This article reviews the principle considerations of PK and PD for the treatment of pneumonia, and highlights potential approaches to optimization and future areas of investigation.

PRINCIPLES OF PHARMACOKINETIC/PHARMACODYNAMIC OPTIMIZATION

With the increasing prevalence of MDR pathogens, the rational use of antibiotics has been emphasized.[19] Antibiotic optimization requires that the pharmacologic properties of antimicrobials be taken into account. PK is the branch of pharmacology that studies the evolution of drug concentrations in different body tissues over time, or, succinctly, what the body does to the drug. A mathematical relationship between the dosing regimen and the resultant plasma concentrations can be established, and it is crucial because the profile of the concentration over time can affect outcomes. In PK models, tissues, or collections thereof, are represented by compartments. For example, a 1-compartment model consists of a single central compartment (eg, the plasma), whereas a multicompartment model consists of a central compartment as well as peripheral compartment(s), which may represent distinct tissue(s), such as adipose or lung tissue. A pharmacokinetic model may also make no assumptions about compartments and treat the body as a single entity.

The drug concentration–time profile is determined by the processes of absorption, distribution, metabolism, and excretion. Absorption describes the rate at which drug is transferred into the central compartment, for example, into the bloodstream from the gastrointestinal tract after oral administration. Distribution describes the transfer among the compartments, which can be a dynamic, bidirectional process. Metabolism describes the chemical transformation of drugs, and elimination describes the excretion of drug from the body.

PKs are also affected by drug physiochemical properties such as aqueous solubility and hydrophilicity. Hydrophilic antibiotics tend to concentrate in the intravascular and extravascular body fluids, whereas lipophilic drugs distribute into lipid tissue and intracellularly.[20] Another chemical characteristic that affects PKs is the degree to which a drug binds protein. Protein-bound drug is not available to distribute out of the central compartment or to interact with a molecular target; thus, for antibiotics, only free drug is microbiologically active.[21] Acidic and pH-neutral drugs primarily bind albumin, whereas basic drugs tend to bind alpha-1 acid glycoprotein. Alterations in the levels of these proteins, such as hypoalbuminemia, which is frequently observed in critically ill patients, can therefore increase the proportion of free drug.

PK models depend on parameters that can help understand the PK properties of a drug. Together, metabolism and elimination determine the clearance (CL), a PK parameter that is defined as the volume of plasma cleared of the drug per unit time. CL can be separated by organ, such as renal CL (CL_R) and hepatic CL (CL_H). Volume of distribution (V_D) is a PK parameter describing the theoretic volume into which a drug has been added. For example, if an intravenous (IV) bolus of 100 mg of a drug yields a concentration of 0.005 mg/mL, the V_D is 20 L. Distribution away from the central compartment results in lower plasma concentrations, yielding a higher V_D. These parameters depend both on the host and the intrinsic properties of the antibiotic. These parameters help to understand antibiotic exposure in plasma and other tissues, providing a pharmacokinetic curve, as illustrated in **Fig. 1**.

The other branch of pharmacology is PD, which assesses the effects of antimicrobial agents, or, colloquially, what the drug does to the body/target. The therapeutic outcome is determined by the antibacterial concentration-time profile at the site of action and the susceptibility of the microorganisms to the antibacterial, expressed as minimum inhibitory concentration (MIC). The pathogen-drug interaction has classically been determined by in vitro methods; however, therapeutic success also depends on the virulence profile, immune response, and the site of infection.[22] Although patients may still succumb to infection despite an optimized antibacterial regimen, using PD principles to maximize antibacterial activity provides the patient with a greater chance of recovery.

PD optimization involves first determining an index, or driver, that predicts inhibition or eradication of bacteria, then establishing a threshold for a desired level of effect, and finally, adjusting dosage to maximize that threshold. Antibiotics have been classified into 3 categories based on the index that best correlates with antibacterial effect: concentration-dependence, time-dependence, or a combination of both[23,24] In brief, antibiotics that are concentration dependent have increasing efficacy with higher concentrations; these antibiotics should be given in higher doses and at longer intervals. On the other hand, antibiotics that demonstrate time-dependence are optimized by maintaining a concentration above a certain threshold, typically the MIC of the pathogen; higher concentrations above the threshold provide no added benefit, and these drugs are best dosed by continuous infusion or by smaller doses given more frequently. For those drugs that exhibit a combination of both, neither concentration nor time clearly correlates better with effect, so the optimization approach is simply to achieve a target exposure, or area under the concentration-time curve (AUC). The PD drivers associated with each of these 3 groups include

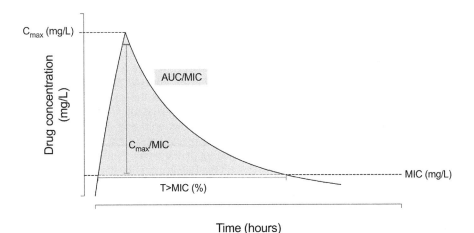

Fig. 1. PK and PD model for antimicrobial efficacy prediction. Schematic profile of IV antibiotic with traditional intermittent infusion. AUC/MIC, area under the curve concentration-time to the MIC; C_{max}/MIC, the ratio of maximum drug concentration to the MIC; T > MIC, percentage of a time period that the drug concentration is above MIC.

the MIC of the organism, as organisms that are less susceptible have higher targets. These PD drivers are as follows: for concentration-dependence, the ratio of maximum free drug concentration to the MIC (fC_{max}/MIC); for time-dependence, the percentage of a time period that the unbound drug concentration is above MIC ($fT > MIC$); and, for drugs that depend on both, the ratio of the area under the free drug concentration-time curve to the MIC ($fAUC_{24h}$/MIC).[23,24] In each case, only free drug is considered, because protein-bound drug cannot exert an antibacterial effect. These drivers also may be reported based on total drug concentrations; however, total drug concentrations have less correlation with effect than free drug concentrations. Importantly, for the treatment of pneumonia, the free drug concentration at the site of infection, for example, the epithelial lining fluid (ELF), may differ significantly from the plasma concentration.

The PD drivers and specific targets for antibacterials used to treat HABP/VABP and CABP are listed in **Table 1**. For β-lactams and macrolides, $fT > MIC$ is the best predictor of bacterial eradication and microbiological response.[25–27] The $fCmax$/MIC most closely predicts the effect of aminoglycosides, fluoroquinolones and polymixins,[28–31] whereas $fAUC$/MIC best predicts the efficacy of vancomycin and the oxazolidinones.[32,33]

A further consideration when optimizing the PD of antibacterials that is not communicated by the PD driver and target is the postantibiotic effect (PAE). This phenomenon was first described following the discovery of penicillin[34] and has been defined as the delay in normal bacterial growth after antibiotic exposure, for example, after a drug is completely eliminated from the target tissue. Aminoglycosides most prominently display this phenomenon, having a prolonged PAE.[35] This effect is due to the mechanism of action of aminoglycosides, which impair protein synthesis in bacteria by irreversibly binding the ribosome, an insult that has lingering effects. For β-lactams except carbapenems, antibiotics do not show an important PAE for gram-negative pathogens. In contrast, significant PAE was reported for gram-positive organisms.[36]

CONSIDERATIONS FOR PNEUMONIA AND CRITICALLY ILL PATIENTS

Measurements of antibacterial concentration in the plasma provide important information and, additionally with the MIC from the clinical isolated strain, aid clinicians in determining the most appropriate dosage regimen to achieve the best outcome. Because unbound drug freely diffuses

into the interstitial space from capillaries, the plasma concentration is considered an estimation of concentrations at the site of infection. Nevertheless, this is not always the case and the pulmonary system has special considerations on the drug distribution that are not reflected by plasma PK data. Moreover, different subcompartments exist in the lung, including the alveolar epithelium, endothelium, interstitial space, and pulmonary alveolar macrophages. Therefore, many factors can influence the penetration and the rate to reach the infected tissue. First, only the unbound drug fraction is considered available to cross the blood-alveolar barrier to get the target lung tissues. As such, the rate of diffusion primarily defines the penetration of the drug into the lungs. This rate is affected by the lipophilicity, polarity, and diffusibility of the molecules and is described by the Fick laws. As mentioned before, lipophilic molecules with low molecular weight (ie, linezolid[37]) penetrate better than hydrophilic compounds (ie, vancomycin[38]). Host factors also affect lung penetration, primarily, inflammation, the pH, or the condensation at the site of infection.[39] Therefore, the plasma concentrations often differ from the local tissue concentrations. Furthermore, even for the same drug, tissue concentrations may differ between healthy patients and those with acute illness. An example of this is provided by a recent study that found significant differences in serum and ELF concentrations of piperacillin between healthy volunteers and critically ill patients.[40] These findings underscore the fact that the lungs are not a uniform tissue, particularly during infection, so the concentration levels can also vary through them.

To overcome this possible discordance with plasma levels, ELF concentrations can be used to more accurately measure penetration in the lungs. ELF is assessed on the interior surface of the alveolar wall and is recovered through bronchoalveolar lavage (BAL). To account for dilution caused by the BAL fluid, the ratio of urea in the lavage fluid to the ratio of urea in the blood is used as a correction factor, as urea freely diffuses between plasma and ELF, yielding the following relation: $V_{ELF} = V_{BAL} * Urea_{BAL}/Urea_{serum}$. Although the measurement of drug concentrations in the ELF is currently the most broadly used technique, it has some limitations. Using this volume correction, we are assuming that urea and antibiotics spread in the tissue at the same rate, which may not be accurate in those with low lung penetration. Moreover, ELF concentrations are useful only to estimate extracellular pathogens' antibiotic exposure, and the lysis of cellular components, such as alveolar macrophages, can be a source

Table 1
Commonly used intravenous antibiotics for the treatment of pneumonia and associated pharmacodynamic characteristics

Antibiotic Class	Antimicrobial Killing Characteristic	Drug	PD Drivers and PD Target
Aminoglycosides	Concentration dependent	Amikacin Tobramycin Gentamicin	$fC_{max}/MIC \geq 10$[30]
β-lactams	Time dependent	Oxacillin	$fT > MIC \geq 50\%$[26]
		Penicillin G	
		Nafcillin	
		Piperacillin/tazobactam	$fT > MIC \geq 50\%$[26]
		Ticarcillin/clavulanic acid	
		Ampicillin/sulbactam	
		Ceftolozane/tazobactam	
		Ceftazidime	$fT > MIC \geq 50\%–70\%$[26]
		Cefepime	
		Ceftriaxone	
		Cefotaxime	
		Ceftaroline	
		Cefazolin	
		Aztreonam	$fT > MIC \geq 50\%–60\%$[108]
		Meropenem	$fT > MIC \geq 40\%$[25]
		Imipenem	
		Doripenem	
		Ertapenem	
Fluoroquinolones	Concentration dependent	Levofloxacin Ciprofloxacin Moxifloxacin	G+ AUC/MIC >125[29] G− fAUC/MIC >30[28]
Glycopeptides	Concentration and time dependent	Vancomycin	AUC/MIC >400[32]
Oxazolidinone	Time dependent	Linezolid Tedizolid	AUC/MIC ≥80–120[33]
Polymyxin	Concentration dependent	Colistin Polymyxin B	$fC_{max}/MIC \geq 12–45$[31,109]
Tetracyclines	Concentration and time dependent	Doxycycline Minocycline	AUC/MIC ≥80[110,a]
Macrolides	Time dependent	Azithromycin Erythromycin Clarithromycin	$fT > MIC \geq 40\%–50\%$[27,a]

Abbreviations: fAUC/MIC, free area under the curve concentration-time to the MIC; fC_{max}/MIC, the ratio of maximum free drug concentration to the MIC; fT > MIC, percentage of a time period that the unbound drug concentration is above MIC; G−, gram-negatives; G+, gram-positives; MIC, minimum inhibitory concentration; PD, pharmacodynamic.
   [a] AUC/MIC targets need to be clinically confirmed with large studies.

of error. In spite of these limitations, ELF determination remains the most useful tool to understand how antibacterials penetrate the lung.

Following physiologic and pharmacologic principles, the relative concentration-time profiles of antibiotics in plasma and ELF can differ. For some antibiotics, lung concentration has a linear relationship with plasma concentration, yielding parallel curves when both are plotted together. For macrolides, oxazolidinones and fluoroquinolones, this relationship is observed, and ELF concentrations are typically higher than plasma concentrations. β-lactams, glycopeptides, and aminoglycosides also show this relationship, but ELF concentrations are typically less than plasma concentrations. In contrast, other antibiotics, such as carbapenems, reveal system hysteresis between ELF and plasma concentrations, which means that ELF and plasma concentrations increase and decrease asynchronously, for example, the ELF concentration may be increasing while the plasma concentration is decreasing, and vice versa.[41] Because of system hysteresis, the penetration ratio changes over time, and therefore it is not possible to accurately estimate the lung concentration at a particular time using the plasma concentration and the mean penetration ratio. To overcome this, nearly all studies determine both ELF and bloodstream concentrations at multiple time points, while mean penetration ratios are determined from the ratio AUC_{plasma}/AUC_{ELF}.

Pharmacokinetic parameters, such as CL and V_D, can be severely altered in patients with pneumonia, especially those that are critically ill. These changes mainly affect PK of hydrophilic drugs, because their tissue distributions are restricted to extracellular and central compartments and are normally cleared by the renal route. For hydrophilic drugs, volume of distribution is closely related to extracellular V_D, which may increase several-fold in critically ill patients.[42,43] Vasodilatation and increased vascular permeability are hallmarks of sepsis.[44] These processes result in the capillary leakage syndrome, which is responsible for the fluid extravasation, causing edema, and hypotension.[45] To maintain systemic pressure, large volumes of fluids are administered. As a result of all of these factors, volume of distribution can increase, yielding lower antibacterial concentrations at the site of infection.[46] Other factors that can contribute to get higher V_D are presence of extracorporeal circuits, surgical drains, or the requirement for mechanical ventilation.[46]

Approximately half of critically ill patients present with a low serum albumin concentration (≤25 g/L).[47] For drugs that bind albumin, hypoalbuminemia leads to increased free drug exposures because fewer binding sites are available.[48] The greater the degree of protein binding, the greater the decrease in free drug exposures will be. Although this may result in a greater pharmacodynamic effect, it also may increase distribution out of the central compartment; therefore, increasing antibacterial V_D.[21] Hypoalbuminemia also affects CL_R, because protein-bound drug is not filtered at the healthy glomerulus, therefore a higher unbound antibiotic fraction results in a greater renal elimination from the vascular component. Ulldemolins and colleagues[48] reported that in hypoalbuminemic condition, protein binding commonly decreases in critically ill patients. The investigators found that increased V_D and CL resulted in reduced $fT > MIC$, leading to therapeutic failure for time-dependent antibacterials. This is especially relevant for highly protein-bound antibiotics, such as ertapenem and ceftriaxone, where V_D and CL increase twofold with in the setting of hypoalbuminemia.

Augmented renal clearance (ARC) occurs in critically ill patients with increased cardiac output, as in early septic shock, which leads to an increase in glomerular filtration rate. It is typically defined as having a creatinine clearance of ≥130 mL/min[49] and primarily affects hydrophilic compounds that are renally eliminated. ARC can have a crucial role in the time-dependent antimicrobials, such as β-lactams, because it is a priority to maintain adequate concentrations in the plasma.[49] Conversely, reduced clearance can also be produced by 2 common ICU complications: acute kidney injury with or without the need for renal replacement therapy, and hepatic dysfunction. For some antibiotics, patients with decreased renal clearance have compensatory pathways for elimination,[50,51] whereas hepatic blood flow may compensate the reduced metabolic capacity due to liver dysfunction. Hepatic impairment leads to accumulation of hepatically metabolized antimicrobials, and may be associated with hypoproteinemia, increasing V_D.[52] For drugs that are eliminated by hepatic and renal clearance, such as fluoroquinolones, clinicians should give special attention when both injuries concurrently occur.

Finally, in addition to the previously described considerations, ICU patients are at higher risk of being colonized by MDR pathogens.[11] As expected, pneumonia caused by MDR bacteria is associated with higher mortality, ICU stay, and worse outcomes.[53] These organisms have higher MICs, which means that higher doses may be necessary to reach PD targets. However, the current clinical data suggest that patients are more frequently underdosed than overdosed.[52]

In summary, the idiosyncrasies of the lung and the wide spectrum of pathophysiological changes in critically ill patients lead to variability in PD target attainment and treatment outcomes. This reveals a need for PK/PD methods to better define and reach PD targets for these patients, especially with all the aforementioned considerations that must be taken into account when treating patients with pneumonia.

APPROACHES TO OPTIMIZATION
Pharmacodynamic Dose Optimization

PK/PD studies are a central part of preclinical and clinical antibiotic development programs; however, labeled dosing recommendations are frequently not specific to the treatment of pneumonia. For example, the approved doses of many IV β-lactams are administered as short infusions, but extending the infusion time to maximize $fT > MIC$ improves outcomes, including those in patients with nosocomial pneumonia.[54,55] Although many antibiotics have several dosing regimens, the use of PK/PD can optimize doses specifically for the treatment of pneumonia. In this section, we discuss the process of using PK/PD studies to determine an optimized dosing regimen to support a clinical trial for pneumonia treatment. As an example, we follow the development of ceftazidime/avibactam.

An overview of the scientific workflow from preclinical development to phase 3 clinical trials is presented in **Fig. 2**. Preclinical animal models of infection are used once an agent has previously demonstrated promising in vitro efficacy. Murine models of pneumonia are most frequently used due to ease, although swine are also used, as they have a pulmonary physiology closer to that of humans and can be mechanically ventilated to study ventilator-acquired pneumonia. Initially, the PK of the drug is studied in the model by measuring tissue concentrations after a range of dosing regimens. For pneumonia, the drug concentration in the ELF can be estimated using the urea ratio between blood and ELF as previously described. Concentration-time profiles are then analyzed to determine PK parameters, such as CL, V_D, and AUC, and data are fit to a PK model. When the PK are known, PD studies are performed to determine the magnitude of effect of the drug, usually measured as a decrease in bacterial density in lung tissue. PD data can then be correlated with different PK measures, such as AUC, maximum concentration achieved, or percentage of time above bacterial MIC, to determine which one best drives efficacy. The magnitude of the PD driver necessary to produce thresholds of efficacy, such as bacteriostasis or bactericidal activity, is then determined. Human dosing regimens can then be designed to meet this PD target.

An instructive example of the use of PK/PD principles to study the efficacy of an antibiotic for pneumonia is found with ceftazidime/avibactam (AvyCaz; Allergan Inc., Jersey City, NJ). Ceftazidime/avibactam is a novel β-lactam/β-lactamase inhibitor combination with activity against extended-spectrum β-lactamases, carbapenemases, AmpC β-lactamases, and OXA-48

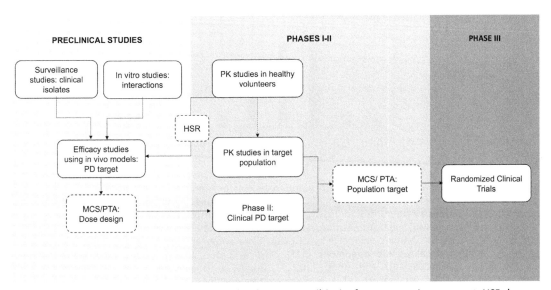

Fig. 2. Stepwise optimization approach to the development antibiotics for pneumonia treatment. HSR, human-simulated regimens. MCS, monte carlo simulation; PTA, probability of target attainment.

enzymes, giving it strong potential for the treatment of HABP due to MDR pathogens. Ceftazidime/avibactam was originally approved by the Food and Drug Administration (FDA) for the treatment of complicated intra-abdominal infection and complicated urinary tract infections at a dose of 2.5 g every 8 hours as a 2-hour infusion, and later received marketing approval for nosocomial pneumonia from both the FDA and the European Medicines Agency. To support an indication for nosocomial pneumonia, it was critical to investigate whether the approved dose would be sufficient to drive efficacy in lung tissue.

Initial surveillance study data demonstrated ceftazidime/avibactam had in vitro activity against more than 19,000 pathogens isolated from patients with HABP, including ventilated patients[56,57] (**Fig. 3**). As expected, ceftazidime-avibactam exhibited high efficacy against *P aeruginosa*, including ceftazidime and meropenem nonsusceptible isolates; $\geq$86.3% of carbapenem-resistant *P aeruginosa* and $\geq$84.6% of *Enterobacteriaceae* isolates were susceptible to ceftazidime/avibactam. In contrast, activity against

A baumannii was poor (susceptibility $\leq$38.5%) due to the lack of activity against metallo- β -lactamases. Still, these data supported CAZ-AVI as a potential therapeutic antimicrobial choice for patients with pneumonia caused by these organisms, for which few treatment options exist.

To predict the efficacy of a given dosing regimen, a PD target must be defined. For cephalosporins, which are time-dependent antibiotics, a free drug time above MIC ($fT > MIC$) of $\geq$50% is predictive of clinical efficacy for VABP.[58] Additionally, the probability that a given dosing regimen will achieve this target also can be determined using a mathematical simulation method known as Monte Carlo simulation (MCS).[59] Briefly, PK models were constructed using serum PK parameters obtained from phase I studies. Then, MCS software creates a hypothetical population of thousands of patients by generating random PK parameters within the distribution of those observed during the phase I study. For each of these hypothetical patients, a concentration-time profile is simulated and the $fT > MIC$ is calculated. The number of patients achieving the target $fT > MIC$ divided by the entire

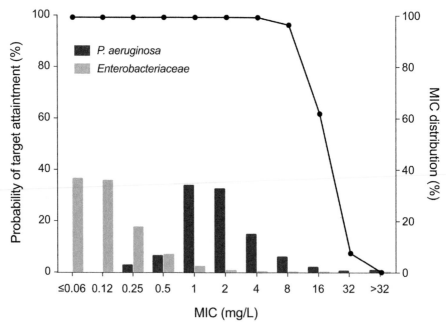

Fig. 3. Distribution of *P aeruginosa* and *Enterobacteriaceae* isolates from HABP patients in US medical centers (2011–2015) in terms of ceftazidime/avibactam MIC level and the PTA of $fT > MIC$ for ceftazidime/avibactam, using 2.5 g every 8 hours as a 2-hour infusion. Histograms represent the distribution frequency of MIC. Lines represent PTA values through MIC level. Distributions of isolates and PTA data were obtained. (*Data from* Sader HS, Castanheira M, Flamm RK. Antimicrobial activity of ceftazidime-avibactam against gram-negative bacteria isolated from patients hospitalized with pneumonia in U.S. Medical Centers, 2011–2015. Antimicrob Agents Chemother 2017;61(4): [pii:e02083-16]; and Zhou LJD, Al Huniti N, Bouchillon S, et al. Pharmacokinetic/pharmacodynamic target attainment (PTA) and cumulative fractions of response (CFR) for ceftazidime, ceftazidime-avibactam, and meropenem against bacteria isolated from patients in Europe in 2012. 24th European Congress of Clinical Microbiology and Infectious Diseases (ECCMID). Barcelona, Spain,13th May, 2014.)

number of simulated patients yields the probability of target attainment (PTA). A PTA of 90% or higher at MIC values of interest is a widely accepted value to support a dose regimen. In our example, the PTA for ceftazidime/avibactam against *P aeruginosa* and *Enterobacteriaceae* at standard regimen of 2.5 g every 8 hours as a 2-hour infusion was greater than 90% for MICs $\leq$8 mg/L[60] (see **Fig. 3**).

Although the serum PK of ceftazidime/avibactam had been described and the dose was highly likely to reach the serum PD target, it was necessary to study the PK in lung tissue specifically. To study the efficacy of the approved human dose for lung infection, a murine dosing regimen simulating the ceftazidime/avibactam serum concentration-time profile in humans was designed.[61] The regimen closely matched the human serum concentration-time profile and showed that ELF penetration was 24% for ceftazidime and 22% for avibactam. Efficacy was achieved against *P aeruginosa* with MICs up to 32 mg/L when serum *f*T > MIC was $\geq$60% and ELF *f*T > MIC was $\geq$12%.

The next step was to link human lung exposures to the PD efficacy target determined from the murine study. To this end, ceftazidime/avibactam lung PK was assessed in healthy volunteers. Two doses of ceftazidime/avibactam, 2.0 g ceftazidime/0.5 g avibactam and 3.0 g ceftazidime/1.0 g avibactam, were studied in 22 and 21 healthy volunteers, respectively.[62] Both regimens were administered every 8 hours as a 2-hour IV infusion. At steady state, plasma samples were collected before the final dose and at multiple time points in the 8 hours thereafter. BAL was performed once per participant at 2, 4, 6, or 8 hours after the last dose. Using PK models, AUC_{ELF}/AUC_{plasma} ratios were similar at 31% to 32% for ceftazidime and 32% to 35% for avibactam. Lung penetration in these patients was greater than that observed with the regimen used in the murine PD study simulating human serum concentrations at a dose of 2.5 g every 8 hours as a 2-hour infusion. The dose demonstrated efficacy in mice and exceeded the lung concentrations achieved in that model, supporting its use in further clinical trials for pneumonia.

The phase III study comparing ceftazidime/avibactam to meropenem in HABP/VABP, has recently been completed[63] (ClinicalTrials.gov, NCT01808092). This multicenter, randomized controlled, double-blind trial included 879 patients with HABP/VABP randomized to receive 2.5 g ceftazidime/avibactam, every 8 hours as a 2-hour infusion or 1.0 g meropenem every 8 hours as a 30-minute infusion. Ceftazidime/avibactam demonstrated noninferiority to meropenem. In the clinically modified intention-to-treat

population, 68.8% of 356 patients in the ceftazidime-avibactam group were clinically cured, compared with 73% of 370 patients in the meropenem group ($P = .0066$). In the clinically evaluable population, 77.4% of 257 participants were clinically cured in the ceftazidime-avibactam group, compared with 78.1% of 270 in the meropenem group ($P = .0007$). Similar results were noted in secondary analysis population. Likewise, all-cause mortality did not statistically differ between treatment groups, but was higher in the ceftazidime/avibactam than in the meropenem group (9% vs 7%). However, ceftazidime/avibactam benefits may have been limited because the population that could most benefit, HABP/VABP patients with carbapenem-resistant isolates, was excluded.

This example shows how a clinical development program can effectively use the principles of PK/PD to optimize an antibiotic for the treatment of pneumonia. In addition to supporting a drug development plan, however, these studies also can be used to investigate subpopulations of interest as phase 4 post-marketing studies.

Local Delivery

Aerosol administration has been investigated as a potential therapeutic optimization to target drug delivery to the lung and avoid the limitations of systemic IV administration.[64] Aerosolized antibiotics could deliver a therapeutically effective drug concentration directly to the respiratory system and rapidly achieve eradication, while reducing drug resistance and systemic exposure to antibiotics.[65] The most recent nebulizers have increased lung deposition of aerosolized antibiotic dose up to 60% compared with old nebulizers.[66,67] The type of nebulizer, the mass median aerodynamic diameter,[68] and the inspiratory flow turbulence[69] are crucial conditions of the final delivery efficiency. Importantly, significant differences were found in a study[70] conducted in mechanically ventilated piglets with pneumonia comparing lung deposition of equivalent doses of ceftazidime administered IV or by an ultrasonic nebulizer (10 ± 3 vs 129 ± 108 µg/g tissue, respectively; $P < .001$). Similar results have been reported when sputum colistin concentration was compared in patients with cystic fibrosis treated with IV versus nebulized colistin.[71]

Aerosolized antibiotics, especially aminoglycosides, have yielded promising results in terms of eradication,[67,72,73] antibiotic delivery,[74,75] and prevention of resistance acquisition.[76] Nevertheless, clinical efficacy was not demonstrated in the 2 most recent clinical trials (IASIS[77] and INHALE). In IASIS (ClinicalTrials.gov, NCT01969799), a phase 3 clinical trial, Kollef and colleagues[77] compared IV meropenem with nebulized combination of 300 mg amikacin and 120 mg fosfomycin every 12 hours versus meropenem alone treatment in patients with gram-negative bacterial VAP. Preliminary data[78] showed extremely high tracheal aspirate concentrations (19,280 ± 13,307 mg*h/L of amikacin and 10,410 ± 7394 mg*h/L of fosfomycin). Despite a decrease in positive tracheal cultures, the study did not demonstrate a significant difference in the primary clinical outcome of change from baseline in the clinical pulmonary infection score during the planned 10-day treatment period, and secondary clinical outcomes including clinical cure, ventilator, and ICU days and mortality. Similar results were observed in the INHALE trial (ClinicalTrials.gov, NCT00805163), in which 725 patients with gram-negative VAP were randomized to receive standard IV therapy plus 400 mg aerosolized amikacin every 12 hours (BAY 41-6551) or aerosolized placebo. Adjunctive aerosolized amikacin was not superior to IV therapy alone, in either the primary outcome of 28 to 32 days' survival or secondary outcomes, including clinical response and ventilator days.[79]

Although the latest studies of aerosolized antibiotic delivery have been designed with the aid of preliminary pharmacologic studies, certain factors make PK optimization of these agents challenging. Certainly, investigators have aimed to reach high lung concentrations to drive efficacy. However, a study of aerosolized delivery of amikacin in swine demonstrates that the extent of drug penetration into the lung tissue is affected by the severity and extent of the infection.[80] It was found that amikacin concentrations were significantly lower in lung parenchyma that was poorly aerated and in sections with a high degree of confluence (197 ± 165 µg/g vs 40 ± 62 µg/g). Therefore, measurements of antibiotic concentration taken from tracheal aspirates may not provide sufficient information about drug delivery into the infected parenchyma. Additional in vivo studies should be performed to elucidate the real antibiotic deposition into confluent areas. Finally, administering higher antibiotic concentrations to improve delivery to infected parenchyma must be balanced against the unclear risk of tissue damage resulting from these concentrations.

Combination Therapy and Synergy

The combination of 2 or more antibiotics as empirical treatment for pneumonia is a standard approach to broaden the initial spectrum of activity against likely pathogens. For most patients, treatment should be subsequently narrowed to appropriate monotherapy once the pathogen and susceptibilities are known. However, combinations of antibiotics also may be used as targeted therapy to exploit synergy, where the total effect of multiple antibiotics used together is greater than the sum of each used individually. This effect increases the rate of bactericidal activity and may be effective at suppressing resistance, particularly for recalcitrant organisms, such as P aeruginosa.[81] Synergy is typically observed from the combination of 2 drugs with complementary mechanisms of action. The classic example of antibiotic synergy is the combination of a β-lactam with an aminoglycoside against gram-negative bacteria: the β-lactam weakens the peptidoglycan layer and permits greater concentrations of the aminoglycoside to reach its target, the ribosome. Contemporary examples of in vitro synergy among agents that may be useful for P aeruginosa pneumonia include combinations of ceftolozane/tazobactam with fosfomycin, colistin, or amikacin.[82,83] However, despite the theoretic benefits of targeted combination therapy, it is not currently supported by clinical data except for patients with a high mortality risk, or against pathogens that are extensively or pan-drug resistant.[15,84]

Multiple in vitro methods are used to measure synergy: time-kill, checkerboard, and gradient diffusion assays. There are several limitations to these methodologies. First, disagreement between methods has been reported.[85,86] Second, the time-consuming nature of these methods and the limited number of bacterial strains tested makes them unsuitable for routine clinical practice.[87] Finally, molecular interaction mechanisms cannot be determined from these studies.[88] Therefore, understanding the mechanisms that drive some antimicrobial combinations to clinical success remains a challenge Consequently, a gold standard method has not been defined yet, but the time-kill assay is considered the most appropriate standard reference technique.

Besides the methodological limitations of in vitro synergy studies, there is a lack of evidence to link these results to clinical outcomes. Further still, discordance between positive in vitro results and negative in vivo outcomes have been reported.[82] Fortunately, during the past decade, some studies assessed this question using animal models and clinical data to correlate with in vitro results.[89–91] Interestingly, Bremmer and colleagues[89] demonstrated that the in vitro combination of minocycline and colistin in the checkerboard platform accurately correlated with microbiological clearance in XDR A baumannii–infected patients. Upcoming studies need to confirm that in vitro data are consistent with in vivo scenarios and correlated with human clinical outcomes.

Therapeutic Drug Monitoring

Therapeutic drug monitoring (TDM) for individual patients can be used to monitor and adjust drug dosing to achieve a target PD driver. Traditionally, TDM has been used in clinical practice to adjust doses of aminoglycosides and glycopeptides, due to the high risk of toxicity associated with these agents.[92–94] This is particularly important when treating pneumonia, as both classes have relatively poor lung penetration.[95,96] For aminoglycosides, which are C_{max}-driven antibiotics, TDM allows for high doses to be maintained, whereas the dosing interval can be extended in patients with reduced renal function. TDM of aminoglycosides is facilitated with the Hartford nomogram, which allows adjustment of the dosing interval based on a single serum concentration.[97] In a study of more than 2000 patients, the nomogram had success in reducing the rate of nephrotoxicity to 1.2% versus 3.0% to 5.0% historically, while maintaining a similar rate of clinical response. TDM is also recommended for vancomycin therapy[98] and can be accomplished with the measurement of trough levels alone, which have been correlated to AUCs known to drive efficacy.

However, the contemporary PK/PD studies[99–101] have shown high interpatient variability in PK among a variety of drugs and have led to the consideration of TDM as a possible optimization approach for other classes of antibiotics, especially the β-lactams, which are often underdosed. In a prospective study, Roberts and colleagues[102] found that 74.2% of critically ill patients required a β-lactam dose adjustment after the first measurement. This study included 89 patients diagnosed with HABP and 47 with CABP. In the HABP cohort, more patients required a dose increase (60%) than a decrease (25%). Among patients with CABP, dose changes were more balanced between increases (32%) and decreases (23%). This disparity could be explained by a difference in comorbidities between the groups. A recent clinical trial[103] randomized 41 patients with normal kidney function receiving meropenem or piperacillin/tazobactam, mostly for pneumonia, to either daily TDM or conventional treatment. The TDM group reached 100% $fT > MIC$ in 94.7% of patients, whereas only 64.8% of patients achieved it in the nonintervention group. TDM has been shown to help patients with continuous renal replacement therapy achieve β-lactam $fT > MIC$ targets.[104] Finally, Patel and colleagues[105] have shown that there is a significant need for TDM among burn patients: 60% of these patients did not achieve target $fT > MIC$.

Despite an abundance of evidence supporting the clinical significance of TDM and increasing implementation in ICUs, an international, multicenter study[106] reveals wide variability among hospitals regarding which patients are selected for TDM, assays used for concentration determination, and target concentrations themselves. This lack of consistency drives the need for guidelines to standardize TDM.

SUMMARY

With the emergence of multidrug resistance worldwide, antibiotic dose optimization guided by the principles of PK/PD is indispensable for the treatment of pneumonia. In this review, we have shown how these principles can be used to increase the probability of successful treatment of pneumonia and suppress the development of resistance. We also have described how this approach is vital for the many antibiotics in preclinical and clinical development. In the context of pneumonia, a robust knowledge of PK/PD specific to the lung is necessary. Without this knowledge, drugs that show promising in vitro activity against the most recalcitrant organisms may fail to successfully treat infections in the lung caused by these organisms, especially when these drugs are used off-label. As some notable failures in the drug development process demonstrate,[107] there are opportunities for improvement in selecting dose regimens. In addition, PK/PD optimization can also limit drug side effects by determining the lowest effective doses and adjusting doses based on serum concentrations to meet PD targets. Although success using these principles has been realized with extended infusions of β-lactams and once-daily aminoglycosides, opportunities remain to bring these principles to the clinic.

REFERENCES

1. World Health Organization. The top 10 causes of death. The 10 leading causes of death in the world, 2000 and 2012. 2014. Available at: http://wwwwhoint/mediacentre/factsheets/fs310/en/. Accessed date May 6, 2018.

2. Martin GS. Sepsis, severe sepsis and septic shock: changes in incidence, pathogens and outcomes. Expert Rev Anti Infect Ther 2012;10(6):701–6.

3. Eber MR, Laxminarayan R, Perencevich EN, et al. Clinical and economic outcomes attributable to health care-associated sepsis and pneumonia. Arch Intern Med 2010;170(4):347–53.

4. Park H, Adeyemi AO, Rascati KL. Direct medical costs and utilization of health care services to treat pneumonia in the United States: an analysis of the 2007-2011 medical expenditure panel survey. Clin Ther 2015;37(7):1466–76.e1.

5. Gibson GJ, Loddenkemper R, Lundback B, et al. Respiratory health and disease in Europe: the new European lung white book. Eur Respir J 2013;42(3):559–63.

6. Almirall J, Bolibar I, Vidal J, et al. Epidemiology of community-acquired pneumonia in adults: a population-based study. Eur Respir J 2000;15(4): 757–63.

7. Kyaw MH, Kern DM, Zhou S, et al. Healthcare utilization and costs associated with S. aureus and P. aeruginosa pneumonia in the intensive care unit: a retrospective observational cohort study in a US claims database. BMC Health Serv Res 2015;15:241.

8. Torio CM, Moore BJ. National inpatient hospital costs: the most expensive conditions by payer, 2013: statistical brief #204. Healthcare Cost and Utilization Project (HCUP) statistical briefs. Rockville (MD): Agency for Healthcare Research and Quality; 2016.

9. Iannella HA, Luna CM. Treatment failure in ventilator associated pneumonia. Curr Respir Med Rev 2012;8(3):239–44.

10. Garcia-Vidal C, Carratala J. Early and late treatment failure in community-acquired pneumonia. Semin Respir Crit Care Med 2009;30(2):154–60.

11. Vincent JL, Rello J, Marshall J, et al. International study of the prevalence and outcomes of infection in intensive care units. JAMA 2009;302(21):2323–9.

12. Jones RN. Microbial etiologies of hospital-acquired bacterial pneumonia and ventilator-associated bacterial pneumonia. Clin Infect Dis 2010; 51(Suppl 1):S81–7.

13. Nicolau DP, Dimopoulos G, Welte T, et al. Can we improve clinical outcomes in patients with pneumonia treated with antibiotics in the intensive care unit? Expert Rev Respir Med 2016;10(8):907–18.

14. Craig WA. The hidden impact of antibacterial resistance in respiratory tract infection. Re-evaluating current antibiotic therapy. Respir Med 2001; 95(Suppl A):S12–9 [discussion: S26–17].

15. Kalil AC, Metersky ML, Klompas M, et al. Management of adults with hospital-acquired and ventilator-associated pneumonia: 2016 clinical practice guidelines by the Infectious Diseases Society of America and the American Thoracic Society. Clin Infect Dis 2016;63(5):e61–111.

16. Kidd JM, Kuti JL, Nicolau DP. Novel pharmacotherapy for the treatment of hospital-acquired and ventilator-associated pneumonia caused by resistant gram-negative bacteria. Expert Opin Pharmacother 2018;19(4):397–408.

17. Bassetti M, Vena A, Castaldo N, et al. New antibiotics for ventilator-associated pneumonia. Curr Opin Infect Dis 2018;31(2):177–86.

18. Liapikou A, Cilloniz C, Torres A. Investigational drugs in phase I and phase II clinical trials for the treatment of community-acquired pneumonia. Expert Opin Investig Drugs 2017;26(11):1239–48.

19. Joint Commission on Hospital Accreditation. APPROVED: new antimicrobial stewardship standard. Jt Comm Perspect 2016;36(7):1, 3–4, 8.

20. Pea F, Furlanut M. Pharmacokinetic aspects of treating infections in the intensive care unit: focus on drug interactions. Clin Pharmacokinet 2001; 40(11):833–68.

21. Roberts JA, Pea F, Lipman J. The clinical relevance of plasma protein binding changes. Clin Pharmacokinet 2013;52(1):1–8.

22. Beceiro A, Tomas M, Bou G. Antimicrobial resistance and virulence: a successful or deleterious association in the bacterial world? Clin Microbiol Rev 2013;26(2):185–230.

23. Craig WA. Pharmacokinetic/pharmacodynamic parameters: rationale for antibacterial dosing of mice and men. Clin Infect Dis 1998;26(1):1–10 [quiz: 11–2].

24. Drusano GL. Antimicrobial pharmacodynamics: critical interactions of 'bug and drug'. Nat Rev Microbiol 2004;2(4):289–300.

25. Ong CT, Tessier PR, Li C, et al. Comparative in vivo efficacy of meropenem, imipenem, and cefepime against Pseudomonas aeruginosa expressing MexA-MexB-OprM efflux pumps. Diagn Microbiol Infect Dis 2007;57(2):153–61.

26. Turnidge JD. The pharmacodynamics of beta-lactams. Clin Infect Dis 1998;27(1):10–22.

27. Craig WA. Does the dose matter? Clin Infect Dis 2001;33(Suppl 3):S233–7.

28. Ambrose PG, Grasela DM, Grasela TH, et al. Pharmacodynamics of fluoroquinolones against Streptococcus pneumoniae in patients with community-acquired respiratory tract infections. Antimicrob Agents Chemother 2001;45(10):2793–7.

29. Forrest A, Nix DE, Ballow CH, et al. Pharmacodynamics of intravenous ciprofloxacin in seriously ill patients. Antimicrob Agents Chemother 1993; 37(5):1073–81.

30. Kashuba AD, Nafziger AN, Drusano GL, et al. Optimizing aminoglycoside therapy for nosocomial pneumonia caused by gram-negative bacteria. Antimicrob Agents Chemother 1999;43(3):623–9.

31. Bergen PJ, Landersdorfer CB, Zhang J, et al. Pharmacokinetics and pharmacodynamics of 'old' polymyxins: what is new? Diagn Microbiol Infect Dis 2012;74(3):213–23.

32. Rybak MJ, Lomaestro BM, Rotschafer JC, et al. Vancomycin therapeutic guidelines: a summary of consensus recommendations from the Infectious

Diseases Society of America, the American Society of Health-System Pharmacists, and the Society of Infectious Diseases Pharmacists. Clin Infect Dis 2009;49(3):325–7.

33. Rayner CR, Forrest A, Meagher AK, et al. Clinical pharmacodynamics of linezolid in seriously ill patients treated in a compassionate use programme. Clin Pharmacokinet 2003;42(15):1411–23.

34. Parker RF, Marsh HC. The action of penicillin on *Staphylococcus*. J Bacteriol 1946;51:181–6.

35. Isaksson B, Nilsson L, Maller R, et al. Postantibiotic effect of aminoglycosides on gram-negative bacteria evaluated by a new method. J Antimicrob Chemother 1988;22(1):23–33.

36. Craig W. Pharmacokinetic and experimental data on beta-lactam antibiotics in the treatment of patients. Eur J Clin Microbiol 1984;3(6):575–8.

37. Honeybourne D, Tobin C, Jevons G, et al. Intrapulmonary penetration of linezolid. J Antimicrob Chemother 2003;51(6):1431–4.

38. Lamer C, de Beco V, Soler P, et al. Analysis of vancomycin entry into pulmonary lining fluid by bronchoalveolar lavage in critically ill patients. Antimicrob Agents Chemother 1993;37(2):281–6.

39. Muller M, dela Pena A, Derendorf H. Issues in pharmacokinetics and pharmacodynamics of anti-infective agents: distribution in tissue. Antimicrob Agents Chemother 2004;48(5):1441–53.

40. Felton TW, Ogungbenro K, Boselli E, et al. Comparison of piperacillin exposure in the lungs of critically ill patients and healthy volunteers. J Antimicrob Chemother 2018;73(5):1340–7.

41. Rodvold KA, George JM, Yoo L. Penetration of anti-infective agents into pulmonary epithelial lining fluid: focus on antibacterial agents. Clin Pharmacokinet 2011;50(10):637–64.

42. Georges B, Conil JM, Seguin T, et al. Population pharmacokinetics of ceftazidime in intensive care unit patients: influence of glomerular filtration rate, mechanical ventilation, and reason for admission. Antimicrob Agents Chemother 2009;53(10): 4483–9.

43. Goncalves-Pereira J, Povoa P. Antibiotics in critically ill patients: a systematic review of the pharmacokinetics of beta-lactams. Crit Care 2011;15(5): R206.

44. van der Poll T. Immunotherapy of sepsis. Lancet Infect Dis 2001;1(3):165–74.

45. Hosein S, Udy AA, Lipman J. Physiological changes in the critically ill patient with sepsis. Curr Pharm Biotechnol 2011;12(12):1991–5.

46. Roberts JA, Lipman J. Pharmacokinetic issues for antibiotics in the critically ill patient. Crit Care Med 2009;37(3):840–51 [quiz: 859].

47. Investigators SS, Finfer S, Bellomo R, et al. Effect of baseline serum albumin concentration on outcome of resuscitation with albumin or saline in patients in intensive care units: analysis of data from the saline versus albumin fluid evaluation (SAFE) study. BMJ 2006;333(7577):1044.

48. Ulldemolins M, Roberts JA, Rello J, et al. The effects of hypoalbuminaemia on optimizing antibacterial dosing in critically ill patients. Clin Pharmacokinet 2011;50(2):99–110.

49. Udy AA, Varghese JM, Altukroni M, et al. Subtherapeutic initial beta-lactam concentrations in select critically ill patients: association between augmented renal clearance and low trough drug concentrations. Chest 2012;142(1):30–9.

50. Wallis SC, Mullany DV, Lipman J, et al. Pharmacokinetics of ciprofloxacin in ICU patients on continuous veno-venous haemodiafiltration. Intensive Care Med 2001;27(4):665–72.

51. Pea F, Viale P, Pavan F, et al. Pharmacokinetic considerations for antimicrobial therapy in patients receiving renal replacement therapy. Clin Pharmacokinet 2007;46(12):997–1038.

52. Blot SI, Pea F, Lipman J. The effect of pathophysiology on pharmacokinetics in the critically ill patient—concepts appraised by the example of antimicrobial agents. Adv Drug Deliv Rev 2014; 77:3–11.

53. Parker CM, Kutsogiannis J, Muscedere J, et al. Ventilator-associated pneumonia caused by multidrug-resistant organisms or *Pseudomonas aeruginosa*: prevalence, incidence, risk factors, and outcomes. J Crit Care 2008;23(1):18–26.

54. Grupper M, Kuti JL, Nicolau DP. Continuous and prolonged intravenous beta-lactam dosing: implications for the clinical laboratory. Clin Microbiol Rev 2016;29(4):759–72.

55. Lal A, Jaoude P, El-Solh AA. Prolonged versus intermittent infusion of beta-lactams for the treatment of nosocomial pneumonia: a meta-analysis. Infect Chemother 2016;48(2):81–90.

56. Flamm RK, Nichols WW, Sader HS, et al. In vitro activity of ceftazidime/avibactam against gram-negative pathogens isolated from pneumonia in hospitalised patients, including ventilated patients. Int J Antimicrob Agents 2016; 47(3):235–42.

57. Sader HS, Castanheira M, Flamm RK. Antimicrobial activity of ceftazidime-avibactam against gram-negative bacteria isolated from patients hospitalized with pneumonia in U.S. Medical Centers, 2011 to 2015. Antimicrob Agents Chemother 2017;61(4) [pii:e02083-16].

58. MacVane SH, Kuti JL, Nicolau DP. Clinical pharmacodynamics of antipseudomonal cephalosporins in patients with ventilator-associated pneumonia. Antimicrob Agents Chemother 2014;58(3):1359–64.

59. Drusano GL, Preston SL, Hardalo C, et al. Use of preclinical data for selection of a phase II/III dose for evernimicin and identification of a preclinical

MIC breakpoint. Antimicrob Agents Chemother 2001;45(1):13–22.

60. Zhou LJD, Al-Huniti N, Bouchillon S, et al. Pharmacokinetic/Pharmacodynamic target attainment (PTA) and cumulative fractions of response (CFR) for ceftazidime, ceftazidime-avibactam, and meropenem against bacteria isolated from patients in Europe in 2012. 24th European Congress of Clinical Microbiology and Infectious Diseases (ECCMID); 2014; Barcelona, Spain, 13th May, 2014.

61. Housman ST, Crandon JL, Nichols WW, et al. Efficacies of ceftazidime-avibactam and ceftazidime against *Pseudomonas aeruginosa* in a murine lung infection model. Antimicrob Agents Chemother 2014;58(3):1365–71.

62. Nicolau DP, Siew L, Armstrong J, et al. Phase 1 study assessing the steady-state concentration of ceftazidime and avibactam in plasma and epithelial lining fluid following two dosing regimens. J Antimicrob Chemother 2015;70(10): 2862–9.

63. Torres A, Zhong N, Pachl J, et al. Ceftazidime-avibactam versus meropenem in nosocomial pneumonia, including ventilator-associated pneumonia (REPROVE): a randomised, double-blind, phase 3 non-inferiority trial. Lancet Infect Dis 2018;18(3): 285–95.

64. Bassetti M, Luyt CE, Nicolau DP, et al. Characteristics of an ideal nebulized antibiotic for the treatment of pneumonia in the intubated patient. Ann Intensive Care 2016;6(1):35.

65. Palmer LB. Aerosolized antibiotics in the intensive care unit. Clin Chest Med 2011;32(3):559–74.

66. Ferrari F, Lu Q, Girardi C, et al. Nebulized ceftazidime in experimental pneumonia caused by partially resistant *Pseudomonas aeruginosa*. Intensive Care Med 2009;35(10):1792–800.

67. Lu Q, Girardi C, Zhang M, et al. Nebulized and intravenous colistin in experimental pneumonia caused by *Pseudomonas aeruginosa*. Intensive Care Med 2010;36(7):1147–55.

68. Brain JD, Valberg PA. Deposition of aerosol in the respiratory tract. Am Rev Respir Dis 1979;120(6): 1325–73.

69. Dolovich MA. Influence of inspiratory flow rate, particle size, and airway caliber on aerosolized drug delivery to the lung. Respir Care 2000;45(6): 597–608.

70. Tonnellier M, Ferrari F, Goldstein I, et al. Intravenous versus nebulized ceftazidime in ventilated piglets with and without experimental bronchopneumonia: comparative effects of helium and nitrogen. Anesthesiology 2005;102(5):995–1000.

71. Yapa SWS, Li J, Patel K, et al. Pulmonary and systemic pharmacokinetics of inhaled and intravenous colistin methanesulfonate in cystic fibrosis patients: targeting advantage of inhalational

administration. Antimicrob Agents Chemother 2014;58(5):2570–9.

72. Goldstein I, Wallet F, Robert J, et al. Lung tissue concentrations of nebulized amikacin during mechanical ventilation in piglets with healthy lungs. Am J Respir Crit Care Med 2002;165(2):171–5.

73. Lu Q, Yang J, Liu Z, et al. Nebulized ceftazidime and amikacin in ventilator-associated pneumonia caused by *Pseudomonas aeruginosa*. Am J Respir Crit Care Med 2011;184(1):106–15.

74. Niederman MS, Chastre J, Corkery K, et al. BAY41-6551 achieves bactericidal tracheal aspirate amikacin concentrations in mechanically ventilated patients with gram-negative pneumonia. Intensive Care Med 2012;38(2):263–71.

75. Luyt CE, Clavel M, Guntupalli K, et al. Pharmacokinetics and lung delivery of PDDS-aerosolized amikacin (NKTR-061) in intubated and mechanically ventilated patients with nosocomial pneumonia. Crit Care 2009;13(6):R200.

76. Palmer LB, Smaldone GC. Reduction of bacterial resistance with inhaled antibiotics in the intensive care unit. Am J Respir Crit Care Med 2014; 189(10):1225–33.

77. Kollef MH, Ricard JD, Roux D, et al. A randomized trial of the amikacin fosfomycin inhalation system for the adjunctive therapy of gram-negative ventilator-associated pneumonia: IASIS Trial. Chest 2017;151(6):1239–46.

78. Montgomery AB, Vallance S, Abuan T, et al. A randomized double-blind placebo-controlled dose-escalation phase 1 study of aerosolized amikacin and fosfomycin delivered via the PARI investigational eFlow(R) inline nebulizer system in mechanically ventilated patients. J Aerosol Med Pulm Drug Deliv 2014;27(6):441–8.

79. Release BLP. Available at: http://press.bayer.com/baynews/baynews.nsf/id/Phase-III-study-program-Amikacin-Inhale-addition-standard-intubated-mechanically-ventilated-patients?OpenDocument&sessionID=1512362907. Accessed November 24, 2017.

80. Elman M, Goldstein I, Marquette CH, et al. Influence of lung aeration on pulmonary concentrations of nebulized and intravenous amikacin in ventilated piglets with severe bronchopneumonia. Anesthesiology 2002;97(1):199–206.

81. Drusano GL, Hope W, MacGowan A, et al. Suppression of emergence of resistance in pathogenic bacteria: keeping our powder dry, part 2. Antimicrob Agents Chemother 2015;60(3):1194–201.

82. Monogue ML, Stainton SM, Baummer-Carr A, et al. Pharmacokinetics and tissue penetration of ceftolozane-tazobactam in diabetic patients with lower limb infections and healthy adult volunteers. Antimicrob Agents Chemother 2017;61(12) [pii: e01449-17].

83. Rico Caballero V, Almarzoky Abuhussain S, Kuti JL, et al. Efficacy of human-simulated exposures of ceftolozane-tazobactam alone and in combination with amikacin or colistin against multidrug-resistant *Pseudomonas aeruginosa* in an in vitro pharmacodynamic model. Antimicrob Agents Chemother 2018;62(5) [pii:e02384-17].

84. Torres A, Niederman MS, Chastre J, et al. International ERS/ESICM/ESCMID/ALAT guidelines for the management of hospital-acquired pneumonia and ventilator-associated pneumonia: guidelines for the management of hospital-acquired pneumonia (HAP)/ventilator-associated pneumonia (VAP) of the European Respiratory Society (ERS), European Society of Intensive Care Medicine (ESICM), European Society of Clinical Microbiology and Infectious Diseases (ESCMID) and Asociacion Latinoamericana del Torax (ALAT). Eur Respir J 2017;50(3) [pii:1700582].

85. Pankey GA, Ashcraft DS, Dornelles A. Comparison of 3 Etest((R)) methods and time-kill assay for determination of antimicrobial synergy against carbapenemase-producing *Klebsiella* species. Diagn Microbiol Infect Dis 2013;77(3):220–6.

86. White RL, Burgess DS, Manduru M, et al. Comparison of three different in vitro methods of detecting synergy: time-kill, checkerboard, and E test. Antimicrob Agents Chemother 1996;40(8):1914–8.

87. Jenkins SG, Schuetz AN. Current concepts in laboratory testing to guide antimicrobial therapy. Mayo Clin Proc 2012;87(3):290–308.

88. Odds FC. Synergy, antagonism, and what the chequerboard puts between them. J Antimicrob Chemother 2003;52(1):1.

89. Bremmer DN, Bauer KA, Pouch SM, et al. Correlation of checkerboard synergy testing with time-kill analysis and clinical outcomes of extensively drug-resistant *Acinetobacter baumannii* respiratory infections. Antimicrob Agents Chemother 2016;60(11):6892–5.

90. Stainton SM, Monogue ML, Nicolau DP. In vitro-in vivo discordance with humanized piperacillin-tazobactam exposures against piperacillin-tazobactam-resistant/pan-beta-lactam-susceptible *Klebsiella pneumoniae* strains. Antimicrob Agents Chemother 2017;61(7) [pii:e00491-17].

91. Monogue ML, Abbo LM, Rosa R, et al. In vitro discordance with in vivo activity: humanized exposures of ceftazidime-avibactam, aztreonam, and tigecycline alone and in combination against New Delhi metallo-beta-lactamase-producing *Klebsiella pneumoniae* in a murine lung infection model. Antimicrob Agents Chemother 2017;61(7) [pii:e00486-17].

92. Touw DJ, Neef C, Thomson AH, et al, Cost-Effectiveness of Therapeutic Drug Monitoring Committee of the International Association for Therapeutic Drug Monitoring and Clinical Toxicology. Cost-effectiveness of therapeutic drug monitoring: a systematic review. Ther Drug Monit 2005;27(1):10–7.

93. Kashuba AD, Bertino JS Jr, Nafziger AN. Dosing of aminoglycosides to rapidly attain pharmacodynamic goals and hasten therapeutic response by using individualized pharmacokinetic monitoring of patients with pneumonia caused by gram-negative organisms. Antimicrob Agents Chemother 1998;42(7):1842–4.

94. Wallace AW, Jones M, Bertino JS Jr. Evaluation of four once-daily aminoglycoside dosing nomograms. Pharmacotherapy 2002;22(9):1077–83.

95. Cruciani M, Gatti G, Lazzarini L, et al. Penetration of vancomycin into human lung tissue. J Antimicrob Chemother 1996;38(5):865–9.

96. Panidis D, Markantonis SL, Boutzouka E, et al. Penetration of gentamicin into the alveolar lining fluid of critically ill patients with ventilator-associated pneumonia. Chest 2005;128(2):545–52.

97. Nicolau DP, Freeman CD, Belliveau PP, et al. Experience with a once-daily aminoglycoside program administered to 2,184 adult patients. Antimicrob Agents Chemother 1995;39(3):650–5.

98. Rybak M, Lomaestro B, Rotschafer JC, et al. Therapeutic monitoring of vancomycin in adult patients: a consensus review of the American Society of Health-System Pharmacists, the Infectious Diseases Society of America, and the Society of Infectious Diseases Pharmacists. Am J Health Syst Pharm 2009;66(1):82–98.

99. Lodise TP, Sorgel F, Melnick D, et al. Penetration of meropenem into epithelial lining fluid of patients with ventilator-associated pneumonia. Antimicrob Agents Chemother 2011;55(4):1606–10.

100. Xiao AJ, Caro L, Popejoy MW, et al. PK/PD target attainment with ceftolozane/tazobactam using Monte Carlo simulation in patients with various degrees of renal function, including augmented renal clearance and end-stage renal disease. Infect Dis Ther 2017;6(1):137–48.

101. Lodise TP Jr, Gotfried M, Barriere S, et al. Telavancin penetration into human epithelial lining fluid determined by population pharmacokinetic modeling and Monte Carlo simulation. Antimicrob Agents Chemother 2008;52(7):2300–4.

102. Roberts JA, Ulldemolins M, Roberts MS, et al. Therapeutic drug monitoring of beta-lactams in critically ill patients: proof of concept. Int J Antimicrob Agents 2010;36(4):332–9.

103. De Waele JJ, Carrette S, Carlier M, et al. Therapeutic drug monitoring-based dose optimisation of piperacillin and meropenem: a randomised controlled trial. Intensive Care Med 2014;40(3):380–7.

104. Economou CJP, Wong G, McWhinney B, et al. Impact of beta-lactam antibiotic therapeutic drug

monitoring on dose adjustments in critically ill patients undergoing continuous renal replacement therapy. Int J Antimicrob Agents 2017;49(5): 589–94.

105. Patel BM, Paratz J, See NC, et al. Therapeutic drug monitoring of beta-lactam antibiotics in burns patients—a one-year prospective study. Ther Drug Monit 2012;34(2):160–4.

106. Wong G, Brinkman A, Benefield RJ, et al. An international, multicentre survey of beta-lactam antibiotic therapeutic drug monitoring practice in intensive care units. J Antimicrob Chemother 2014;69(5):1416–23.

107. Ambrose PG. Antibacterial drug development program successes and failures: a pharmacometric explanation. Curr Opin Pharmacol 2017;36:1–7.

108. Mouton JW. Impact of pharmacodynamics on breakpoint selection for susceptibility testing. Infect Dis Clin North Am 2003;17(3):579–98.

109. Dudhani RV, Turnidge JD, Coulthard K, et al. Elucidation of the pharmacokinetic/pharmacodynamic determinant of colistin activity against *Pseudomonas aeruginosa* in murine thigh and lung infection models. Antimicrob Agents Chemother 2010; 54(3):1117–24.

110. Bowker KE, Noel AR, Macgowan AP. Pharmacodynamics of minocycline against *Staphylococcus aureus* in an in vitro pharmacokinetic model. Antimicrob Agents Chemother 2008; 52(12):4370–3.

New Antibiotics for Pneumonia

Matteo Bassetti, MD, PhD*, Elda Righi, MD, PhD, Alessandro Russo, MD,
Alessia Carnelutti, MD

KEYWORDS

- Pneumonia • Multidrug-resistant bacteria • *K pneumoniae* • *P aeruginosa* • *A baumannii*
- Methicillin-resistant *Staphylococcus aureus* • New antimicrobial options

KEY POINTS

- Antimicrobial resistance among patients with pneumonia represents a major challenge for clinicians, considering the high rates of morbidity and mortality and subsequent health care costs.
- Gram-negative pathogens, like *Pseudomonas aeruginosa*, *Acinetobacter baumanii*, and *Klebsiella pneumoniae*, represent the most important etiologies associated with unfavorable outcome, especially in specific settings like ICUs.
- Methicillin-resistant *Staphylococcus aureus*, however, has an important role in the etiology of pneumonia, accounting for up to 30% of cases of hospital-acquired pneumonia.
- Due to the progressive increase in antimicrobial resistance, many new antibiotics have been developed during recent years for treatment of pneumonia and have been approved or are currently under evaluation in phase II or phase III clinical trials.
- These new drugs are characterized by a broad spectrum of activity against multidrug-resistant pathogens, in particular extended-spectrum β-lactamase–producing and carbapenem-resistant Enterobacteriaceae.

INTRODUCTION

The progressive increase in antimicrobial resistance among patients with pneumonia represents a major challenge for clinicians, mainly due to the high reported rates of delayed prescription of an adequate antibiotic treatment, leading to increased mortality, prolonged length of hospital stay, and substantial increase in health care costs.[1,2]

In countries burdened by high resistance rates, a major threat in treating pneumonia is currently represented by infections caused by multidrug-resistant (MDR) gram-negative pathogens, in particular *Pseudomonas aeruginosa*, *Acinetobacter baumanii*, and *Klebsiella pneumoniae*, which frequently display resistance to all β-lactam antibiotics (including carbapenems), leading to high rates of inappropriateness of empiric antibiotic therapy, particularly in IXU patients.[3–5] Until recently, due to the lack of novel therapeutic options, when a carbapenem-resistant pathogen was suspected or confirmed, combination therapies (often including high-dose carbapenems, colistin or aminoglycosides or fosfomycin) were widely use, although the

Conflict of Interest: M. Bassetti has participated in advisory boards and/or received speaker honoraria from Achaogen, Angelini, Astellas, AstraZeneca, Bayer, Basilea, Cidara, Gilead, Menarini, MSD, Paratek, Pfizer, Roche, The Medicine Company, Shionogi, Tetraphase, VenatoRx and Vifor. The remaining authors have no conflicts of interest.
Infectious Diseases Clinic, Department of Medicine, University of Udine, Azienda Sanitaria Universitaria, Presidio Ospedaliero Universitario Santa Maria della Misericordia, Colugna Street, Udine 33100, Italy
* Corresponding author. Infectious Diseases Clinic, Azienda Sanitaria Universitaria, Presidio Ospedaliero Universitario Santa Maria della Misericordia, 50, Colugna Street, Udine 33100, Italy.
E-mail address: matteo.bassetti@asuiud.sanita.fvg.it

Clin Chest Med 39 (2018) 853–869
https://doi.org/10.1016/j.ccm.2018.08.007

results were not satisfactory and mortality rates remained high.[6]

Another problem is represented by methicillin-resistant *Staphylococcus aureus* (MRSA), which is the most common resistant pathogen involved in pneumonia both in the community (in particular among patients presenting with specific risk factors, such as previous MRSA infection or colonization, recent antimicrobial treatment, and having recent contact with a health care system) and in the nosocomial setting, accounting for up to 30% of cases in hospital-acquired pneumonia (HAP).[7,8] Although vancomycin still represents a widely used antibiotic for the treatment of MRSA pneumonia, its role has been questioned during recent years due to its limited pulmonary penetration, the need for therapeutic drug monitoring to achieve adequate plasma concentrations, the risk of nephrotoxicity, and the lack of an oral formulation, not allowing the treatment of outpatients.[9,10] Linezolid represents a valid option for the treatment of MRSA pneumonia and was found superior to vancomycin for the treatment of MRSA HAP in a recent phase IV, randomized controlled trial.[11] Linezolid is characterized by a good pulmonary penetration and is available as an oral formulation, allowing oral de-escalation and treatment of outpatients. Linezolid is affected by some limitations in clinical practice, however, in particular the risk of hematological side effects with anemia and thrombocytopenia (particularly in patients with underlying hematologic alterations and when renal impairment is present) and the potential for drug interactions with selective serotonin reuptake inhibitors and other compounds with serotonergic activity, due to the inhibition of the monoamine oxidase pathway.[12]

Due to the progressive increase in antimicrobial resistance, many new antibiotics have been developed during recent years and have been approved for the treatment of pneumonia or are currently under evaluation in phase II or phase III clinical trials.

This article reviews the characteristics of newly approved and investigational options for the treatment of respiratory tract infections due to MDR pathogens, including their spectrum of activity, current approval status or state of development, and potential role in daily clinical practice.

β-LACTAMS AND β-LACTAMS/β-LACTAMASE INHIBITORS
Novel Cephalosporins

Ceftobiprole
Ceftobiprole is a new-generation broad-spectrum cephalosporin that exhibits potent in vitro activity against gram-positive and gram-negative pathogens and has been approved in Europe for the treatment of adults with HAP (excluding ventilator-associated pneumonia [VAP]) or community-acquired pneumonia (CAP).[13] Ceftobiprole shows broad-spectrum in vitro activity against pathogens that cause HAP and CAP, including MRSA, *Haemophilus influenzae* (including β-lactamase–producing strains), *Moraxella catarrhalis*, *Escherichia coli*, and *K pneumoniae,* and also *P aeruginosa.* Ceftobiprole has demonstrated in vitro activity against *Staphylococcus aureus* strains that were resistant to vancomycin and those that are not susceptible to linezolid. Ceftobiprole shows limited activity against *Acinetobacter* spp and is susceptible to hydrolysis by enzymes (eg, extended-spectrum β-lactamases [ESBLs]) produced by Enterobacteriaceae. Similar to other β-lactams, ceftobiprole exerts its antibacterial activity by binding to penicillin binding proteins (PBPs) and inhibiting their transpeptidase activity,[14] which is essential for the synthesis of the peptidoglycan layer of bacterial cell walls. Based on pharmacokinetics (PK)/pharmacodynamics (PD) studies, a 500-mg every-8-hour dosage was considered optimal to providing coverage against gram-positive bacteria.[15] The clinical efficacy of intravenous ceftobiprole for the treatment of adult patients with HAP or CAP has been evaluated in 2 trials.[16,17] In phase III trials, ceftobiprole was noninferior to ceftazidime plus linezolid in patients with HAP and to ceftriaxone with or without linezolid in patients with severe CAP. In patients with HAP, noninferiority of ceftobiprole to ceftazidime plus linezolid was not demonstrated in a subset of patients with VAP, and then this indication was excluded. Most common treatment-related adverse events occurring in patients treated with ceftobiprole in HAP or CAP trials in patients included nausea, diarrhea, infusion site reactions, vomiting, hepatic enzyme elevations, and hyponatremia.

Ceftaroline
Ceftaroline is a cephalosporin with an in vitro spectrum of activity that includes most of the common bacterial pathogens associated with CAP. The prodrug ceftaroline fosamil has been approved in the United States in 2010 for the treatment of CAP and acute bacterial skin and skin structure infections (ABSSSIs). The approval of ceftaroline for the treatment of CAP was based on 2 phase 3 multinational, randomized controlled trials conducted in hospitalized patients, FOCUS 1 (Clinicaltrials.gov, identifier NCT00621504) and FOCUS 2 (Clinicaltrials.gov,

identifier NCT00509106), in which ceftaroline fosamil, 600 mg every 12 hours, demonstrated noninferiority compared with ceftriaxone, 1 g every 24 hours, with differences in clinical cure rates at the test-of-cure visit favoring ceftaroline fosamil in both trials.[18,19] In a subsequent phase 3 randomized controlled trial in Asian patients with PORT class 3 to 4 CAP (Clinicaltrials.gov, identifier NCT01371838), ceftaroline fosamil, 600 mg every 12 hours, demonstrated superiority to ceftriaxone (2 g every 24 hours).[20] Based on these data, ceftaroline should be considered as an alternative to ceftriaxone for the cephalosporin component of empirical antibiotic regimens in adult patients hospitalized with CAP, with a reasonable safety profile. These findings have been also supported by real-world observational data from the CAPTURE study.[21,22] The CAPTURE program assessed the outcomes of patients who were excluded in the original phase 3 trials in a noncomparative fashion. The CAPTURE registry has provided valuable insights into ceftaroline use in special populations including the elderly, critically ill, those with renal dysfunction, and those with MRSA CAP.

Cefiderocol

Cefiderocol is a novel parenteral siderophore cephalosporin based on the mechanism of bacterial cell entry binding to ferric iron. Cefiderocol is then actively transported into bacterial cells through the outer membrane via the bacterial iron transporters and by passive diffusion through porin channels into the periplasmatic space.[23] Cefiderocol demonstrated in vitro activity against ESBL-producing Enterobacteriaceae, carbapenem-resistant Enterobacteriaceae (CRE) and meropenem (MER)-resistant P aeruginosa, Stenotrophomonas maltophilia, and A baumannii. Furthermore, cefiderocol showed activity against classes A, B, and D carbapenemase-producing isolates, comprising metallo-β-lactamase (MBL)–producing Enterobacteriaceae. Strains of MDR P aeruginosa and A baumannii, including class B metallo-β-lactamase producers, were susceptible to cefiderocol.[24] Cefiderocol is in phase 3 of clinical development. Two clinical trials are ongoing for various infections, including VAP. The APEKS-NP trial is a clinical study on nosocomial pneumonia. The aim of the trial was to compare cefiderocol versus MER (both in association with linezolid) in adults with HAP, VAP, and health care–associated pneumonia (HCAP) caused by gram-negative pathogens (Clinicaltrials.Gov, identifier NCT03032380). In addition, a phase 3 trial (CREDIBLE-CR) has been initiated in 2017 to provide evidence of efficacy of cefiderocol in patients

with serious infections (HCAP, HAP, VAP, complicated urinary tract infections[cUTIs], and bloodstream infections [BSIs]) caused by carbapenem-resistant gram-negative bacteria. In this trial, cefiderocol is compared with best available therapy, including up to 3 antibacterial agents for carbapenem-resistant gram-negative bacteria with either a polymyxin-based or non–polymyxin-based regimen (ClinicalTrials.Gov, identifier NCT02714595). Considering its profile, cefiderocol is a promising cephalosporin with an important potential for the treatment of pneumonia due to carbapenem-resistant GNB, including CRE, MDR P aeruginosa, and A baumannii.

β-Lactams/β-Lactamase Inhibitors

Ceftazidime/avibactam

Ceftazidime is a third-generation cephalosporin, administered intravenously or intramuscularly, binding to a variety of PBPs including the PBP3 of gram-negative bacteria, such as P aeruginosa. Avibactam is a semisynthetic, non–β-lactam, β-lactamase inhibitor and differs from other β-lactamase inhibitors (such as clavulanic acid, sulbactam, and tazobactam) in structure, mechanism of inhibition, and spectrum of inhibition.[25] Avibactam inhibits the in vitro activity of Ambler class A (ESBL and K pneumoniae carbapenemase [KPC]), Ambler class C (AmpC), and some Ambler class D (OXA-48) enzymes, but it is not active against MBLs or against Acinetobacter OXA–type carbapenemases.[26]

Clinical indications for ceftazidime/avibactam (CAZ-AVI) use include HAP and VAP both in empiric and targeted therapy.[27] The role of CAZ-AVI has been reported in recent real-world studies in the setting of severe infections due to CRE. CAZ-AVI, therefore, may be considered a reasonable alternative to colistin in the treatment of KPC-producing infections and in patients with documented bacteremia.[28,29] In vitro and in vivo data about PK/PD of CAZ-AVI confirmed that penetration of CAZ-AVI in the epithelial lining fluid (ELF) represents approximately 30% of the plasma concentrations. Clinical studies documented that CAZ-AVI, 2000 mg/500 mg every 8 hours, is the optimal dose regimen to achieve the PK/PD target attainment in patients with HAP. Thus, CAZ-AVI could represent an option to treat HAP caused by MDR gram-negative bacilli.[30] Data regarding the safety of CAZ-AVI include experience from phase I and phase II trials and recent phase III trials. In phase II studies, adverse events were similar in both treatment arms. CAZ-AVI can be considered well tolerated: the most common adverse events reported included headache, gastrointestinal symptoms (eg, abdominal pain, vomiting, nausea, and constipation), and infusion-site reactions.[31] Most of these adverse events were mild to moderate and some could be attributable to other comorbidities or concomitant metronidazole therapy.[32]

Ceftolozane/tazobactam

Ceftolozane/tazobactam is a β-lactam/β-lactamase inhibitor combination that exhibits bactericidal activity through inhibition of bacterial cell wall biosynthesis, mediated through PBPs. Ceftolozane is a potent PBP3 inhibitor and has a higher affinity for PBP1b compared with other β-lactam agents; for these reasons, ceftolozane/tazobactam differs from other cephalosporins due to its increased activity against some AmpC β-lactamases, especially P aeruginosa.[33] The addition of tazobactam provides enhanced activity against ESBL-producing Enterobacteriaceae.[34]

Ceftolozane/tazobactam is not currently approved for pneumonia but seems promising in this indication due to its specific action in severe infections caused by MDR and extensively drug-resistant[35,36] P aeruginosa, the high cure rates displayed in patients with pulmonary exacerbation of cystic fibrosis, and for the good profile of tolerability.[37] Moreover, ceftolozane/tazobactam displays a good ELF penetration, implying a potential role for the treatment of respiratory infections. PK/PD studies, however, suggested that an increased dosage (3 g every 8 hours, intravenous) might be necessary for the treatment of pneumonia.[38] A phase III trial (ASPECT-NP) to assess the safety and efficacy of ceftolozane/tazobactam (3 g every 8 hours) compared with MER (1 g every 8 hours) for the treatment of VAP or ventilated HAP caused by P aeruginosa is ongoing (Clinicaltrials. gov, identifier NCT02070757). Recently, a retrospective study including 21 patients treated with ceftolozane/tazobactam for MDR P aeruginosa infections has been published. Most infections (18 of 21) involved the respiratory tract, and ceftolozane/tazobactam was successful in 71% of patients.[39] Based on data from clinical trials, adverse effects due to ceftolozane/tazobactam did not considerably differ from other cephalosporins, the most common being nausea, diarrhea, headache, and pyrexia. In a phase 3 trial investigating intraabdominal infections, patients with moderate renal impairment (CrCl 30–50 mL/min) showed numerically lower cure rates in the ceftolozane/tazobactam plus metronidazole arm compared with the MER arm (11 of 23 [48%] vs 9 of 13 [69.2%], respectively). A decreased cure rate in patients aged greater than or equal to 65 years compared with younger ones (69% vs 82%, respectively)

was also believed secondary to changes in renal clearance. On this basis, the Food and Drug Administration (FDA) included a warning in the package insert of ceftolozane/tazobactam to monitor renal function at least daily in patients with changing CrCl and to adjust ceftolozane/tazobactam dosing as needed.[40]

Aztreonam/avibactam

Aztreonam is the first member of the monobactam class. Aztreonam is active against a broad spectrum of gram-negative pathogens, except Enterobacter spp, although it is inactive against gram-positive aerobic and anaerobic bacteria, including Bacteroides fragilis.[41] Aztreonam is the only β-lactam stable to hydrolysis by MBLs; however, it is easily hydrolyzed by class A and class C β-lactamases.[41] Avibactam has broad-spectrum activity against Ambler class A and AmpC β-lactamases and certain class D β-lactamases and acts by formation of a highly stable covalent bond with the enzyme's active serine; the covalent adduct formation inactivates the β-lactamases.[42]

A recent study aimed to define the inhibitory profile of aztreonam/avibactam across a global collection of Enterobacteriaceae collected from hospitalized patients in 208 hospitals from 40 countries between 2012 and 2015. Overall, more than 99.9% of all Enterobacteriaceae and 99.8% of MER-nonsusceptible isolates were inhibited by aztreonam/avibactam at a concentration of 8 μg/mL. Specifically, against MBL-producing Enterobacteriaceae, aztreonam/avibactam was 8-fold to 32-fold more potent than MER, with minimum inhibitory concentration (MICs) of 8 μg/mL and a MIC$_{90}$ of 1 μg/mL. Limited activity has been shown against A baumannii or P aeruginosa compared with aztreonam alone.[43]

In a similar study conducted across 84 medical centers in the United States, aztreonam/avibactam was tested against 10,451 Enterobacteriaceae, including 116 Metallo-β-lactamases- and/or OXA-48-like–producing isolates. All isolates were inhibited at aztreonam/avibactam MICs of less than or equal to 8 μg/mL, with highest aztreonam/avibactam reported MIC of 4 μg/mL.[44]

A phase 1 study investigating the safety and tolerability of aztreonam/avibactam in healthy subjects (Clinicaltrials.gov, identifier NCT01689207) and a phase 2 study evaluating PK, safety, and tolerability of aztreonam/avibactam for the treatment of complicated intra-abdominal infection (cIAI) in hospitalized adults (REJUVENATE) have been recently completed (Clinicaltrials.gov, identifier NCT02655419). A phase 3 comparative study to determine the efficacy, safety, and tolerability of aztreonam/avibactam with or without metronidazole versus MER (with or without colistin) for the treatment of serious infections (including HAP and VAP) due to gram-negative bacteria is ongoing (Clinicaltrials.gov, identifier NCT03329092).

Ceftaroline/avibactam

Ceftaroline belongs to the new fifth-generation cephalosporin group and is characterized by a unique activity against MRSA due to its high binding affinity for PBP2a.[45] Ceftaroline provides an attractive broad spectrum, bactericidal activity against both gram-positive (with the exception of Enterococci) and gram-negative bacteria, with the exception of ESBL-producing Enterobacteriaceae and carbapenemase-producing Enterobacteriaceae.[46–50] Ceftaroline has been approved by FDA and the European Medicines Agency for the treatment of ABSSSI and CAP.

The combination of ceftaroline and avibactam further extends the antimicrobial spectrum to include ESBL-producing Enterobacteriaceae and KPC-producing Enterobacteriaceae as well as anaerobes. Conversely, limited activity was demonstrated against P aeruginosa and A baumanii.[36–39]

Safety, tolerability, and PK of ceftaroline/avibactam were evaluated in a phase 1 study conducted in 60 healthy adult subjects. No appreciable accumulation of either drug occurred with multiple intravenous doses of ceftaroline/avibactam, and PK parameters for ceftaroline and avibactam were similar at days 1 and 10. Ceftaroline/avibactam was well tolerated at total daily doses of up to 1800 mg of each compound, and all adverse events were mild to moderate in severity and were represented by diarrhea, dry mouth, and headache. Infusion-site reactions were the most common events reported with multiple dosing.[51] Moreover, no association between ceftaroline/avibactam administration and QT/QTc prolongation was observed.[52]

A phase 2 study comparing treatment with ceftaroline/avibactam versus doripenem for the treatment of adult patients with cUTI has recently been completed (Clinicaltrials.gov, identifier NCT01281462). Although no studies investigating the role of ceftaroline/avibactam for the treatment of respiratory tract infections are currently available, ceftaroline/avibactam represents a potential option for the treatment of respiratory tract infections, particularly when ESBL-producing Enterobacteriaceae , KPC-producing Enterobacteriaceae, or MRSA is suspected or confirmed.

Imipenem/relebactam

Relebactam (REL) (formerly known as MK-7655) is a novel, intravenous, class A and class C

β-lactamase inhibitor and is currently under evaluation in combination with imipenem/cilastatin (IMI) for the treatment of resistant gram-negative infections.[53] In vitro studies have demonstrated REL to restore imipenem's activity against KPC-producing CRE, including K pneumoniae, and to lower imipenem MICs in P aeruginosa, particularly in strains with depressed OprD expression and increased AmpC expression.[54] Conversely, the addiction of REL to IMI seems not to provide any adjunctive benefit against A baumanii and Stenotrophomonas maltophilia.[54,55]

A phase 3 study evaluating the efficacy and safety of IMI/REL (200/100 mg to 500/250 mg depending on renal function) compared with colistimethate sodium for the treatment of IMI-resistant bacterial infections, including HAP, VAP, cIAI and cUTI, has recently been completed and results are pending (Clinicaltrials.gov, identifier NCT02452047).

A noninferiority, phase 3 trial evaluating the efficacy and safety of IMI/REL compared with piperacillin/tazobactam for the treatment of HAP and VAP (Clinicaltrials.gov, identifier NCT02493764) is ongoing.

Data regarding safety and tolerability come from 2 phase 2 trials (Clinicaltrials.gov, identifier NCT01506271, and Clinicaltrials.gov, identifier NCT01505634) investigating the role of IMI/REL in the setting of cIAI and cUTI. IMI/REL was well tolerated, with diarrhea, nausea, vomiting, and headache the most commonly reported adverse events.[66,67]

Meropenem/vaborbactam

Vaborbactam (formerly known as RPX7009) (VAB) belongs to novel class A and class C β-lactamase inhibitors. VAB in combination with MER has been studied for the treatment of infections due to resistant gram-negative pathogens.[58] VAB is a cyclic boronic acid pharmacophore and is a potent inhibitor of serine β-lactamases due to the high affinity between the serine-based active sites of β-lactamases and boronates, leading to the formation of a covalent complex and inhibition of β-lactamase enzymes.[59,60] In particular, VAB was found effective in lowering MER MIC_{50} from 32 μg/mL to 0.06 μg/mL and MIC_{90} from 32 μg/mL to 1 μg/mL in a study encompassing 991 isolates of KPC-producing Enterobacteriaceae collected between 2014 and 2015.[59]

Safety, tolerability, and PK of VAB after single and multiple ascending doses were evaluated in a phase 1 study in healthy adult subjects (Clinicaltrials.gov, identifier NCT01751269). Overall, VAB showed a favorable tolerability profile, with no serious reported adverse events. Mild adverse events were mainly represented by headache and catheter site complications.[61]

MER/VAB has been approved by the FDA on August 2017 for the treatment of cUTIs based on the results of the TANGO1 trial, showing the superiority of MER/VAB (2 g/2 g every 8 hours) compared with piperacillin/tazobactam (4 g/0.5 g every 8 hours) for the treatment of cUTI and acute pyelonephritis in adult patients (Clinicaltrials.gov, identifier NCT02166476).

A phase 3 study evaluating efficacy, safety, and tolerability of MER/VAB compared with best available therapy for the treatment of infections due to CRE has recently been completed and results are awaited (Clinicaltrials.gov, identifier NCT02168946).

NON–β-LACTAM ANTIBIOTICS
Plazomicin

Plazomicin is a semisynthetic aminoglycoside inhibiting bacterial protein synthesis with exhibition of a dose-dependent bactericidal activity. Plazomicin has shown potent activity against gram-positive bacteria such as MRSA. Plazomycin shows the peculiar mechanism of resistance to aminoglycoside-modifying enzymes, typical of CRE[62]; then it has activity against Enterobacteriaceae but is less active against nonfermenting gram-negative bacteria. Plazomicin shows a similar activity against MDR P aeruginosa but has a significantly improved activity against OXA-producing A baumannii, compared with other aminoglycosides.[63] PK/PD properties of plazomicin revealed a linear and dose-proportional profile, making plazomicin a promising candidate for the treatment of nosocomial pneumonia.[64] The phase III CARE study (Clinicaltrials.gov, identifier NCT01970371) evaluated the efficacy and safety of plazomicin versus colistin for the treatment of serious infections due to CRE and has been recently completed. Each drug was combined with a second antibiotic, either MER or tigecycline. The CARE trial enrolled 29 BSI and 8 patients with HAP/VAP. A lower rate of mortality or serious disease-related complications was observed for plazomicin compared with colistin (23.5 vs 50.0%, respectively).[65] In addition, plazomicin showed a favorable safety profile and was associated with a lower incidence of drug-related adverse events, including serum creatinine elevations. There were no events associated with potential ototoxicity and no study drug–related deaths in either cohort.

Eravacycline

Eravacycline is a novel fluorocycline in phase 3 clinical development for cIAI and cUTI.

Eravacycline is structurally similar to tigecycline but is not subjected to the mechanisms that are responsible for tetracycline resistance, such as efflux pumps and ribosomal protection proteins.[66] The most attractive characteristic of eravacycline is the broad-spectrum activity against both gram-positive and gram-negative resistant pathogens, including MRSA, enterococci (included vancomycin-resistant Enterococci), and Enterobacteriaceae expressing resistance genes from different classes of β-lactamases (in particular ESBL, KPC, and OXA), with a 2-fold to 4-fold greater activity than tigecycline.[67,68] Moreover, eravacycline currently represents the most potent antibiotic against MDR A baumanii, with a 4-fold higher activity compared with tigecycline, including strains resistant to sulbactam, imipenem/MER, levofloxacin, and amikacin/tobramycin.[69] Eravacycline exerts also a potent activity against anaerobic pathogens.[70] As tigecycline, eravacycline is not effective against P aeruginosa.[71]

Together with the broad-spectrum activity, another attractive characteristic of eravacycline is the availability of both intravenous and oral formulations, making eravacycline a potential option for early oral shift and early discharge in patients with infections due to MDR gram-negative bacteria.[72] In a recent phase 3, randomized, double-blind, multicenter study, eravacycline was found noninferior compared with ertapenem for the treatment of patients with cIAI (Clinicaltrials.gov, identifier NCT01844856).[73] No studies investigating eravacycline efficacy for the treatment of respiratory tract infections are ongoing; however, a phase 1 study conducted in 20 healthy adult volunteers analyzed eravacycline safety and pulmonary concentration after the administration of 1 mg of eravacycline per kilogram intravenously every 12 hours for a total of 7 doses over 4 days. Eravacycline was found to achieve 6-fold and a 50-fold higher concentrations in the ELF and alveolar macrophages than in plasma respectively, supporting its potential role for the treatment of respiratory tract infections. Moreover, eravacycline was well tolerated, with no serious adverse events and no treatment discontinuations.[74] Promising data for the use of eravacycline for the treatment of pneumonia come from a study by Grossman and colleagues,[75] showing eravacycline as effective as linezolid in a neutropenic MRSA mouse lung infection model. These data make eravacycline an attractive option for the treatment of respiratory tract infections due to resistant pathogens, including MRSA; β-lactamase–producing Enterobacteriaceae; and MDR A baumanii and for oral step-down therapy.

Omadacycline

Omadacycline (OMC) is the first aminomethylcycline in late-stage clinical development. Aminomethylcyclines are semisynthetic antibiotics related to the tetracycline.[76] Modifications in the chemical structure of OMC allow it to overcome the 2 main mechanisms of tetracycline resistance, efflux pumps and ribosomal protection. OMC demonstrated potent, broad-spectrum in vitro activity against common gram-positive aerobes (including methicillin-resistant and penicillin-resistant strains), gram-negative aerobes, anaerobes, and atypical bacterial pathogens.[77]

The Omadacycline for Pneumonia Treatment In the Community (OPTIC) study compared the efficacy and safety of intravenous to once-daily oral OMC and intravenous to once-daily oral moxifloxacin in patients with CAP. In the phase 3 OPTIC study, OMC adacycline was effective and noninferior to moxifloxacin for the treatment of CAP.[78] According to FDA endpoints, the clinical response rates were high, and OMC was generally safe and well tolerated and had an overall safety profile similar to that of moxifloxacin but with a lower incidence of diarrhea (and no cases of Clostridium difficile). In conclusion, omadacycline is clinically effective and can be considered an attractive once-daily option for the treatment of CAP.

Iclaprim

Iclaprim is an investigational dihydrofolate reductase inhibitor antibiotic that is effective against gram-positive MDR bacteria, such as MRSA. Iclaprim also has activity against some gram-negative bacteria (like H influenzae and M catarrhalis). The peculiarity of this drug is based on a mechanism overcoming trimethoprim-resistance with an increased potency without the need for coadministration of sulfonamides reducing sulfonamide-associated toxicity. A randomized, double-blind phase 2 study compared the efficacy of iclaprim with vancomycin in patients with HAP caused by gram-positive pathogens.[79] Seventy patients were randomized to receive 0.8 mg/kg intravenous every 12 hours (n = 23) or 1.2 mg/kg every 8 hours (n = 24) of iclaprim or vancomycin, 1 g every 12 hours (n = 23), all administered twice daily for 7 days to 14 days. There were no cases of VAP in the study. Cure rates in the intention-to-treat (ITT) population were 73.9% (17 of 23), 62.5% (15 of 24), and 52.2% (12 of 23) in the iclaprim, every 12 hours; iclaprim every 8 hours; and vancomycin groups, respectively. The mortality rates at 28 days were 8.7% (2 of 23), 12.5% (3 of 24), and 21.7% (5 of 23) for iclaprim, every 12 hours; iclaprim, every 8 hours; and vancomycin

groups, respectively, with no statistically significant differences. The adverse event profiles of both iclaprim dosing regimens were similar to that of vancomycin.

Solithromycin

Solithromycin is a fluoroketolide, classified as a fourth-generation macrolide antibiotic. Phase 2 and phase 3 trials have been conducted assessing solithromycin for use in CAP due to Streptococcus pneumoniae, H influenzae, and atypical pathogens, including those resistant to other macrolide antibiotics. A phase 2, randomized, double-blind, controlled trial was conducted comparing 5 days of solithromycin (800 mg once on day 1, 400 mg once daily thereafter) to 5 days of levofloxacin (750 mg once daily) in patients with CAP[80]; moreover, a phase 3 trial, SOLITAIRE-ORAL, was performed comparing the same 5-day regimen of solithromycin to 7 days of moxifloxacin, 400 mg once daily.[81] Moxifloxacin was chosen as a comparator for its role in the guidelines as monotherapy and similar spectrum of activity to solithromycin. Early clinical response in the ITT population was observed in 333 of 426 (78.2%) patients in the solithromycin group and 338 of 434 (77.9%) patients in the moxifloxacin group with a demonstrated noninferiority. Early clinical response in the clinically evaluable population also showed noninferiority (solithromycin 326 [80.9%], moxifloxacin 330 [81.1%], difference −0.19; 95% CI, 5.8–5.5). Of importance, in the trial there was a significant rate of aminotransferase elevations reported: alanine aminotransferase (ALT) was elevated greater than 3 times upper limit of normal in 22 (5.4%) patients receiving solithromycin and only in 14 (3.3%) patients receiving moxifloxacin; aspartate aminotransferase (AST) was elevated greater than 3 times upper limit of normal in 10 (2.5%) patients receiving solithromycin compared with 8 (1.9%) patients receiving moxifloxacin. Finally, in SOLITAIRE-IV (a phase III, randomized, double-blind, controlled study) comparing solithromycin to moxifloxacin,[82] prescribers had the option to switch to oral therapy based on predefined criteria. Intravenous doses for both drugs were 400 mg once daily; oral therapy was the same as in SOLITAIRE-ORAL, including the 800-mg loading dose given as the first dose. The criteria for noninferiority were confirmed, but solithromycin was associated with elevations in ALT and AST. In conclusion, if safety concerns about solithromycin and hepatotoxicity are resolved, solithromycin may find a place as a first-line therapy for CAP or as a second-line therapy for patients who fail to show early clinical response to other first-line therapies.

Tedizolid

Tedizolid belongs to the class of oxazolidinones and is currently approved for the treatment of ABSSSIs. Tedizolid is characterized by a potent in vitro activity against gram-positive pathogens, with a 4-fold to 8-fold greater activity than linezolid; moreover, tedizolid is active against linezolid-nonsusceptible strains.[83]

Tedizolid might represent a promising option for the treatment of MRSA pneumonia because of many advantages over linezolid, including lower risk of myelotoxicity[84,85]; lower risk of drug-drug interactions with selective serotonin reuptake inhibitors, compounds with serotonergic activity, and adrenergic agents due to its weak and reversible in vitro inhibition of the monoamine oxidase pathway[86]; and high bioavailability (>80%), with in vivo half-life value approximately 2-fold greater compared with linezolid, allowing once daily administration.[87]

Moreover, PK/PD studies showed that tedizolid achieves approximately 40-fold higher concentration in ELF relative to free plasma ones, supporting the use of tedizolid in the setting of pneumonia.[88]

The role of tedizolid for the treatment of MRSA respiratory tract infections is only investigational so far. Promising data supporting the use of tedizolid for the treatment of respiratory infections, however, come from a study conducted in an in vivo murine pneumonia model, showing tedizolid as effective as linezolid and more effective than vancomycin for the treatment of MRSA pneumonia.[89]

A phase 4 study designed to characterize the PK of intravenous and oral tedizolid in patients with cystic fibrosis is ongoing (Clinicaltrials.gov, identifier NCT02444234).

A phase 3, randomized, double-blind study comparing tedizolid (200-mg intravenous once daily for 7 days or 14 days in bacteremia) versus linezolid (600 mg intravenous every 12 hours for 10 days or 14 days for bacteremia) for the treatment of patients with presumed gram-positive HAP or VAP is recruiting (Clinicaltrials.gov, identifier NCT02019420).

Telavancin

Telavancin belongs to the class of new lipoglycopeptides and exerts a rapid, concentration-dependent, bactericidal activity against a broad-spectrum of gram-positive pathogens, including MRSA and S pneumoniae.[90,91] This drug is characterized by the presence of a lipophilic side chain that attaches to the bacterial membrane, showing increased affinity compared with old glycopeptides. Telavancin acts through 2 different mechanisms of action: inhibition of bacterial wall synthesis (transglycosylation and transpeptidation) and disruption of bacterial membrane function.[92]

PK/PD studies demonstrated that telavancin achieves good concentrations in ELF in healthy volunteers, with a median area under the curve $(AUC)_{ELF}$ approximately 75% of the free AUC_{plasma}.[93]

Noninferiority of telavancin (10 mg/kg every 24 hours) versus vancomycin (1 g every 12 hours) for the treatment of HAP has been demonstrated in 2 phase 3, randomized, double-blind studies (ATTAIN studies).[94] A systematic review and meta-analysis of data coming from ABSSSI and HAP studies on telavancin, however, suggested a higher risk of nephrotoxicity and serious adverse events among telavancin-treated patients compared with vancomycin.[95] In particular, an increased mortality in patients with HAP and moderate-to-severe renal impairment treated with telavancin compared with vancomycin was reported.[96] A post hoc analysis of data from the 2 phase 3 ATTAIN trials demonstrated that, in the subset of patients without severe renal impairment or preexisting acute renal failure, clinical and safety outcomes were similar in the telavancin and vancomycin treatment groups.[97] Telavancin is currently approved by the European Medicines Agency for the treatment of adult patients with HAP (including VAP) only for MRSA known or suspected infections and when other alternative treatments are not suitable. Moreover, it is strongly suggested to restrict the use of telavancin only to patients with normal renal function.[98]

Delafloxacin

Delafloxacin belongs to the class of fluoroquinolones and exerts a potent anti-MRSA activity together with a broad-spectrum activity against both gram-positive (including penicillin-sensitive, penicillin-resistant, and levofloxacin-resistant S pneumoniae, Streptococcus pyogenes, and Enterococci) and gram-negative pathogens (E coli, Klebsiella spp, H influenzae, M catharralis, and quinolone-susceptible P aeruginosa).[99–101] Moreover, delafloxacin is active against anaerobes and atypical respiratory tract pathogens (eg, Legionella, Chlamydia, and Mycoplasma).[102–104]

Due to the peculiar dual mechanism of DNA target inhibition (DNA gyrase and topoisomerase IV), delafloxacin is characterized by a reduced probability for the selection of resistant in vitro mutants.[105]

In a neutropenic murine lung infection model, delafloxacin demonstrated a high penetration into the lung compartment, because ELF concentrations were substantially higher than plasma ones.[106] The potential role of delafloxacin for the treatment of respiratory tract infection has been evaluated in 2 phase 2 studies, with promising results. In a double-blind, randomized, phase 2 study, 309 outpatients affected by CAP were treated with once-daily oral administration of delafloxacin at different dosages (100 mg, 200 mg, and 400 mg) for 7 days, with overall clinical and bacteriologic cure rates demonstrated in up to 87% of patients. Furthermore, pathogen eradication rates were higher than 90% for *H influenzae*, *H parainfluenzae*, and other atypical bacteria and achieved 100% for *Staphylococcus aureus* and *S pneumoniae*.[107] The second study investigated the safety and efficacy of delafloxacin in patients with acute bacterial exacerbation of chronic bronchitis. Four different regimens were tested (100 mg, 200 mg, 400 mg, and 500 mg, given orally every 24 hours); clinical response was similar in the 4 treatment groups, with clinical and microbiological cure rates higher than 70%.[108] Data coming from studies on the use of delafloxacin for the treatment of ABSSSI demonstrate that delafloxacin at the dose of 300 mg every 12 hours is well tolerated, with diarrhea the most common adverse event.[109] Moreover, in healthy volunteers, doses up to 900 mg were well tolerated, without any effect on QTc prolongation.[110]

Due to the broad-spectrum activity, including MRSA, the availability of an oral formulation, the reduced probability for resistance selection, and the good tolerability profile, delafloxacin could represent a promising option for the treatment of respiratory tract infections.

A phase 3 study comparing delafloxacin to moxifloxacin for the treatment of adult patients with CAP (DEFINE-CABP) is ongoing (Clinicaltrials.gov, identifier NCT02679573).

Murepavidin

Murepavadin (formally known as POL7080) represents the first in class of Outer Membrane Protein Targeting Antibiotics and acts through a novel mechanism of action by binding to the lipopolysaccharide transport protein D, leading to lipopolysaccharide alterations in the outer membrane of the bacterium and inducing cell death.[111] In vitro, murepavadin exhibits a specific and potent antimicrobial activity against *P aeruginosa*, whereas murepavadin was shown inactive against other gram-negative species, including other *Pseudomonas* species (eg, *P luteola* and *P oryzihabitans*), *Stenotrophomonas maltophilia*, *Burkholderia cepacia*, Enterobacteriaceae, and *A baumannii*, or against gram-positive bacteria.[112]

PK/PD studies found murepavadine ELF penetration approximately 100% relative to the free plasma concentration in healthy subjects, supporting a potential role for murepavadine for the treatment of respiratory tract infections.[113] A phase 2 study investigating PK, safety, and efficacy of murepavidin for the treatment of VAP due to *P aeruginosa* has recently been completed and results are pending (Clinicaltrials.gov, identifier NCT02096328).

A multicenter, open-label, randomized, phase 3 study comparing murepavidin combined with 1 antipseudomonal antibiotic versus 2 antipseudomonal antibiotics in adult subjects with bacterial VAP suspected or confirmed to be due to *P aeruginosa* is ongoing (Clinicaltrials.gov, identifier NCT03409679).

Lefamulin

Lefamulin is a novel pleuromutilin antibiotic currently undergoing FDA review for treatment of CAP as intravenous and oral formulations. Lefamulin exhibits a unique mechanism of action through inhibition of protein synthesis by binding to the peptidyl transferase center of the 50s bacterial ribosome, thus preventing the binding of transfer RNA for peptide transfer. Lefamulin displays activity against gram-positive and atypical pathogens typically associated with CAP, like *S pneumoniae*, *H influenzae*, *Mycoplasma pneumonia*, *Legionella pneumophila*, and *Chlamydophila pneumoniae*; its activity also includes MRSA and vancomycin-resistant *Enterococci*. Phase 2 trials indicate that lefamulin is well tolerated at an intravenous dose of 150 mg twice daily or an oral dose of 600 mg twice daily. The Lefamulin Evaluation Against Pneumonia 1 (LEAP 1) trial was a multinational phase 3 study that compared the efficacy and safety of lefamulin to moxifloxacin with or without linezolid in CAP (Clinicaltrials.gov, identifier NCT02559310). Lefamulin was found noninferior. The LEAP 2 trial was completed in 2018 and compare the safety and efficacy of oral lefamulin to oral moxifloxacin monotherapy (Clinicaltrials.gov, identifier NCT02813694).

SUMMARY

Several new drugs for the treatment of pneumonia have been recently approved or are in advanced stage of development (**Table 1**). The most attractive characteristic of new drugs is represented by

Table 1
Characteristics of new antibiotics for pneumonia and development phase

Drug	Spectrum of Activity	Administration	Development Phase for Pneumonia
Cefiderocol	Enterobacteriaceae ESBL, CRE (including MBL), MDR *Pseudomonas*, MDR *Acinetobacter*, *Stenotrophomonas maltophilia*	2 g q8h IV	Phase III for HAP/VAP, HCAP (NCT03032380); Phase III for VAP (NCT02714595)
CAZ-AVI	Gram negatives, including, ESBL, KPC, and OXA-producing strains, some MDR *Pseudomonas* strains	2.5 g q8h IV	Completed phase III trial for HAP/VAP (NCT01808092)
Tedizolid	Gram-positive (including MRSA) and some linezolid-resistant strains	200 mg q24h IV, oral	Phase III for HAP/VAP (NCT02019420)
Ceftolozane/ tazobactam	Gram negatives, including ESBL, MDR *Pseudomonas*	1.5 g q8h; 3 g q8h (VAP) IV	Phase III trial for HAP/VAP (NCT02070757)
MER/VAB	Gram negatives, including ESBL, KPC. No activity against MBL and OXA	2 g/2 g q8h IV	Completed phase II trial in CRE pneumonia Phase III trial for HAP/VAP (NCT03006679)
Imipenem/REL	Gram negatives, including AmpC, ESBL, KPC no activity against MBL and OXA	500 mg/250–125 mg q6h IV	Phase III for HAP/VAP (NCT02452047) Phase III for VAP, HAP (NCT02493764)
Plazomicin	Gram positives (including MRSA) and gram negatives, including, ESBL, CRE (most KPCs, OXA; no NDMs), MDR *Pseudomonas*, MDR *Acinetobacter*, and aminoglycosides resistant isolated	15 mg/kg q24h IV	Phase III for HAP/VAP (NCT01970371)
OMC	Gram-positive aerobes (including methicillin-resistant and penicillin-resistant strains), gram-negative aerobes, anaerobes, and atypical bacterial pathogens	IV: 100 mg q12h for 2 doses, followed by 100 mg q24h Oral: 300 mg q24h	No ongoing trials
Cetftobiprole	MRSA, *H influenzae* (including β-lactamase–producing strains), *M catarrhalis*, *E coli*, *K pneumoniae*, and *P aeruginosa*	500 mg q8h IV	Phase III for CAP and HAP in pediatric patients (NCT03439124)

(continued on next page)

Table 1
(continued)

Drug	Spectrum of Activity	Administration	Development Phase for Pneumonia
Ceftaroline	MRSA, methicillin-resistant *Staphylococcus epidermidis*, penicillin-resistant *S pneumoniae*, and vancomycin-resistant *Enterococcus faecalis* (not *E faecium*), gram-negative pathogens no ESBL-producing	600 mg q12h, IV	No ongoing trials
Iclaprim	MRSA, gram-negative bacteria (like *H influenzae* and *M catarrhalis*)	80 mg q12h	Planned
Solithromycin	*S pneumoniae*, *H influenzae*, and atypical pathogens	IV: 800 mg q24h on day 1 followed by 400 mg q24h Oral: 400 mg q24h	Phase II and III for CAP (NCT02605122)
Aztreonam/avibactam	Enterobacteriaceae, including OXA48-producing and MBL-producing. Limited activity against *A baumannii* and *P aeruginosa*	6500 mg ATM/2167 mg AVI q24h on day 1 followed by 6000 mg ATM/2000 mg AVI q24h, IV	Phase III for HAP/VAP (NCT03329092)
Ceftaroline/avibactam	MRSA, ESBL-producing Enterobacteriaceae, and KPC-producing Enterobacteriaceae	600/600 mg q24h, IV	No ongoing trials
Eravacycline	MRSA, *Enterococci* (including vancomycin-resistant) and Enterobacteriaceae expressing ESBL, KPC, and OXA	1 mg/kg q12h IV	No ongoing trials
Telavancin	MRSA and *S pneumoniae*	10 mg/Kg q24h IV	No ongoing trials
Delafloxacin	MRSA, penicillin-sensitive, penicillin-resistant, and levofloxacin-resistant *S pneumoniae*, *Streptococcus pyogenes* and *Enterococci*. Gram-negative pathogens, including quinolone-susceptible *P aeruginosa*. Anaerobes	IV: 300 mg q12h Oral: 450 mg q12h	Phase III for CAP (NCT02679573)

(continued on next page)

Table 1
(continued)

Drug	Spectrum of Activity	Administration	Development Phase for Pneumonia
Murepavadin	*P aeruginosa, Stenotrophomonas maltophilia, Burkholderia cepacia,* Enterobacteriaceae, *A baumannii*, gram-positive bacteria	Not defined	Phase III for VAP (NCT03409679)
Lefamulin	gram-positive and atypical organisms, including MRSA and vancomycin-resistant *Enterococci*	IV: 150 mg q12h Oral: 600 mg q12h	No ongoing trials

Abbreviations: ATM, aztreonam; AVI, avibactam; IV, intravenous; NDM, New Delhi metallo-betalactamase; OXA, oxacillinase; SSTI, skin and soft tissue infection.

the broad spectrum of activity against MDR pathogens, in particular ESBL-producing Enterobacteriaceae and CRE, which still represent a major threat in clinical practice due to the lack of therapeutic options. Moreover, new compounds in most cases are characterized by favorable toxicity profiles compared with old drugs currently used in clinical practice. Some of the new antimicrobials will be also available as oral formulations, with the potential for oral shift even in infections due to resistant pathogens.

REFERENCES

1. Kollef MH, Bassetti M, Francois B, et al. The intensive care medicine research agenda on multidrug-resistant bacteria, antibiotics, and stewardship. Intensive Care Med 2017;43(9):1187–97.
2. Bassetti M, Welte T, Wunderink RG. Treatment of Gram-negative pneumonia in the critical care setting: is the beta-lactam antibiotic backbone broken beyond repair? Crit Care 2016;20:19.
3. Gross AE, Van Schooneveld TC, Olsen KM, et al. Epidemiology and pre- dictors of multidrug-resistant community-acquired and healthcare-associated pneumonia. Antimicrob Agents Chemother 2014;58:5262–8.
4. Delle Rose D, Pezzotti P, Fortunato E, et al. Clinical predictors and microbiology of ventilator-associated pneumonia in the intensive care unit: a retrospective analysis in six Italian hospitals. Eur J Clin Microbiol Infect Dis 2016;35:1531–9.
5. Claeys KC, Zasowski EJ, Trinh TD, et al. Antimicrobial stewardship opportunities in critically ill patients with gram-negative lower respiratory tract infections: a multicenter cross-sectional analysis. Infect Dis Ther 2018;7:135–46.
6. Bassetti M, De Waele JJ, Eggimann P, et al. Preventive and therapeutic strategies in critically ill patients with highly resistant bacteria. Intensive Care Med 2015;41:776–95.
7. Teshome BF, Lee GC, Reveles KR, et al. Application of a methicillin-resistant *Staphylococcus aureus* risk score for community-onset pneumonia patients and outcomes with initial treatment. BMC Infect Dis 2015;15:380.
8. Koulenti D, Lisboa T, Brun-Buisson C, et al. EU-VAP/CAP Study Group. Spectrum of practice in the diagnosis of nosocomial pneumonia in patients requiring mechanical ventilation in European intensive care units. Crit Care Med 2009;37:2360–8.
9. Cruciani M, Gatti G, Lazzarini L, et al. Penetration of vancomycin into human lung tissue. J Antimicrob Chemother 1996;38:865–9.
10. Ye ZK, Li C, Zhai SD. Guidelines for therapeutic drug monitoring of vancomycin: a systematic review. PLoS One 2014;9:e99044.
11. Wunderink RG, Niederman MS, Kollef MH, et al. Linezolid in methicillin-resistant Staphylococcus aureus nosocomial pneumonia: a randomized, controlled study. Clin Infect Dis 2012;54:621–9.
12. Bassetti M, Baguneid M, Bouza E, et al. European perspective and update on the management of complicated skin and soft tissue infections due to methicillin-resistant Staphylococcus aureus after more than 10 years of experience with linezolid. Clin Microbiol Infect 2014;20(Suppl 4):3–18.
13. Basilea Pharmaceutica International Ltd. Basilea's antibiotic ceftobiprole obtains regulatory approval in Europe for pneumonia [media release]. 2018. Available at: http://www.basilea.com/chameleon/public/584f9d1e-4298-e47c0475a5e5e5288ded/5825. Accessed March 21, 2018.

14. Hebeisen P, Heinze-Krauss I, Angehrn P, et al. In vitro and in vivo properties of Ro 63-9141, a novel broad-spectrum cephalosporin with activity against methicillin-resistant staphylococci. Antimicrob Agents Chemother 2001;45(3):825–36.

15. Murthy B, Schmitt-Hoffmann A. Pharmacokinetics and pharmacodynamics of ceftobiprole, an anti-MRSA cephalosporin with broad-spectrum activity. Clin Pharmacokinet 2008;47:21–33.

16. Awad SS, Rodriguez AH, Chuang YC, et al. A Phase 3 randomized double-blind comparison of ceftobiprole medocaril versus ceftazidime plus linezolid for the treatment of hospital acquired pneumonia. Clin Infect Dis 2014;59(1):51–61.

17. Nicholson SC, Welte T, File TM Jr, et al. A randomised, doubleblind trial comparing ceftobiprole medocaril with ceftriaxone with or without linezolid for the treatment of patients with community-acquired pneumonia requiring hospitalisation. Int J Antimicrob Agents 2012;39:240–6.

18. File TM, Low DE, Eckburg PB, et al. FOCUS 1: a randomized, double blinded, multicentre, Phase III trial of the efficacy and safety of ceftaroline fosamil versus ceftriaxone in community-acquired pneumonia. J Antimicrob Chemother 2011;66(Suppl 3):iii19–32.

19. Low DE, File TM, Eckburg PB, et al. FOCUS 2: a randomized, doubleblinded, multicentre, Phase III trial of the efficacy and safety of ceftaroline fosamil versus ceftriaxone in community-acquired pneumonia. J Antimicrob Chemother 2011;66(Suppl 3): iii33–44

20. Zhong NS, Sun T, Zhuo C, et al. Ceftaroline fosamil versus ceftriaxone for the treatment of Asian patients with community-acquired pneumonia: a randomised, controlled, double-blind, Phase 3, non-inferiority with nested superiority trial. Lancet Infect Dis 2015;15:161–71.

21. Huang X, Jandourek A, Cole P, et al. Current use of ceftaroline for community-acquired bacterial pneumonia (cabp) in us hospitals: length of stay and total cost from the capture study. Chest J 2013;144: 259.

22. Maggiore C, Pasquale T, Jandourek A, et al. Experience with ceftaroline fosamil as monotherapy and combination therapy with vancomycin in acute bacterial skin and skin structure infections and community-acquired bacterial pneumonia. ASHP Midyear Meeting 2013. Orlando (FL): American Society of Health-System Pharmacists; 2013. p. 5–112.

23. Portsmouth S, Van Veenhuyzen D, Echols R, et al. Clinical response of cefiderocol compared with imipenem/cilastatin in the treatment of adults with complicated urinary tract infections with or without pyelonephritis or acute uncomplicated pyelonephritis: results from a multicenter, doubleblind, randomized study (APEKS-cUTI). Open Forum Infect Dis 2017;4(Suppl_1):S537–8.

24. Boyd S, Anderson K, Albrecht V, et al. In vitro activity of cefiderocol against multi-drug resistant carbapenemase-producing gram-negative pathogens. Open Forum Infect Dis 2017;4(suppl_1): S376.

25. Sader HS, Castanheira M, Flamm RK, et al. Antimicrobial activity of ceftazidime-avibactam against Gram-negative organisms collected from U.S. medical centers in 2012. Antimicrob Agents Chemother 2014;58:1684–92.

26. Keepers TR, Gomez M, Celeri C, et al. Bactericidal activity, absence of serum effect, and time–kill kinetics of ceftazidime-avibactam against b-lactamase-producing Enterobacteriaceae and Pseudomonas aeruginosa. Antimicrob Agents Chemother 2014;58:5297–305.

27. Torres A, Zhong N, Pachl J, et al. Ceftazidime-avibactam versus meropenem in nosocomial pneumonia, including ventilator-associated pneumonia (REPROVE): a randomised, double-blind, Phase 3 non-inferiority trial. Lancet Infect Dis 2018;18(3): 285–95.

28. van Duin D, Lok JJ, Earley M, et al, Antibacterial Resistance Leadership Group. Colistin versus ceftazidime-avibactam in the treatment of infections due to carbapenem-resistant enterobacteriaceae. Clin Infect Dis 2018;66:163–71.

29. Shields RK, Nguyen MH, Chen L, et al. Ceftazidime-avibactam is superior to other treatment regimens against carbapenem-resistant klebsiella pneumoniae bacteremia. Antimicrob Agents Chemother 2017;61(8) [pii:e00883-17].

30. Bassetti M, Vena A, Castaldo N, et al. New antibiotics for ventilator-associated pneumonia. Curr Opin Infect Dis 2018;31:177–86.

31. Vazquez JA, Gonzá lez Patzán LD, Stricklin D, et al. Efficacy and safety of ceftazidime-avibactam versus imipenem-cilastatin in the treatment of complicated urinary tract infections, including acute pyelonephritis, in hospitalized adults: results of a prospective, investigator-blinded, randomized study. Curr Med Res Opin 2012;28:1921–31.

32. Lucasti C, Popescu I, Ramesh MK, et al. Comparative study of the efficacy and safety of ceftazidime/avibactam plus metronidazole versus meropenem in the treatment of complicated intra-abdominal infections in hospitalized adults: results of a randomized, double-blind, Phase II trial. J Antimicrob Chemother 2013;68:1183–92.

33. Tato M, García-Castillo M, Bofarull AM, et al, CENIT Study Group. In vitro activity of ceftolozane/tazobactam against clinical isolates of Pseudomonas aeruginosa and Enterobacteriaceae recovered in Spanish medical centres: results of the CENIT study. Int J Antimicrob Agents 2015;46:502–10.

34. Armstrong ES, Farrell DJ, Palchak M, et al. In vitro activity of ceftolozane-tazobactam against anaerobic organisms identified during the ASPECT-cIAI Study. Antimicrob Agents Chemother 2015;60: 666–8.

35. Xipell M, Bodro M, Marco F, et al. Successful treatment of three severe MDR or XDR *Pseudomonas aeruginosa* infections with ceftolozane/tazobactam. Future Microbiol 2017;12:1323–6.

36. Munita JM, Aitken SL, Miller WR, et al. Multicenter evaluation of ceftolozane/tazobactam for serious infections caused by carbapenem-resistant *Pseudomonas aeruginosa*. Clin Infect Dis 2017;65(1): 158–61.

37. Monogue ML, Pettit RS, Muhlebach M, et al. Population pharmacokinetics and safety of ceftolozane-tazobactam in adult cystic fibrosis patients admitted with acute pulmonary exacerbation. Antimicrob Agents Chemother 2016;60:6578–84.

38. Xiao AJ, Miller BW, Huntington JA, et al. Ceftolozane/tazobactam pharmacokinetic/pharmacodynamic-derived dose justification for Phase 3 studies in patients with nosocomial pneumonia. J Clin Pharmacol 2016;56:56–66.

39. Haidar G, Philips NJ, Shields RK, et al. Ceftolozane–tazobactam for the treatment of multidrug-resistant Pseudomonas aeruginosa infections: clinical effectiveness and evolution of resistance. Clin Infect Dis 2017;65:110–20.

40. Solomkin J, Hershberger E, Miller B, et al. Ceftolozane/tazobactam plus metronidazole for complicated intra-abdominal infections in an era of multidrug resistance: results from a randomized, double-blind, Phase 3 trial (ASPECT-cIAI). Clin Infect Dis 2015;60:1462–71.

41. Brogden RN, Heel RC. Aztreonam. A review of its antibacterial activity, pharmacokinetic properties and therapeutic use. Drugs 1986;31:96–130.

42. Lahiri SD, Mangani S, Durand-Reville T, et al. Structural insight into potent broad-spectrum inhibition with reversible recyclization mechanism: avibactam in complex with CTX-M-15 and Pseudomonas aeruginosa AmpC b-lactamases. Antimicrob Agents Chemother 2013;57:2496–505.

43. Karlowsky JA, Kazmierczak KM, de Jonge BLM, et al. In vitro activity of aztreonam-avibactam against enterobacteriaceae and pseudomonas aeruginosa isolated by clinical laboratories in 40 countries from 2012 to 2015. Antimicrob Agents Chemother 2017;61 [pii:e00472-17].

44. Sader HS, Mendes RE, Pfaller MA, et al. Antimicrobial activities of aztreonam-avibactam and comparator agents against contemporary (2016) clinical enterobacteriaceae isolates. Antimicrob Agents Chemother 2017;62(1) [pii:e01856-17].

45. Saravolatz LD, Stein GE, Johnson LB. Ceftaroline: a novel cephalosporin with activity against methicillin-resistant Staphylococcus aureus. Clin Infect Dis 2011;52:1156–63.

46. Castanheira M, Jones RN, Sader HS. Activity of ceftaroline and comparator agents tested against contemporary Gram-positive and -negative (2011) isolates collected in Europe, Turkey, and Israel. J Chemother 2014;26:202–10.

47. Werth BJ, Rybak MJ. Ceftaroline plus avibactam demonstrates bactericidal activity against pathogenic anaerobic bacteria in a one-compartment in vitro pharmacokinetic/pharmacodynamic model. Antimicrob Agents Chemother 2014;58:559–62.

48. Castanheira M, Sader HS, Farrell DJ, et al. Activity of ceftaroline-avibactam tested against Gram-negative organism populations, including strains expressing one or more β-lactamases and methicillin-resistant Staphylococcus aureus carrying various staphylococcal cassette chromosome mec types. Antimicrob Agents Chemother 2012;56:4779–85.

49. Flamm RK, Farrell DJ, Sader HS, et al. Antimicrobial activity of ceftaroline combined with avibactam tested against bacterial organisms isolated from acute bacterial skin and skin structure infections in United States medical centers (2010-2012). Diagn Microbiol Infect Dis 2014;78:449–56.

50. Sader HS, Flamm RK, Jones RN. Antimicrobial activity of ceftaroline-avibactam tested against clinical isolates collected from U.S. Medical Centers in 2010-2011. Antimicrob Agents Chemother 2013;57:1982–8.

51. Riccobene TA, Su SF, Rank D. Single- and multiple-dose study to determine the safety, tolerability, and pharmacokinetics of ceftaroline fosamil in combination with avibactam in healthy subjects. Antimicrob Agents Chemother 2013;57:1496–504.

52. Das S, Armstrong J, Mathews D, et al. Randomized, placebo-controlled study to assess the impact on QT/QTc interval of supratherapeutic doses of ceftazidime-avibactam or ceftaroline fosamil-avibactam. J Clin Pharmacol 2014;54:331–40.

53. Thaden JT, Pogue JM, Kaye KS. Role of newer and re-emerging older agents in the treatment of infections caused by carbapenem-resistant Enterobacteriaceae. Virulence 2017;8:403–16.

54. Livermore DM, Warner M, Mushtaq S. Activity of MK-7655 combined with imipenem against Enterobacteriaceae and Pseudomonas aeruginosa. J Antimicrob Chemother 2013;68:2286–90.

55. Lapuebla A, Abdallah M, Olafisoye O, et al. Activity of imipenem with relebactam against gram-negative pathogens from New York City. Antimicrob Agents Chemother 2015;59:5029–31.

56. Lucasti C, Vasile L, Sandesc D, et al. Phase 2, dose-ranging study of relebactam with imipenem-cilastatin in subjects with complicated

intra-abdominal infection. Antimicrob Agents Chemother 2016;60:6234–43.

57. Sims M, Mariyanovski V, McLeroth P, et al. Prospective, randomized, double-blind, Phase 2 dose-ranging study comparing efficacy and safety of imipenem/cilastatin plus relebactam with imipenem/cilastatin alone in patients with complicated urinary tract infections. J Antimicrob Chemother 2017;72:2616–26.

58. Castanheira M, Huband MD, Mendes RE, et al. Meropenem-vaborbactam tested against contemporary gram-negative isolates collected worldwide during 2014, including carbapenem-resistant, kpc-producing, multidrug-resistant, and extensively drug-resistant enterobacteriaceae. Antimicrob Agents Chemother 2017;61 [pii:e00567-1].

59. Hackel MA, Lomovskaya O, Dudley MN, et al. In vitro activity of meropenem-vaborbactam against clinical isolates of KPC-positive Enterobacteriaceae. Antimicrob Agents Chemother 2017;62 [pii:e01904-17].

60. Sun D, Rubio-Aparicio D, Nelson K, et al. Meropenem-vaborbactam resistance selection, resistance prevention, and molecular mechanisms in mutants of KPC-producing Klebsiella pneumoniae. Antimicrob Agents Chemother 2017;61 [pii: e01694-17].

61. Griffith DC, Loutit JS, Morgan EE, et al. Phase 1 study of the safety, tolerability, and pharmacokinetics of the β-lactamase inhibitor vaborbactam (RPX7009) in healthy adult subjects. Antimicrob Agents Chemother 2016;60:6326–32.

62. Wright H, Bonomo RA, Paterson DL. New agents for the treatment of infections with Gram-negative bacteria: restoring the miracle or false dawn? Clin Microbiol Infect 2017;23:704–12.

63. Cass R, Kostrub CF, Gotfried M, et al. A double-blind, randomized, placebo controlled study to assess the safety, tolerability, plasma pharmacokinetics and lung penetration of intravenous plazomicin in healthy subjects. 23rd European Congress on Clinical Microbiology and Infectious disease, Berlin, April 27–30, 2013. 1637.

64. McKinnell JA, Connoly LE, Pushkin R, et al. Improved outcomes with plazomicin (PLZ) compared with colistin (CST) in patients with bloodstream infections (BSI) Caused by carbapenem-resistant enterobacteriaceae (CRE): results from the CARE study. Open Forum Infect Dis 2017;4: S531–1531.

65. Li H, Estabrook M, Jacoby GA, et al. In vitro susceptibility of characterized beta-lactamase producing strains tested with avibactam combinations. Antimicrob Agents Chemother 2015;59: 1789–93.

66. Clark RB, Hunt DK, He M, et al. Fluorocyclines. 2. Optimization of the C-9 side-chain for antibacterial activity and oral efficacy. J Med Chem 2012;55: 606–22.

67. Abdallah M, Olafisoye O, Cortes C, et al. Activity of eravacycline against Enterobacteriaceae and Acinetobacter baumannii, including multidrug-resistant isolates, from New York City. Antimicrob Agents Chemother 2015;59:1802–5.

68. Zhanel GG, Baxter MR, Adam HJ, et al. In vitro activity of eravacycline against 2213 Gram-negative and 2424 Gram-positive bacterial pathogens isolated in Canadian hospital laboratories: CANWARD surveillance study 2014-2015. Diagn Microbiol Infect Dis 2018;91(1):55–62.

69. Seifert H, Stefanik D, Sutcliffe JA, et al. In-vitro activity of the novel fluorocycline eravacycline against carbapenem non-susceptible Acinetobacte baumannii. Int J Antimicrob Agents 2018;51:62–4.

70. Snydman DR, McDermott LA, Jacobus NV, et al. Evaluation of the in vitro activity of eravacycline against a broad spectrum of recent clinical anaerobic isolates. Antimicrob Agents Chemother 2018;62(5) [pii:e02206-17].

71. Sutcliffe JA, O'Brien W, Fyfe C, et al. Antibacterial activity of eravacycline (TP-434), a novel fluorocycline, against hospital and community pathogens. Antimicrob Agents Chemother 2013;57:5548–58.

72. Bassetti M, Righi E. Eravacycline for the treatment of intra-abdominal infections. Expert Opin Investig Drugs 2014;23:1575–84.

73. Solomkin J, Evans D, Slepavicius A, et al. Assessing the efficacy and safety of eravacycline vs ertapenem in complicated intra-abdominal infections in the investigating gram-negative infections treated with eravacycline (IGNITE 1) trial: a randomized clinical trial. JAMA Surg 2017;152:224–32.

74. Connors KP, Housman ST, Pope JS, et al. Phase I, open-label, safety and & pharmacokinetic study to assess bronchopulmonary disposition of intravenous eravacycline in healthy men and women. Antimicrob Agents Chemother 2014;58:2113–8.

75. Grossman TH, Murphy TM, Slee AM, et al. Eravacycline (TP-434) is efficacious in animal models of infection. Antimicrob Agents Chemother 2015;59: 2567–71.

76. Honeyman L, Ismail M, Nelson ML, et al. Structure-activity relationship of the aminomethylcyclines and the discovery of omadacycline. Antimicrob Agents Chemother 2015;59:7044–53.

77. Macone AB, Caruso BK, Leahy RG, et al. In vitro and in vivo antibacterial activities of omadacycline, a novel aminomethylcycline. Antimicrob Agents Chemother 2014;58:1127–35.

78. Sun H, Ting L, Machineni S, et al. Randomized, open-label study of the pharmacokinetics and safety of oral and intravenous administration of omadacycline to healthy subjects. Antimicrob Agents Chemother 2016;60:7431–5.

79. Huang DB, File TM Jr, Torres A, et al. A phase II randomized, double-blind, multicenter study to evaluate efficacy and safety of intravenous Iclaprim versus vancomycin for the treatment of nosocomial pneumonia suspected or confirmed to be due to gram-positive pathogens. Clin Ther 2017;39:1706–18.

80. Oldach D, Clark K, Schranz J, et al. Randomized, double-blind, multicenter phase 2 study comparing the efficacy and safety of oral solithromycin (CEM-101) to those of oral levofloxacin in the treatment of patients with community-acquired bacterial pneumonia. Antimicrob Agents Chemother 2013;57(6):2526–34.

81. Barrera CM, Mykietiuk A, Metev H, et al, SOLITAIRE-ORAL Pneumonia Team. Efficacy and safety of oral solithromycin versus oral moxifloxacin for treatment of community-acquired bacterial pneumonia: a global, double-blind, multicentre, randomised, active-controlled, non-inferiority trial (SOLITAIRE-ORAL). Lancet Infect Dis 2016;16(4):421–30.

82. File TM Jr, Rewerska B, Vucinic-Mihailovic V, et al. SOLITAIRE-IV: a randomized, double-blind, multicenter study comparing the efficacy and safety of intravenous-to-oral solithromycin to intravenous-to-oral moxifloxacin for treatment of community-acquired bacterial pneumonia. Clin Infect Dis 2016;63(8):1007–16.

83. Li S, Guo Y, Zhao C, et al. In vitro activities of tedizolid compared with other antibiotics against Gram-positive pathogens associated with hospital-acquired pneumonia, skin and soft tissue infection and bloodstream infection collected from 26 hospitals in China. J Med Microbiol 2016;65:1215–24.

84. Lodise TP, Fang E, Minassian SL, et al. Platelet profile in patients with acute bacterial skin and skin structure infections receiving tedizolid or linezolid: findings from the Phase 3 ESTABLISH clinical trials. Antimicrob Agents Chemother 2014;58:7198–204.

85. Shorr AF, Lodise TP, Corey GR, et al. Analysis of the Phase 3 ESTABLISH trials of tedizolid versus linezolid in acute bacterial skin and skin structure infections. Antimicrob Agents Chemother 2015;59:864–71.

86. Shaw KJ, Barbachyn MR. The oxazolidinones: past, present, and future. Ann N Y Acad Sci 2011;1241:48–70.

87. Flanagan S, Passarell J, Lu Q. Tedizolid population pharmacokinetics, exposure response, and target attainment. Antimicrob Agents Chemother 2014;58:6462–70.

88. Lodise TP, Drusano GL. Use of pharmacokinetic/pharmacodynamic systems analyses to inform dose selection of tedizolid phosphate. Clin Infect Dis 2014;58(Suppl 1):S28–34.

89. Tessier PR, Keel RA, Hagihara M, et al. Comparative in vivo efficacies of epithelial lining fluid exposures of tedizolid, linezolid, and vancomycin for methicillin-resistant Staphylococcus aureus in a mouse pneumonia model. Antimicrob Agents Chemother 2012;56:2342–6.

90. Smith JR, Barber KE, Hallesy J, et al. Telavancin demonstrates activity against methicillin-resistant Staphylococcus aureus isolates with reduced suscept-ibility to vancomycin, daptomycin, and linezolid in broth microdilution MIC and one-compartment pharmacokinetic/pharmacodynamic models. Antimicrob Agents Chemother 2015;59:5529–34.

91. Pfaller MA, Mendes RE, Sader HS, et al. Telavancin activity against Gram-positive bacteria isolated from respiratory tract specimens of patients with nosocomial pneumonia. J Antimicrob Chemother 2010;65:2396–404.

92. Zhanel GG, Calic D, Schweizer F, et al. New lipoglycopeptides: a comparative review of dalbavancin, oritavancin and telavancin. Drugs 2010;70:859–86 [Erratum appears in Drugs 2011;71:526].

93. Lodise TP Jr, Gotfried M, Barriere S, et al. Telavancin penetration into human epithelial lining fluid determined by population pharmacokinetic modeling and Monte Carlo simulation. Antimicrob Agents Chemother 2008;52:2300–4.

94. Rubinstein E, Lalani T, Corey GR, et al, ATTAIN Study Group. Telavancin versus vancomycin for hospital-acquired pneumonia due to gram-positive pathogens. Clin Infect Dis 2011;52:31–40.

95. Polyzos KA, Mavros MN, Vardakas KZ, et al. Efficacy and safety of telavancin in clinical trials: a systematic review and meta-analysis. PLoS One 2012;7:e41870.

96. Barriere SL. The ATTAIN trials: efficacy and safety of telavancin compared with vancomycin for the treatment of hospital-acquired and ventilator-asso- ciated bacterial pneumonia. Future Microbiol 2014;9:281–9.

97. Torres A, Rubinstein E, Corey GR, et al. Analysis of Phase 3 telavancin nosocomial pneumonia data excluding patients with severe renal impairment and acute renal failure. J Antimicrob Chemother 2014;69:1119–26.

98. Masterton R, Cornaglia G, Courvalin P, et al. The clinical positioning of telavancin in Europe. Int J Antimicrob Agents 2015;45:213–20.

99. Almer LS, Hoffrage JB, Keller EL, et al. In vitro and bactericidal activities of ABT-492, a novel fluoroquinolone, against Gram-positive and Gram- negative organisms. Antimicrob Agents Chemother 2004;48:2771–7.

100. Gunderson SM, Hayes RA, Quinn JP, et al. In vitro pharmacodynamic activities of ABT-492, a novel quinolone, compared to those of levofloxacin

against Streptococcus pneumoniae, Haemophilus influenzae, and Moraxella catarrhalis. Antimicrob Agents Chemother 2004;48:203–8.

101. Pfaller MA, Sader HS, Rhomberg PR, et al. In vitro activity of delafloxacin against contemporary bacterial pathogens from the United States and Europe, 2014. Antimicrob Agents Chemother 2017;61 [pii: e02609-16]. [Erratum appears in: Antimicrob Agents Chemother 2018;62(2)].

102. Goldstein EJ, Citron DM, Merriam CV, et al. In vitro activities of ABT-492, a new fluoroquinolone, against 155 aerobic and 171 anaerobic pathogens isolated from antral sinus puClinicalTrials.Gov, IdentifierNCTure specimens from patients with sinusitis. Antimicrob Agents Chemother 2003;47: 3008–11.

100. Hammerschlag MR, Roblin PM. The in vitro activity of a new fluoro- quinolone, ABT-492, against recent clinical isolates of Chlamydia pneumoniae. J Antimicrob Chemother 2004;54:281–2.

104. Waites KB, Crabb DM, Duffy LB. Comparative in vitro susceptibilities and bactericidal activities of investigational fluoroquinolone ABT- 492 and other antimicrobial agents against human mycoplasmas and ureaplasmas. Antimicrob Agents Chemother 2003;47:3973–5.

105. Remy JM, Tow-Keogh CA, McConnell TS, et al. Activity of delafloxacin against methicillin-resistant Staphylococcus aureus: resistance selection and characterization. J Antimicrob Chemother 2012; 67:2814–20.

106. Thabit AK, Crandon JL, Nicolau DP. Pharmacodynamic and pharmacokinetic profiling of delafloxacin in a murine lung model against community-acquired respiratory tract pathogens. Int J Antimicrob Agents 2016;48:535–41.

107. Longcor J, Hopkins S, Wickler M, et al. A Phase 2 study of the safety and eficacy of oral delafloxacin (DLX) in community acquired pneumonia (CAP). Presented at ID Week 2012; San Diego, CA, October 17–21, 2012.

108. Longcor J, Hopkins S, Wickler M, et al. A Phase 2 safety and efficacy study of oral delafloxacin (DLX) in subjects with acute bacterial exacerbation of chronic bronchitis (ABECB). Presented at ID Week 2012; San Diego, CA, October 17–21, 2012.

109. O'Riordan W, Mehra P, Manos P, et al. A randomized Phase 2 study comparing two doses of delafloxacin with tigecycline in adults with complicated skin and skin-structure infections. Int J Infect Dis 2015;30:67–73.

110. Litwin JS, Benedict MS, Thorn MD, et al. A thorough QT study to evaluate the effects of therapeutic and supratherapeutic doses of delafloxacin on cardiac repolarization. Antimicrob Agents Chemother 2015;59:3469–73.

111. Werneburg M, Zerbe K, Juhas M, et al. Inhibition of lipopolysaccharide transport to the outer membrane in Pseudomonas aeruginosa by peptidomimetic antibiotics. Chembiochem 2012;13:1767–75.

112. Martin-Loeches I, Dale GE, Torres A. Murepavadin: a new antibiotic class in the pipeline. Expert Rev Anti Infect Ther 2018;21:1–10.

113. Winter E, Boetsch C, Brennan B, et al. Penetration of POL7080/RO7033877 into Epithelial lining fluid and alveolar macrophages of healthy volunteers. 2015. Presented. Joint 55th Interscience Conference on Antimicrobial Agents and Chemotherapy and 28th International Congress of Chemotherapy, San Diego, CA. September 17–21, 2015.

Personalizing the Management of Pneumonia

Samir Gautam, MD, PhD, Lokesh Sharma, PhD,
Charles S. Dela Cruz, MD, PhD*

KEYWORDS

- Pneumonia • Personalized • Precision • Individualized • Immunomodulation • Antibiotic resistance

KEY POINTS

- The current approaches to diagnosing pneumonia and identifying pathogens rely on antiquated methods that have poor test characteristics.
- Treatment strategies are similarly crude because they rely on broad-spectrum empiric antibiotics, which promotes antimicrobial resistance, and in some cases steroids, which have numerous unwanted side effects.
- Emerging genomic methods have the capability to improve microbiologic diagnosis and assessment of host immune responses.
- This information may enable the formulation of personalized treatment of patients, featuring highly selective antimicrobials and targeted immunomodulation.

INTRODUCTION

Lower respiratory tract infections (LRTIs) are the leading cause of death in developing countries and account for more than 4 million deaths per year worldwide.[1] They result in the loss of 103,000 disability-adjusted life years annually, making pneumonia the single greatest contributor to human disease burden.[2,3] It is astonishing, therefore, that diagnosis of pneumonia in most cases (even at academic centers) still relies on decades-old and highly unreliable clinical criteria such as the chest radiograph,[4] which has a sensitivity less than 50% and positive predictive value less than 30%.[5] The difficulty only increases in patients with underlying cardiopulmonary disease or immunosuppression; two of the populations at highest risk of death from LRTI. Microbiological culture, another pillar of pneumonia diagnosis, is

similarly faulty, as it reveals a pathogen in less than half of cases.[6,7]

In the absence of dependable diagnostic guideposts, clinicians faced with any suspicion of pneumonia have traditionally resorted to treating with empiric broad-spectrum antibiotics 'just to be safe'. However, this time-worn adage is finally being questioned, as data have accumulated to show the danger of indiscriminate antimicrobial use both to society and to individual patients. On a population level, antibiotic administration for suspected respiratory infection is now appreciated as a major driver of antibiotic resistance,[2,8,9] which in turn has been identified by the World Health Organization (WHO) as one of the biggest global threats to human health.[10] Meanwhile, the harm of inappropriate antibiotics to patients is also becoming recognized.[11] In addition to the risk of allergy and drug toxicity,

Disclosure: This work was supported by grants from the NHLBI (HL126094 and HL103770 to CSD and T32-HL007778 to SG).
Pulmonary Critical Care and Sleep Medicine, Center for Pulmonary Infection Research and Treatment, Yale University, 300 Cedar Street, TACS441, New Haven, CT 06520-8057, USA
* Corresponding author.
E-mail address: charles.delacruz@yale.edu

Clin Chest Med 39 (2018) 871–900
https://doi.org/10.1016/j.ccm.2018.08.008
0272-5231/18/Published by Elsevier Inc.

antibiotics produce profound and lasting alterations in the microbiome of the gut and lung (dysbiosis),[12] which manifest overtly through secondary infections such as *Clostridium difficile* infection (CDI) but also more subtly through alterations in host response to infection and contributions to diabetes mellitus, atherosclerosis, inflammatory bowel disease, and asthma.[13,14] It is likely that these direct hazards to the patient will serve as a greater deterrent to antibiotic overuse than less tangible risks such as breeding resistance.

If the current methods for diagnosing and managing pneumonia are inadequate, what are the alternatives? In general, there are 2 strategies. The first relies on guidelines, such as those put forth by the Infectious Diseases Society of America (IDSA) and American Thoracic Society (ATS) for community-acquired pneumonia (CAP) and for hospital-acquired pneumonia (HAP) and ventilator-acquired pneumonia (VAP).[15,16] These guidelines synthesize the best available data into an evidence-based approach for the management of pneumonia, with goals of simplicity and the ability to generalize. These goals are in part born of necessity, because guidelines must be accessible to nonspecialists, but it is also an inescapable consequence of the large, unstratified patient populations in studies that inform the guidelines. Recommendations are similarly monolithic and therefore have limited relevance for uncommon infections and unique hosts, such as those with compromised immune or cardiopulmonary function. Diagnosis and management become significant challenges in these patients, especially during critical illness. In such cases especially, an alternative strategy is needed, one that combines greater diagnostic granularity with individually tailored therapy: so-called personalized medicine.

The first step toward personalized medicine is refinement of diagnostic categories. For pneumonia, this requires subclassification of the syndrome, which is currently defined broadly by (1) evidence of systemic infection (leukocytosis, fevers, or chills), (2) respiratory symptoms (dyspnea, cough, sputum), and (3) new radiographic infiltrates.[17] This highly inclusive entity could, for instance, be divided into viral pneumonia, bacterial pneumonia, and noninfectious respiratory disease using additional diagnostic techniques (eg, biomarkers)- a preliminary degree of endotyping referred to as stratified medicine.[18] Such subgroups remain large enough to enable well-powered clinical trials and, thus, endotyping at this level may leverage conventional evidence-based medicine to guide management.

However, the full realization of personalized medicine requires a complete delineation of disease mechanisms, advanced diagnostics for interrogating these mechanisms in patients, and targeted therapies for modulating them. The closest approximation to this vision is in oncology, where tumors are sequenced to identify driver mutations for selective targeting (eg, with tyrosine kinase inhibitors), and the host immune response is assessed to determine candidacy for checkpoint inhibitors. Thus, the field is beginning to adopt a "tissue-agnostic" approach, wherein therapy is guided not by histologically defined tissue of origin but by the molecular biology and immunology of the tumor and host; a dramatic departure from traditional oncologic management.

Respiratory infection has much to learn from this paradigm. For pneumonia, personalization would require a comprehensive molecular description of the pathogen, the host, and the immunologic phenomena that stem from their interaction. This description will allow management decisions to be determined by not only data from empiric trials but also basic microbiological and immunologic principles. Examples include delivery of highly selective antimicrobials based on pathogen taxonomy and susceptibility, and rational manipulation of dysregulated host responses to promote pathogen clearance and limit immunopathology.

A useful framework for understanding the complex interplay of host and pathogen, based on the concepts of resistance and tolerance, has been defined by Ayres and Schneider[19,20] (graphically represented in **Fig. 1**). Resistance refers to the host's ability to clear microbes, whereas tolerance is a term borrowed from ecological immunology that describes the host's ability to endure a microbial insult. Resistance comprises the host's defenses against an invading pathogen, including intrinsic epithelial mechanisms, innate immunity, adaptive responses, and others as described later. Tolerance is influenced by a more varied set of factors, including the pathologic consequences of immune effectors (eg, reactive oxygen species [ROS] released from infiltrating neutrophils) as well as mechanisms unrelated to resistance (eg, myocardial infarction in patients with influenza infection).[21] To eliminate confusion with the traditional concept of immunologic tolerance, this article refers instead to resilience, following the example of Mizgerd and colleagues.[22] Using this this framework, 4 phases in the personalized diagnosis and management of pneumonia can be described (summarized in **Fig. 1**).

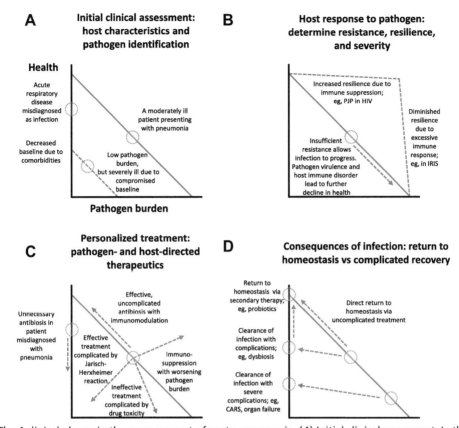

Fig. 1. The 4 clinical phases in the management of acute pneumonia. (*A*) Initial clinical assessment. In this phase, the patient's baseline level of health and immunologic competency are assessed. Simultaneously, rapid identification of pathogen is pursued. Health (dependent variable) is a conceptual term that reflects the clinical status of the patient: a composite of criteria including hemodynamic stability and organ function. With increasing pathogen burden (independent variable), health declines. (*B*) Host response to pathogen. The slope of the curve is determined by tissue resilience, which depends on characteristics of the host, the pathogen, and their interaction. For instance, host resilience to *Pneumocystis jiroveci* pneumonia (PJP) is substantially increased in AIDS, permitting a high pathogen burden with little disorder but dramatically decreases in the setting of immune reconstitution. Pathogen virulence also affects resilience and therefore the slope of the curve. The rapidity of decline along the curve (over time) is determined by the adequacy of host resistance. (*C*) Personalized therapy. Based on a comprehensive characterization of the host, pathogen, and their interaction, a treatment regimen consisting of antimicrobials and immunomodulators is administered. Antimicrobial therapy may have several consequences, including uncomplicated resolution of infection, pathogen killing complicated by immunologic disorder (eg, the Jarisch-Herxheimer reaction), and drug toxicity. Pathogen killing and drug toxicity diminish health independently from the pathogenesis of infection, thus leading to deviation from the original curve. Immunosuppression alone may improve health but increase pathogen burden. (*D*) Consequences of infection. In patients who survive infection, pathogen burden returns to zero, but the effects of illness and treatment may produce a new, compromised state of health, which may manifest as permanent dysfunction (eg, scarring of lung parenchyma), potentially treatable conditions (such as dysbiosis), and/or increased susceptibility to secondary infection (compensatory anti-inflammatory response syndrome [CARS]). IRIS, immune reconstitution inflammatory syndrome. (*Data from* Ayres JS, Schneider DS. Tolerance of infections. Annu Rev Immunol 2012:30;271–94.)

PHASE I: CHARACTERIZATION OF HOST AND PATHOGEN
Characterization of Host

Physiologic reserve
One of the clinician's first priorities when encountering a patient with pneumonia (or any patient) is to estimate the patient's baseline level of health, which in turn helps determine the likelihood of their ability to survive the disease. This physiologic reserve (depicted as the Y intercept in **Fig. 1**A), is a composite of several parameters, including age and premorbid organ function. For instance, decreased FEV$_1$ (forced expiratory volume in 1 second) diminishes the patient's ability to withstand an additional insult to lung mechanics. Likewise, impaired cardiac

performance or coronary artery patency predisposes to heart failure and myocardial infarction, respectively. Such compromise of physiologic reserve should prompt more aggressive care, but this often manifests as broader-spectrum and less-judicious administration of antibiotics, a mistake partly based on the faulty assumption of antibiotic safety. The authors propose that aggressive care should instead translate into more comprehensive diagnostic characterization of host and microbe, which in turn enables a more highly individualized therapeutic plan that maximizes efficacy and minimizes side effects. The initial clinical assessment also includes an appraisal of disease severity, as this guides clinical triage and immediate management. However, since this is a manifestation of the host response to pathogen, it is dealt with in relation to phase II.

Resistance

As defined earlier, resistance refers to the host's ability to clear a pathogen load. This term comprises not only the innate and adaptive immune mechanisms enumerated in **Box 1** but numerous other parameters, including adequacy of cough, ciliary clearance, mucus quality (influenced by periciliary pH and mucins), release of antimicrobial peptides and opsonins, ROS production, and the barrier function that prevents invasive infection.[25] Opportunities to therapeutically modulate these mechanisms are touched on in relation to phase III and reviewed elsewhere.[25] Graphically, inadequate resistance leads to a more rapid decline down the curve depicted in **Fig. 1**B.

Swift recognition of an immunocompromised state is critical, because it informs triage and empiric antibiotic therapy against unique pathogens to which a host may be susceptible. This

---

Box 1
Innate immune responses in pneumonia

Innate immunity in the lung (reviewed in detail elsewhere[23]) mediates both host defense and immunopathology; as such, a description of its basic mechanisms is essential to understand the targets of host-directed diagnostics and therapeutics, fundamental components of personalized pneumonia management. In brief, alveolar macrophages and respiratory epithelial cells collaborate to clear low levels of pathogens. When these defenses are overwhelmed, danger-associated molecular patterns (DAMPs) released from damaged parenchyma and pathogen-associated molecular patterns (PAMPs) activate innate immune signaling pathways via PRRs, which are expressed by both epithelial and immune cells. This process leads to the release of chemokines and cytokines, which induce the extravasation of neutrophils and exudative fluid into the interstitium and airspaces.

Innate immune signaling: Viral nucleic acids activate PRRs in dendritic cells, macrophages, and alveolar epithelial cells, including the cytosolic RIG-I-like receptors and AIM-like receptors, as well as endosomal TLRs (eg, 3, 7, 8, and 9). Recognition of viral PAMPs by plasmacytoid dendritic cells (DCs) leads to production of type I IFNs, which promote antiviral defenses, whereas macrophages and conventional DCs generate cytokines such as tumor necrosis factor (TNF)-α, IL-1β, IL-6, IL-12, and IL-23, which stimulate type I and III innate lymphoid cells (ILCs) and initiate T helper (Th) 1 and Th17 adaptive responses. Type I ILCs (similar to Th1 cells) are characterized by robust production of IFNγ, whereas type III ILCs (similar to Th17 cells) generate IL-17 and IL-22.

In contrast, PAMPs derived from extracellular bacteria (eg, lipopolysaccharide) and fungi (eg, β-glucan) activate cell-surface PRRs, including TLRs (1, 2, 4, and 6) and C-type lectin receptors (eg, dectin-1, dectin-2, and mincle), leading to production of an overlapping set of cytokines (including TNFα, IL-1β, IL-6, IL-12, and IL-23) but less type I IFN. Similar signals derive from the NOD-like receptors, which mediate cytosolic recognition of bacterial PAMPs.

Sequelae of pulmonary inflammation: Ideally, recruitment of neutrophils and other immune effectors leads to pathogen clearance with little collateral damage. However, overexuberant neutrophilic responses can be deleterious because they may induce parenchymal destruction per se (eg, via ROS and protease release), alveolar edema, and progression to acute respiratory distress syndrome.[24] Therefore, the acute inflammatory phase must be tightly controlled in terms of both severity and duration. Several mechanisms mediate the resolution of lung inflammation, including a switch from proinflammatory to antiinflammatory innate signaling (thereby limiting further leukocyte recruitment) and clearance of apoptotic neutrophils via efferocytosis (see the text concerning phase IV).

It is worth noting that the pathogen may benefit from immune-mediated tissue destruction because it provides critical nutrients for further proliferation; this may help explain the presence of pathologic immune responses in certain infections, which would otherwise serve as an advantage to neither the host nor the pathogen.

point is most dramatically shown by the 1-hour door-to-needle time recommended for administration of antipseudomonal antibiotics in patients with neutropenic fever, who may rapidly decompensate and die within hours from gram-negative rod bacterial infection if not treated promptly (discussed later).[26] However, subtler examples include hypogammaglobulinemic patients, who may require adjunctive therapies such as intravenous immunoglobulin,[27] and those with altered immune responsiveness caused by pathogen recognition receptor (PRR) polymorphisms. This section describes some of the mechanisms that lead to impaired host resistance, both genetic and acquired. Characterizing these defects in individual patients would facilitate personalized therapy for acute pneumonia in several ways: through predicting severity of disease course, indicating pneumonia susceptibilities that will guide empiric antimicrobial coverage, and identifying deficient host immune pathways that may be therapeutically enhanced.

Genetic determinants of reduced resistance

The study of rare patients with primary immunodeficiencies helps to elucidate the pathogenesis of human infections, as shown by the case of a young child with interferon (IFN) regulatory factor 7 (IRF7) deficiency and severe influenza.[28] This finding confirmed the putative role of the IRF7 pathway in the generation of protective type I IFN during influenza infection suggested by prior animal studies. However, to explain the interindividual variability of pneumonia severity observed in the general population, it is more valuable to identify common and benign genetic variants that influence disease susceptibility.[29] Polymorphisms linked to influenza and legionella infections that take particularly variable clinical courses are highlighted here.

The best-studied genetic determinant of influenza susceptibility is IFN-induced transmembrane protein 3 (IFITM3), which associates with the endosome to block cytosolic delivery of the genome of RNA viruses, a necessary step in their replication.[30] IFITM3 also plays a role in IRF3 activation and persistence of memory T cells within the lung.[31] Through these mechanisms, IFITM3 polymorphisms impair tissue resistance, leading to higher viral burdens and worse clinical outcomes.[32] For instance, the C allele produces severe disease when homozygous[33] and is fairly prevalent, especially in Asian people, where it is observed in more than 50% of the Han Chinese and Japanese populations.[29,34] Several smaller studies have identified additional disease-associated single nucleotide polymorphisms

(SNPs; reviewed elsewhere[35]), but their clinical significance is not yet clear; it is likely that influenza susceptibility is a complex trait influenced by several of these loci.

Legionella susceptibility has been linked to STING (Stimulator of IFN Genes, encoded by *TMEM173/STING*), an adaptor protein downstream of cGAS and IFI16, innate immune sensors of cytosolic DNA. Activation of this pathway elicits a type I IFN response important for host defense against viruses and certain bacteria, including *Legionella*.[36] Human *TMEM173/STING* shows considerable interindividual variability; for instance, 20% of the population in the 1000 Human Genome Project database express the HAQ allele, which contains 3 nonsynonymous substitutions.[37] Recently, Ruiz-Moreno and colleagues[38] showed that carriage of this variant is associated with heightened susceptibility to legionella pneumonia in humans. Mutations in toll-like receptors (TLRs) have also been shown to affect *Legionella* susceptibility, as TLR5 truncation (affecting a surprising ~10% of individuals) and TLR2 mutation lead to increased risk,[39,40] whereas certain TLR4 polymorphisms are protective.[41]

Genetic risk modifiers for CAP (irrespective of etiology) have also been described. For instance, a genome-wide association study (GWAS) identified several common variants in the *FER* gene (a cytosolic tyrosine kinase that contributes to neutrophil recruitment and endothelial permeability) that afford marked protection from death from pneumonia.[42] A deleterious polymorphism in interleukin (IL)-6 and a protective SNP within IL-10 have been recognized as well.[40] Regarding noninfluenza viral pathogens, susceptibility to severe rhinovirus infection in children has been linked to a variant of cadherin-related family member 3 (CDHR3; the receptor for rhinovirus-C),[43–45] and several genetic risk factors have been identified for pediatric respiratory syncytial virus (RSV) infection; because the focus is on adult disease here, readers are referred to recent reviews on these topics.[46,47] In addition, although not all are specifically related to pneumonia, a plethora of additional polymorphisms in PRRs have been shown to predispose to viral, mycobacterial, and fungal infections (reviewed in Refs.[48,49]).

The potential clinical utility of identifying susceptibility loci in patients with pneumonia is significant. In the acute setting, as noted earlier, such data could improve prognostication, guide the individualization of empiric antibiosis, and identify therapies that can augment defective resistance mechanisms. Furthermore, identification of high-risk patients could inform preventive strategies, including more aggressive vaccination, counseling on exposure avoidance, and prompter administration of antimicrobial prophylaxis after exposure (eg, oseltamivir for influenza). These measures are considered later in relation to phase III.

Acquired defects in resistance

Certain forms of acquired immunocompromise, such as hypogammaglobulinemia, neutropenia, hematologic malignancy, steroid use, and acquired immunodeficiency syndrome (AIDS), are readily recognized on history and basic laboratory studies and cue clinicians to consider pertinent clinical syndromes, such as *Pneumocystis jiroveci* pneumonia (PJP) in AIDS. This level of personalized therapy is well established in clinical practice and needs no further elaboration here. However, more common conditions, such as diabetes, chronic kidney disease (CKD), cirrhosis, alcoholism, smoking, and advanced age (immunosenescence), also increase risk of pneumonia but in less definable ways. Predisposition to LRTI is also influenced by transient risk factors, such as air pollution,[50] intercurrent viral infections,[51] sepsis (discussed later relation to phase IV), and antibiotic use. In addition, omission of vaccination and/or waning immunity caused by remote vaccination represent, in effect, missed opportunities to improve resistance.

Is it possible for clinicians to comprehensively catalog all of the resistance deficits present in a given patient, quantify their individual effects, integrate their collective impact, and use this information to meaningfully guide clinical management? At present, the answer is clearly no, but this a priori approach is not the only means of assessing a patient's immunocompetence. An alternative, or complementary, strategy is to interrogate patient immune responsiveness directly, using in vivo or ex vivo assays. A well-known example of the former is the tuberculin hypersensitivity test, which reports on T-cell reactivity.[52] Quantifying surface markers of T-cell exhaustion, a phenomenon observed in sepsis that predisposes to secondary infection (discussed further in relation to phase IV), has also been explored as a method for assessing adequacy of T-cell immunity in the clinical setting.[53] Another conceivable approach is transcriptomic analysis of local immune responses at the respiratory epithelium. This approach may be particularly useful in the context of active infection, as defective resistance mechanisms could be identified in situ and targeted for therapy. Functional assays such as these effectively integrate genetic and acquired defects in resistance and may provide clinicians with more concrete data than patient history alone to guide empiric antibiosis, immunomodulation, and preventive strategies.

Characterization of Pathogens

First introduced in the nineteenth century, plate-based microbiological culture remains the gold standard for identifying bacterial and fungal pathogens in the lung and for determining their antimicrobial sensitivity. However, it has 2 major drawbacks: long turnaround times (>36–48 hours) and poor sensitivity.[54] The former requires at least 2 days of empiric antibiotics, with all of the attendant risks enumerated later in relation to phase III, and even then antimicrobial coverage may miss the offending pathogen (eg, in the case of an unexpected multi-drug resistant [MDR] organism). The prolonged incubation times required for fungal cultures (often >2 weeks) create further risks for inadequate antibiotic therapy, as empiric antifungal agents are rarely used outside of neutropenia.[55]

The inadequate sensitivity of culture was shown by a landmark study in patients with CAP, which showed that conventional culture failed to provide a diagnosis in more than 60% of patients despite addition of an extensive list of infectious biomarkers.[6] Similarly dismal numbers exist for patients with VAP, in whom more than 50% lack an identifiable pathogen.[7] Reasons for this poor sensitivity include failure of culture to detect fastidious organisms and inadequate sampling methods (eg, underuse of invasive techniques). Clearly, improved microbiologic diagnostics are needed.

Invasive sampling

Despite decades of debate, the question of when to obtain invasive cultures has not yet been answered. With regard to VAP, the European and American guidelines are at odds; the former favor quantitative distal sampling, whereas the latter recommend semiquantitative endotracheal aspiration.[16,56] Two of the more commonly cited randomized control trials (RCTs) addressing this question are Fagon and colleagues'[57] demonstration that bronchoscopy increased antibiotic-free days, and the Canadian Critical Care Trial Group's[58] study showing no benefit. This discrepancy may be attributable in part to a lack of patient endotyping, and criteria for identifying appropriate patients for bronchoscopy should be pursued. However, methodological advances since the time of these trials should also be considered. For instance, combining invasive sampling with nucleic acid–based or mass spectrometry–based diagnostics (described later) might allow more effective assessment of pathogen identification, burden, and antibiotic sensitivity, and therefore increase the efficacy of bronchoscopy. More recent studies have shown the utility of this approach (reviewed in Ref.[59]).

Nonbronchoscopic sampling (via blind catheterization of the lower airways) is an alternative that addresses many drawbacks of the bronchoscopic approach.[60] These drawbacks include expense, risk to the patient, and the need for highly trained operators, which often produces delays that compromise the yield of cultures due to antibiotic exposure before bronchoscopy. Although not guided specifically toward diseased portions of the lung, nonbronchoscopic methods still correlate well with their bronchoscopy in a range of patient populations and microbiological tests.[61–66] Again, the utility of such methods is bound to increase when combined with rapid molecular diagnostics.

Bronchoscopy to diagnose pneumonia in the nonintubated immunocompromised population is another source of controversy; although it remains standard of care, evidence for this practice remains sparse. A good example comes from patients with hematological malignancies who present with pulmonary symptoms and/or infiltrates. A multicenter RCT showed that a noninvasive work-up in such patients (including imaging, traditional culture, and biomarkers) was noninferior to bronchoscopy with respect to rates of pathogen identification.[67] The reliance on bronchoscopy in this population is called further into question by the impact of invasive procedures on patients' quality of life, particularly at the end stages of disease; a host-specific aspect of personalized medicine that is often neglected. However, if combined with molecular microbiological testing, the yield of bronchoscopy in the immunocompromised may improve substantially.

A theoretic argument against invasive sampling comes from the cystic fibrosis literature, in which it has been shown that pathogens from different parts of the lung may express completely different resistance patterns, such that sampling error alone may lead to inappropriate antibiotic selection.[68] Similar differences in microanatomic bacterial communities have been described for patients with advanced chronic obstructive pulmonary disease (COPD).[69] Although the results relate less to acute pneumonia, prolonged residence in an intensive care unit (ICU), and the consequent acquisition of multiple MDR strains, could conceivably produce similar spatial heterogeneity.

Matrix-assisted laser desorption ionization time of flight mass spectrometry

In contrast with the conventional approach to microbial recognition using colony appearance on culture plates, matrix-assisted laser desorption ionization time of flight mass spectrometry (MALDI-TOF MS) identifies pathogens via proteomic profiling. The technique is both (requiring only minutes) and inexpensive on a per-sample basis.[70] Furthermore, it identifies not only pathogens but also certain resistance mechanisms by detecting products of β-lactam hydrolysis,[71] fluoroquinolone acetylation,[72] and proteins that mediate resistance (eg, penicillin binding protein 2a [PBP2a], encoded by *MecA*, which mediates methicillin resistance in *Staphylococcus aureus*).[73] Additional techniques are being developed to allow direct assessment of antibiotic sensitivity via measurement of stable isotope-labeled amino acid incorporation into proteins[74]; a surrogate of microbial growth with much faster kinetics than traditional growth curves.

Biomarkers

Pathogen-associated biomarkers are the most widely used complement to traditional culture techniques. Although they remain limited in the number of pathogens they can detect and cannot offer insight into antimicrobial resistance, they are widely available, rapid (because they require no microbial culture), inexpensive, and in some cases highly specific for their targets. The list includes *Legionella* and pneumococcal urinary antigens, *Mycoplasma* and *Chlamydia* antibodies, *Histoplasma* urine antigen, galactomannan (associated with aspergillosis), and β-glucan (a nonspecific fungal marker). An example of recent progress comes from Wunderink and colleagues,[75] who showed a doubling in detection rate of pneumococcal CAP with the use of a second urinary antigen compared with a conventional assay alone (9.7% vs 5.4%). Although encouraging, it nevertheless reveals that the standard urinary pneumococcal antigen assay (one of the best and widely biomarkers) still misses at least 40% of diagnoses, highlighting the need for further work in this area.

Quantitative polymerase chain reaction

Simple, rapid assays using quantitative polymerase chain reaction (qPCR) may be used to identify pathogens and resistance mechanisms using primers designed according to sequenced genomes. Polymerase chain reaction (PCR) is extremely effective for diagnosis of viral infection and is in common use for detecting respiratory viruses in the upper respiratory tract; a surrogate for LRTI. Several caveats of this technique exist, including the potential dissociation between upper respiratory tract infection and LRTI and the poor sensitivity for Herpesviridae (eg, herpes simplex virus [HSV] and cytomegalovirus [CMV]). The latter is an important weakness given the potential pathogenic role of these viruses even in immunocompetent hosts (discussed later in relation to phase III).

PCR has valuable application in the diagnosis of bacterial infections as well, for instance in identifying the MecA gene in S aureus. qPCR can be used to assess relative microbial burdens and pathogen dominance; an important indicator of potential pathogenicity, as discussed later. This assessment may be achieved by normalizing the amount of pathogen to the total bacterial community, which is assessed using general bacterial primers.

The rapidity of PCR is one of its greatest strengths, and could help to remove the need for empiric antibiotics in pneumonia. The present guidelines recommend antibiotic therapy within 4 hours based on data showing increased mortality with delays in therapy (although even these data have been questioned[76])[77]; thus, the prompt performance of a PCR-based diagnostic, which takes ~2 hours, may allow immediate delivery of targeted antimicrobial therapy.

Metataxonomics and metagenomics

An important limitation of qPCR is its inapplicability to microbes and resistance genes not yet fully sequenced. High-throughput techniques, including 16s (metataxonomics) and whole-genome sequencing (WGS; shotgun metagenomics), which offer the ability to define the respiratory microbiome in a comprehensive and unbiased manner, overcome this hurdle. They also allow the identification of fastidious organisms such as mycobacteria that grow poorly using conventional culture.[78,79]

16s sequencing relies on the use of primers against highly conserved sequences in the ribosomal RNA of bacteria to amplify the variable region of the gene, which in turn is used to identify individual taxa. Semiquantitative relative abundance may also be assessed. The technique is rapid and inexpensive compared with WGS but provides no insight into nonribosomal genes, including those that mediate resistance and virulence. WGS, which completely characterizes the genomes of recovered microbes, holds the promise of predicting antimicrobial susceptibility, but it is not yet approved for this application.[80] The reason is that the effects of subtle genetic variants (eg, SNPs in antibiotic target genes) on resistance have not yet been characterized. To address this issue, research groups are pursuing large GWAS analyses on thousands of clinical isolates to create a comprehensive catalog of resistance loci; this will serve as both a reference for patient WGS and a basis for developing models that predict resistance in novel variants.[81–83]

An additional challenge to overcome, which affects both high-throughput sequencing techniques, is distinguishing colonizer from true pathogen. This challenge is a general caveat for any microbiological diagnostic, even with the far-less-sensitive plate-based culture; an isolated microbe may represent anything from beneficial commensal to harmful microbiota, to colonizing pathogen, to disease-causing pathogen. One fairly straightforward method of defining a pathogen is to demonstrate its ecological dominance in the recovered bacterial population. For instance, Wunderink and colleagues[84] proposed the following criteria for discriminating pathogen from colonizer on bronchoalveolar lavage (BAL) or tracheal aspirate: total bacterial density of greater than 10^4 colony-forming units (CFU)/mL, high total bacterial DNA burden, low community diversity, and a high abundance of the pathogen.[85,86]

However, complexities arise from interspecies interactions, which are known to critically affect the virulence of a given pathogen. For example, a dominant pathogen may be detectable but not the source of disease because it is held in check by 1 or more cocolonizers (protective microbiota).[87] An alternative is to assess for expression of genes, including virulence factors, which are expressed only after a microbe makes the phenotypic switch from colonizer to pathogen.[88,89] Triggers for this switch include interaction with commensals, viral infections, cigarette smoking, and air pollution.[2] As an example, Molyneaux and colleagues[90] showed a significant increase in overall bacterial burden as well as an outgrowth of Haemophilus influenzae specifically in patients with COPD after rhinovirus infection.

Additional complications of metaomics include turnaround time, risks of contamination, inability to discriminate live from dead microbes, the extremely low abundance of microbial DNA compared with host, and cost. For now, this approach may only be applicable to the ICU patients, whose condition is tenuous enough and care is costly enough to justify the additional expense. Patients with chronic respiratory infections represent another potential target.

PHASE II: CHARACTERIZE THE HOST RESPONSE TO PATHOGEN

As described in **Box 1**, the central host response to lung infection is neutrophilic infiltration. This response explains not only the histopathologic hallmark (neutrophilic alveolitis) but also the classic clinical symptoms (dyspnea, cough, purulent sputum), signs (fever and hypoxemia), laboratory abnormalities (leukocytosis and bandemia), and radiographic findings (infiltrates). However, the poor specificity of each of these clinical features leads to the frequent overdiagnosis of pneumonia and unnecessary administration of antibiotics. Identification of respiratory microbes by means of the diagnostics described in relation to phase I is helpful but only indicates the presence of potential pathogen; it does not prove that it is causing a clinically meaningful infection. In addition, microbiologic cultures, still the gold standard diagnostic, take days to mature. Thus, it is essential to develop more sophisticated methods for interrogating host responses that will (1) enable accurate and rapid identification of patients with pneumonia; and (2) discriminate between bacterial, viral, and other pathogen classes to guide empiric antibiosis. The first is a sine qua non of pneumonia management, whereas the second is the first step toward personalization (ie, endotyping).

The Use of Host Response to Diagnose Pneumonia

Protein biomarkers
Biomarkers (often present in serum, quantitative, rapidly processed, and potentially amenable to point-of-care testing) represent a highly attractive diagnostic modality. In the context of pneumonia diagnosis, biomarkers are used as reporters of the inflammatory neutrophilic response in the lung parenchyma. Balk and colleagues provide a more complete description in this issue, but the 2 most commonly used biomarkers, procalcitonin (PCT) and C-reactive protein (CRP), are briefly discussed here.

The biology of PCT is still incompletely understood, but it is known to be produced by immune and parenchymal cells in most tissues in response to stimulation with pathogen-associated molecular patterns (PAMPs), danger-associated molecular patterns (DAMPs), and inflammatory cytokines (see **Box 1**). PCT appears in serum at about 4 hours and peaks at 6 hours, making it an effective early indicator of pneumonia.[91] One of the principal advantages of PCT is that its expression is suppressed by type I IFN, which increases its specificity for bacterial rather than viral infection. Very low PCT values are helpful in ruling out bacterial infection and withholding antibiotics, as shown by Christ-Crain and colleagues,[92] but the current guidelines do not recommend its use in this capacity. A drawback to PCT is its low expression in atypical infections (ie, Legionella, Mycoplasma, and Chlamydophila)[93,94] and in bacterial pneumonia following viral infection.[95]

CRP is synthesized by the liver in response to IL-6, making it a less-specific marker for lung infection. Like CRP, it appears quickly (at ~6 hours) but peaks much more slowly (at 36–50 hours) and its clearance is delayed.[96] CRP levels correlate with pulmonary bacterial loads (measured by quantitative tracheal aspirates) in VAP[97] and are more useful than PCT in the detection of atypical infections.

Inclusion of additional cytokine biomarkers in the laboratory evaluation of pneumonia, including tumor necrosis factor (TNF)-α, IL-6, IL-8, and IL-10, mildly improves discrimination of bacterial from viral infections and can be used to increase suspicion for particular bacterial pathogens (eg, Enterobacteriaceae elicit more IL-8), but these cytokines are not yet used in common practice.[94,98–100] Notably, few studies have examined IFN-stimulated genes (ISGs), which could increase the positive predictive value for viruses, as transcriptomic studies have suggested (discussed later).

To conclude, there is ample evidence to show that the biomarkers in current use aid in the diagnosis of pneumonia, but they are not yet reliable enough to identify patients with nonbacterial causes and permit withholding of antibiotics; a critical "litmus test" for pneumonia diagnostics. One of the principal limitations of biomarkers in current use is their poor specificity; CRP and PCT levels are increased during inflammation from virtually any source, acute and chronic alike, including neoplastic, rheumatologic, necrotic (eg, pancreatitis or trauma), and infectious (with little discrimination between pathogen classes). Thus, they are indicators of systemic inflammation, not of pneumonia, and as such largely remain a complement to the similarly nonspecific markers of neutrophilic alveolitis in common use, such as fever, cough, sputum, leukocytosis, and radiographic infiltrates.

Neutrophilia in lower airway secretions
Sputum neutrophilia is the quintessential surrogate for the alveolar purulence that characterizes bacterial pneumonia. In immunocompromised and intubated patients, tracheal aspirates or direct alveolar assessment via invasive sampling has proved particularly useful. For instance, in a population consisting mostly of patients with hematologic malignancy and solid organ transplants, BAL neutrophilia was shown to have better area under the curve (AUC) for diagnosing pneumonia than either PCT or CRP, using quantitative culture as a gold standard.[101] More recently, Choi and colleagues[102] showed that BAL neutrophil count greater than 510/μL was a highly effective predictor of bacterial pneumonia, with an odds ratio of 13.5. BAL neutrophil count also effectively

discriminated bacterial from viral pneumonia, with an AUC of 0.855; its performance further improved when combined with CRP.

Transcriptomics

In contrast with the focused interrogation of clinically available biomarkers, transcriptomics provides a global view of differential gene expression in response to infection. Clustering analysis is used to identify distinct RNA expression patterns that correlate with presence or absence of infection, different classes of pathogens, disease severity, and prognosis. Given the inclusion of tens or even hundreds of genes in such immune response signatures, their potential sensitivity and specificity is far more robust than biomarker-based diagnostic strategies.

Early transcriptomic studies established that much of the immune response in pneumonia is consistent across pathogen classes, but specificity can be found in the activation of distinct signaling pathways downstream of particular PRRs (eg, TLR4 activation by extracellular gram-negative bacteria vs TLR3 activation by RNA viruses).[103] An example of is the transcriptomic analysis performed by Ramilo and colleagues,[104] who examined blood from 36 pediatric patients acutely infected with influenza A and 16 with *Streptococcus pneumoniae* (mostly pneumonia) and identified a 35-gene panel that discriminated viral from bacterial infection with 95% accuracy in an independent cohort. Similarly, Zaas and colleagues[105] were able to establish a 30-gene viral signature based on blood transcriptomes from human volunteers subjected to viral challenge with rhinovirus, RSV, and influenza A. This finding was validated in an independently acquired data set, showing 100% accuracy for identifying viral infection and 93% for bacterial infection. Tang and colleagues[106] subsequently assayed whole blood from ICU patients in respiratory failure caused by influenza, bacterial pneumonia, and presumed sterile systemic inflammatory response syndrome (SIRS). Again, they showed an ability to robustly identify viral infection throughout the 5 days of follow-up, largely based on upregulation of ISGs and inhibition of innate inflammatory cytokines, which indicates a profound state of immunosuppression in influenza. However, they were unable to establish a bacterial signature that could distinguish between bacterial infection and sterile SIRS. Of note, there was surprisingly little concordance between viral signatures in the 3 studies, perhaps because of differences in training cohorts or in bioinformatic techniques. However, the few common genes were all IFN-inducible.

Although these studies laid important groundwork for the application of transcriptomics in pneumonia endotyping, their utility was limited by 2 issues. First, gene panels were too extensive (>25 transcripts) to permit analysis in standard clinical laboratories. Second, they had not addressed the fundamental problem of how to identify patients who need antibiotics.

The first issue was addressed in a follow-up study by Zaas and colleagues,[107] who were able to translate their viral signature into a real-time PCR-based assay using commercially available probes. Landry and Foxman[108] studied nasopharyngeal swabs from patients and showed that a set of only 3 transcripts in these samples (*CXCL10*, *IFIT2*, and *OASL*) could predict viral infection with 97% accuracy. More recently, Tang and colleagues[109] reported a single serum biomarker capable of discriminating influenza from bacterial infection with an AUC of 91% in a large, newly enrolled cohort: *IFI27*, an ISG that is upregulated in plasmacytoid dendritic cells (DCs) in response to TLR7 activation. These studies represent some of the best examples to date of the translation of transcriptomic analysis into the development of robust but technically feasible clinical assays.

Substantial progress toward solving the second problem was made by Tsalik and colleagues,[110] who assessed host expression profiles in patients with confirmed viral infection, bacterial infection, coinfection, and sick but noninfected controls. The use of this last control was a unique and important feature of the study because it helped to directly address the question of how to identify patients with sterile respiratory illness. Although the 4 signatures each required large numbers of probes (up to 71), they had superb test characteristics with AUCs between 90% and 99% in external validation analyses. A similar aim guided Ramilo and colleagues[104] in their study of an analogous set of patients with viral and bacterial monoinfections, coinfection, and controls. Using advanced bioinformatics techniques, they identified a parsimonious 10 gene classifier with a sensitivity of 95% for bacterial infection (compared with 38% sensitivity of PCT); another step toward establishing a rule-out test to guide withholding of antibiotics. Note that 7 of these 10 genes overlap with the biosignature identified independently by Zaas's group using unique analytical methods,[111] suggesting the field may be converging on a common classifier. Further studies will be necessary to confirm the utility of this probe set in larger cohorts and in the immunocompromised, a population that is particularly prone to overtreatment with antimicrobials.

A final study worth mentioning compared the immune response in patients with sepsis caused by peritonitis versus pneumonia. There was little to distinguish between these two cohorts, suggesting that transcriptomic analysis is unable to delineate the anatomic source of infection, at least when applied to peripheral leukocytes in late-stage sepsis (see **Fig. 1**A).[112]

Use of Host Response to Define Severity at Presentation and Guide Prognostication

As mentioned earlier, the severity of clinical presentation in pneumonia primarily depends on the host response to the pathogen and the associated bystander immunopathology (**Fig. 2**). The existing measures of severity, including CURB-65 (confusion, urea, respiratory rate, blood pressure, age ≥65 years) and pneumonia severity index (PSI), are clinical scoring scales used to assess the end-organ consequences of this inflammatory response (eg, renal dysfunction) and are principally used for triage. PSI additionally accounts for comorbidities and therefore incorporates the concept of physiologic reserve described in relation to phase I. In contrast, biomarkers report directly and quantitatively on the inflammatory tone of the host in response to infection. They have been used to gain insight into additional clinical parameters, including acute stability and

prognosis, as well as response to infection, as discussed in relation to phase III. The use of biomarkers in this context is discussed briefly here and in detail by Balk and colleagues elsewhere in this issue (also see Torres and colleagues'[113] recent review).

As might be predicted, systemic levels of inflammatory cytokines (including IL-6, IL-10, and IFNγ) are significantly higher in patients with severe CAP than in patients with nonsevere CAP and in healthy individuals.[98,114] Furthermore, IL-6 correlates with clinical scoring scales[115,116] and predicts 30-day mortality in hospitalized patients with CAP.[98,114] Addition of CRP to a composite clinical index including both PSI and CURB-65 improves 30-day mortality prediction, achieving an AUC of 0.88.[114] PCT on its own shows similar prognostic accuracy to CURB-65 and scales with severity.[117] Van Vught and colleagues[118] provided an important caveat to these findings, showing that systemic cytokines do not correlate with PSI in the elderly.

Given that the progression to sepsis (discussed further in relation to phase IV) portends a worse outcome in patients with pneumonia, it is of prognostic value to detect this transition. Protracted, smoldering inflammation marks the later phase of sepsis; evidence of this in patients recovering from acute pneumonia, as marked by increased levels of IL-6 and IL-10, was shown to correlate with increased mortality at 1 year.[119] In contrast,

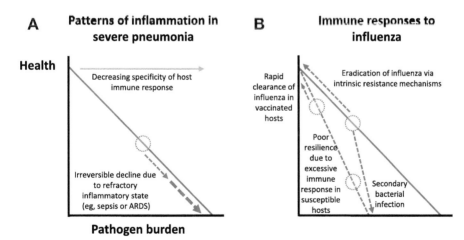

Fig. 2. Host response to pathogen. (*A*) Patterns of inflammation in severe pneumonia. Failure of resistance mechanisms allows progression of infection (in the absence of antibiotics). However, when the severity of infection reaches a threshold, it may lead to an irreversible decline caused by uncontrollable inflammatory syndromes such as sepsis or ARDS. The specificity of host immune signatures decreases at these end stages of infection because the inflammatory response degenerates to a common pattern regardless of microbe class and initial site of infection. (*B*) Immune responses to influenza. Influenza represents a useful example of host response during infection, given its highly variable course. In most patients, influenza is cleared effectively, with or without antiviral medication. In some, however, secondary bacterial infection complicates the illness. Still others are predisposed to excessive immune responses (poor resilience) and therefore follow the more precipitous clinical course depicted by the dotted line on the left. Such patients would benefit from vaccination, which leads to rapid clearance after exposure (*top left arrow*).

local immune responses at the respiratory epithelium, as revealed by sputum cytokine profiles, are blunted in severe CAP despite exaggerated inflammation in the periphery.[120] This discordance between lung and systemic immune compartments highlights the importance of site selection when assessing host responses. In influenza infection, Oshansky and colleagues[121] showed the potential for using mucosal-specific host responses to predict clinical outcomes, showing that a nasal cytokine profile characterized by increased monocyte chemoattractant protein-3 (MCP-3) and IFN-α2 could predict progression to severe disease independently of age, viral load, and neutralizing antibody titers.

Assessment of Resilience

As mentioned in the context of host resistance, there is remarkable interindividual variability in the severity of pneumonia caused by a given pathogen, ranging from mild infection treated in the outpatient setting to fulminant sepsis requiring ICU admission. Physiologic reserve, pathogen burden, and resistance contribute substantially to this variability, but host resilience, defined as the host's ability to tolerate a pathogen load, also plays a critical role. Simply put, 2 patients with similar baseline health and pathogen load may develop widely discordant disease severities, a phenomenon largely attributable to the host's predisposition toward immunopathology. A unique example is shown in **Fig. 1**B, which shows the increased resilience to PJP observed in patients with AIDS; although driven by a pathologic process (ie, severe immunocompromise), the patient is able to tolerate an extraordinary pathogen burden with minimal pulmonary inflammation.

The data presented by Oshansky and colleagues[121] exemplify the more common pattern observed in practice: decreased host resilience leading to more severe disease. Despite similar physiologic reserve (indicated by age in these otherwise healthy children), host resistance (indicated by neutralizing antibodies), and pathogen burden (indicated by viral load), a subset of patients progressed to severe influenza, suggesting an underlying immunologic susceptibility. Although the investigators focused on the prognostic value of the signature, it is notable the biomarkers (eg, IFN-α2) are known components of the cytokine storm that mediates immunologic disorder, organ dysfunction, and death in extreme cases.[122,123] Therefore, these markers could potentially function as theranostics in influenza, both guiding initiation of immunosuppression and indicating response to therapy.

Substantial efforts have been made to identify the genetic underpinnings of susceptibility to influenza infection and other forms of pneumonia (see **Fig. 2**). The topic has been reviewed elsewhere,[46,124] and more extensively in the context of sepsis,[125] but, in these analyses, susceptibility loci are not clearly stratified by mechanism (ie, whether they affect resistance or resilience). One genetic variant that seems to specifically compromise resilience affects CD55, which protects the respiratory epithelium from complement deposition, a process implicated in the immunopathogenesis of severe influenza.[126] A second study used an integrated genomic approach to identify susceptibility loci in patients with CAP that progressed to sepsis.[127] First, unsupervised transcriptomic analysis divided the study cohort into 2 endotypes using a 7-gene classifier; one expressing sepsis response signature 1 (SRS1, marked by an immunosuppressed phenotype and increased 14-day mortality), and the other expressing SRS2. Next, genetic analysis identified a set of approximately 4000 quantitative trait loci that predisposed to the higher-risk phenotype, SRS1.

At present, the clinical utility of disease-associated SNPs is limited, but several potential applications can be envisioned as the list expands and host genomics come into more routine clinical practice. For instance, identification of variants that compromise resilience may prompt more aggressive immunosuppression. Also, from a research perspective, disease-associated SNPs give mechanistic insight into human infection and represent future therapeutic targets.

In closing, we propose that personalized analysis of host immune responses should ideally (1) confirm true infection; (2) identify bacterial processes that require antibiotics; (3) estimate severity to guide triage and prognostication; (4) assess host resistance, as discussed in relation to phase I; and (5) characterize host resilience. The last 2 should be performed with sufficient granularity to identify specific pathways for modulation as described in relation to phase III. In addition, as indicated by studies, including that by Oshansky and colleagues,[121] test performance may improve with integration of local respiratory epithelial and systemic immune responses.

PHASE III: PERSONALIZED TREATMENT AND ASSESSMENT OF THERAPEUTIC RESPONSE

Armed with a clinical dataset that confirms the presence of pneumonia, identifies the offending pathogen and its susceptibilities, and describes the host's immune competence and immunopathologic diatheses, clinicians are prepared to devise a treatment plan. This plan will have the following aims: (1) to reduce pathogen burden, both through direct attack on the microbe (eg, with antibiotics) and through support of host-intrinsic resistance mechanisms; and (2) to optimize host resilience, largely through suppression of hyperactive and maladaptive immune pathways.

A key principle that informs the following discussion is that clearance of bacteria in patients treated for pneumonia is a collaboration between host resistance and antimicrobials (**Fig. 3**A). Some patients with pneumonia may have sufficiently robust immunity to eradicate the infection without therapy (**Fig. 3**B). On the other end of the spectrum are neutropenic patients dependent on antibiotics until count recovery (**Fig. 3**C). The remainder of patients are somewhere in between these extremes, and clinicians are responsible for personalizing an antibiotic regimen that balances the patient's reliance on antibiotics against the substantial hazards of these drugs. Antibiotic choice, dose, and duration are considered, as are so-called antibiotic-sparing interventions, including nonantimicrobial pharmaceutics (eg, recombinant antimicrobial peptides).

Antibiotic Therapy for Bacterial and Fungal Pneumonia

Hazards of antibiotics

As mentioned at the outset, there is a widespread misconception that antibiotics are benign medications, but the risks of antibiotic use are myriad, with none more ominous than the growing specter of resistance (see **Fig. 1**C).[128]

The clinical use of antimicrobials, an estimated 50% of which is unnecessary,[129] leads to the spread of resistance in a fairly well-described sequence. First, antibiosis creates a selection pressure that leads to enrichment of microflora and pathogens with preexisting resistance, as well as generation of de novo resistance.[130] Subsequent transfer of resistance determinants between organisms in vivo and human-to-human transmission of resistant organisms (eg, by the fecal-oral route in the community and via clinicians' hands in hospital) leads to dissemination within a population.[131] If this process continues unchecked, the WHO warns,[132] a postantibiotic era will soon begin, with an estimated loss of 10 million lives to antimicrobial resistance per year by 2050.[133] Even rapid deescalation of antibiotics (in cases in which a pathogen is isolated) carries a substantial risk of selecting resistant bacteria because their macrobiotic effects are rapid and persist for months after exposure.[12,134]

Additional hazards of antibiotics include their adverse drug-drug interactions and class-specific toxicities, such as the nephrotoxicity observed with vancomycin, aminoglycosides, amphotericin, and polymyxins; a particular concern in the ICU.[135,136] Furthermore, new mechanisms of toxicity continue to emerge, such as the ability to induce mitochondrial dysfunction and

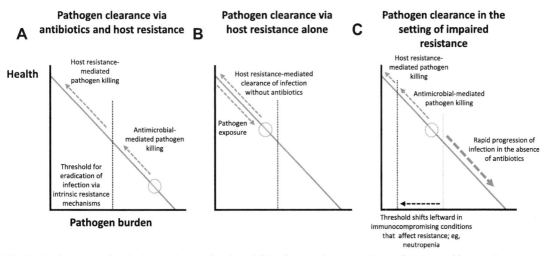

Fig. 3. Mechanisms of reducing pathogen burden. (*A*) Pathogen clearance via antibiotics and host resistance. In healthy hosts, brief antibiosis reduces pathogen burden to a level that allows eradication by immune mechanisms. (*B*) Pathogen clearance via host resistance alone. If the inoculum is small enough, healthy hosts can clear pathogens without specific therapy. (*C*) Pathogen clearance in the setting of impaired resistance. When immunocompromise affects resistance mechanisms against particular pathogens, antimicrobial therapy is essential, as is exemplified by neutropenic patients infected with pyogenic bacteria. Impaired resistance also leads to rapid progression of infection. This finding contrasts with the immunocompromise observed in patients with AIDS with opportunistic infections, which affects resilience (see **Fig. 1**B).

ROS damage,[137] indicating the field's incomplete knowledge on the subject. Antibiotics may also induce potentially catastrophic hypersensitivity reactions, such as anaphylaxis, toxic epidermal necrolysis, and drug rash with eosinophilia and systemic symptoms (DRESS) in susceptible hosts.

In addition, antimicrobial agents destabilize the microbiome, producing a state known as dysbiosis. As mentioned earlier, this may affect the development and course of various disease, including diabetes, atherosclerosis, and asthma.[13,14] However, more immediate for patients is the risk of CDI, which accounts for roughly 29,000 deaths per year in the United States.[138] All antibiotics, even low-risk classes, predispose to CDI, and their effects are cumulative with respect to number of agents, dose, and duration.

Based on abundant mouse data, it is likely that gut dysbiosis predisposes to pneumonia as well[139–144]; consistent with this is clinical evidence that oral probiotics protect ICU patients from VAP, as described in relation to phase IV. Furthermore, antibiotic use may lead to secondary pneumonia courtesy of pathobionts: normally benign flora that may overgrow and cause infection in the setting of dysbiosis, analogously to C difficile.[145] In addition, it has been shown in humans that carriage of certain taxa within the nasal microbiome correlates with improved adaptive immunity to respiratory pathogens, namely responses to influenza A vaccination.[146] Antimicrobials may compromise this component of the microbiota as well.

Considering this litany of potential hazards, it is not surprising that the unnecessary use of antibiotics has been shown to increase mortality in certain patient populations, including those with sepsis in the ICU.[147]

Antibiotic selection
Selection of a particular antibiotic is guided largely by susceptibilities, but, except in cases of MDRs, a fair breadth of choice usually remains. Personalizing this decision should first take into account potential adverse reactions, perhaps in the future using pharmacogenomic techniques to predict toxicity,[148] although this approach may find more use in the context of chronic lung infections, which require more prolonged courses of therapy.[149] Second, clinicians must decide between bacteriostatic versus bactericidal agents, although, as argued by Spellberg and colleagues,[150] the distinction is arbitrary and in general populations there seems to be no advantage to bactericidal drugs despite the folklore belief. Nevertheless, there are specific circumstances in which each may be desirable. Drawing on the example of

endocarditis and meningitis, for which bactericidal drugs are recommended based on the relative paucity of immune effectors at these sites of infection, heavily immunosuppressed patients may benefit more from bactericidal drugs. In contrast, bacteriostatic drugs that inhibit protein synthesis may improve immune resilience; for instance in postviral pneumonia.[151,152] In addition, an argument has been made for the use of bacteriostatic drugs in pneumococcal pneumonia because lytic agents increase the generation of pneumolysin, a proinflammatory toxin with numerous harmful effects, including myocardial toxicity.[153]

Antibiotic dosing
In recent years, some of the basic assumptions on which current dosing protocols are based have been called into question.[154–156] For instance, the practice of administering antibiotics at their maximum tolerable dose is based on the prevailing notion that low doses create selection pressure for the emergence of resistance, whereas high doses of antibiotics kill microbes before resistance can develop.[157] Among others, Read and colleagues[155] have challenged this belief, arguing that, when MDRs are present at the start of infection, they are likely held in check by other microbiota not affected by resistance mechanisms that compromise microbial fitness; in the presence of antibiotics, these protective microbiota are killed, allowing the resistant organisms to flourish unabated, a phenomenon called competitive release. In contrast, when MDRs are absent at the outset, they recommend a high-dose regimen for preventing development of resistance according to the conventional argument.

The implications of this model for patients with pneumonia are potentially practice-changing. Patients with severe infection or immunocompromise would still be given the conventional high-dose protocol, but, for those with robust physiologic reserve and fairly mild disease, outpatient therapy with the lowest clinically effective dose may be the optimal regimen. However, close follow-up to monitor for underdosing and treatment failure (a particular concern in drug hypermetabolizers) would be essential. Given this risk, and that subtherapeutic antibiosis may promote resistance,[158] navigating this lower bound of the therapeutic window would require great vigilance if adopted into clinical practice.

Duration of therapy
Determining the optimal duration of therapy is a crucial feature of personalizing pneumonia management. Antibiotic courses have shortened to as little as 5 days, and effort has been made to

dentify biomarkers that may guide even earlier cessation. For instance, protocols such as stopping therapy when PCT decreases to 20% of its peak have been shown to reduce antibiotic days.[159] Taking abbreviated courses to the extreme, it has been shown that even a single day of antibiotics can have significant clinical effect, as a dose of ceftriaxone given before a course of linezolid substantially improved cure rates.[160] Besides minimizing antibiotic exposure, an additional theoretic benefit of short courses is suggested by models showing that brief therapeutic pulses may reduce the risk of inducing resistance without compromising pathogen killing.[161]

Conceptually, the optimal duration is a function of pathogen burden, adequacy of host resistance, and efficiency of chemotherapeutic killing. Rather than attempting to predict this a priori, it may be preferable to use a theranostic strategy that follows an indicator of microbial persistence, either indirectly using host response (eg, PCT) or directly using a microbial marker (eg, serum galactomannan and β-glucan in aspergillosis).[162] CAP guidelines do incorporate a fair degree of personalization, as the recommended length of therapy varies depending on host response indicators. Given the success of the current guideline-based approach, as shown in a large RCT by Uranga and colleagues,[163] the bar would be high for any potential alternatives.

Antimicrobial Therapy for Viral Pneumonia

The administration of neuraminidase inhibitors such as oseltamivir for influenza is well established in clinical practice, but management of other forms of viral pneumonia is less clear despite their substantial clinical burden. In one series of patients in the ICU with severe CAP, 36% had a viral cause without bacterial coinfection on BAL, and, within this group, rhinovirus, parainfluenza, and human metapneumovirus were all more frequently recovered than influenza.[164] HSV may be an additional contributor to severe respiratory disease, even in immunocompetent hosts, as it has been shown that 21% of nonimmunocompromised patients on prolonged mechanical ventilation have evidence of HSV bronchopneumonitis by high viral titer on BAL-specific and HSV-specific nuclear inclusions in cells recovered on BAL or biopsy.[165] Likewise, CMV may have pathogenic effects in previously immunocompetent critically ill patients.[166]

In immunocompromised populations, these pathogens are routinely treated,[167] but it may be advantageous to treat in select immunocompetent patents as well. For instance, ribavirin is highly effective therapy for upper and lower respiratory tract infection from RSV in hematological malignancy and carries few side effects, particularly in the oral formulation.[168–170] Given these features, as well at its additional activity against parainfluenza and human metapneumovirus, ribavirin may prove useful in immunocompetent patients with severe viral pneumonia, although data to this end are currently lacking.

Nonantibiotic Pathogen-Directed Therapies for Pneumonia

An alternative, or complement, to chemotherapy-based regimens for pneumonia is a diverse collection of therapeutics that includes synthetic antimicrobial peptides,[171] engineered bacteriophage lysins,[172] neutralizing antibodies (eg, against influenza),[173] and antibodies targeting pathogen-associated toxins (eg, pneumolysin).[174] These therapeutics are reviewed by Czaplewski and colleagues[175] but are also mentioned here for their utility in personalized therapy.

Lytic bacteriophages epitomize this class of 'antibiotic alternatives'.[176] Reemerging after their initial description in the preantibiotic era, these viruses have potent bactericidal effects on actively replicating cells and are highly specific for particular bacterial species, so their dysbiotic effects are minimal. In addition, they have low potential for generating antimicrobial resistance or host toxicity. Although still largely the purview of basic research, this approach may eventually translate to the clinic, perhaps as a last resort for respiratory pathogens with extended drug resistance.

Host-Directed Therapies for Improving Host Resistance

Most of the measures discussed earlier promote pathogen clearance predominantly through direct toxic effects on the microbe. However, some function by blunting virulence (eg, antibodies that target bacterial toxins or neutralize viruses), leaving host resistance mechanisms to clear the attenuated pathogen. A third strategy, not mutually exclusive with the others, is to bolster host resistance directly using immunotherapeutics.[177] To this point, the clinical application of such therapy has largely been restricted to chronic infections with mycobacteria and aspergillus unresponsive to antimicrobials.[178,179] The use of such strategies as chimeric antigen receptor-T therapy and supplemental cytokine therapy in this context provides an instructive model for acute pneumonia. A notable example from this literature is the administration of recombinant IL-2 to a patient with idiopathic CD4+ lymphopenia and antibiotic-refractory *Mycobacterium avium-intracellulaire* lung disease, with resultant resolution of infection.[180]

Another concept worth exploring is the use of supportive therapies that promote nonimmunologic aspects of host resistance, such as secretion clearance, including routine chest physiotherapy, which has been shown to decrease the incidence of VAP.[181] Along similar lines, cough augmentation may be useful in a select group of patients to prevent or manage VAP, although meta-analyses show that it does not seem to improve time to extubation in the general ICU population.[182] An as-yet unexplored direction would be to counteract the known defects in mucociliary clearance in critically ill[183] and intubated[184] patients by improving mucus rheology. One approach to doing so is the use of cystic fibrosis (CF) transmembrane regulator (CFTR) modulators such as ivacaftor, which has been shown to potentiate the function of CFTR in patients without CF.[185,186]

Host-Directed Therapies for Improving Resilience

As stated earlier, the principal determinant of severity in most cases of pneumonia is the immunopathology associated with the host response, not the virulence of the pathogen. A portion of this immunopathology is attributable to collateral damage from essential immunological defense mechanisms, while another is simply due to excessive inflammation. Ideally, immunosuppressive agents should selectively target the latter, but in practice, medications like glucocorticoids potently inhibit both. However, when simultaneously treating with antibiotics, resistance mechanisms play a less pivotal role in eradication of microbes, and therefore the impaired resistance induced by immunosuppressive therapy may be an acceptable sacrifice for the reduction of pathologic inflammation. Macrolides represent a unique example among antibiotics in that they simultaneously clear pathogen and dampen inflammation. The latter effect was strikingly revealed by a meta-analysis that showed a mortality benefit in CAP even in patients with macrolide-resistant bacteria.[187] Similar dissociation of clinical efficacy from microbicidal activity was shown in CF.[188]

Antimicrobial therapy also has the potential to exacerbate immunologic disorders. This exacerbation occurs via release of PAMPs from lysed pathogens; the so-called Jarisch-Herxheimer reaction (see **Fig. 1**C). Often observed in the early stages of treatment of cellulitis and spirochetal disease, this phenomenon is best known for its role in PJP therapy in patients with AIDS. In such patients, the insufficiency of host defenses permits the proliferation of fungi to high levels within the lungs. On initiation of antimicrobial therapy, fungal lysis leads to a massive bloom of cell wall components, including β-glucan, which elicits an intense inflammatory response through dectin-1 that may result in ARDS.[189] It is therefore common practice to treat these patients simultaneously with steroids to avert the potential immunopathologic response. More targeted approaches have also been explored, such as cotreatment with β-glucan synthesis inhibitors (echinocandins), which has shown efficacy in mouse models.[189] What role the Jarisch-Herxheimer reaction might play in other causes of pneumonia has not been explored in detail.

A more heated debate surrounds the use of immunosuppression in non-PJP pneumonia. Torres and colleagues[190] were able to solve this problem using a fairly simple endotyping strategy as they limited administration of steroids to patients with a hyperinflammatory phenotype, as indicated by CRP level greater than 150 mg/dL. A contemporaneous study similarly showed a benefit to steroid use in severe pneumonia; unsurprisingly, the mean CRP in the study cohort was also greater than 150 mg/dL.[191] These successes highlight the value of personalizing therapy, even if to a rudimentary degree. As the sophistication of host diagnostics increases, it should be possible to endotype in much finer detail, enabling more effective prediction of response to immunosuppression.

Another possible explanation for the failure of steroids in early trials relates to the immunologic nonspecificity of these agents. In this sense, steroids might be considered antipersonalized therapy because they indiscriminately inhibit immune pathways across the spectrum from protective to pathologic. Instead, patient stratification according to immune pathway dysregulation should be used to target immunotherapy and minimize side effects. One such targeted therapeutic strategy is the use of PRR antagonists,[192] which could in principle halt the inflammatory paroxysm at its source. However, the TLR4 antagonist, eritoran, failed to improve outcomes in sepsis (even in a subgroup analysis of the 50% with pneumonia)[193] despite its demonstrated protection against endotoxemia in healthy volunteers.[194] It may be that PRR antagonism is most effective early in the disease process (as suggested by animal models as well[195]), and that advanced disease requires a very different approach (including immunostimulation, for instance), as explored in relation to phase IV.

PHASE IV: SECONDARY THERAPIES TO ADDRESS THE CONSEQUENCES OF INFECTION AND TREATMENT
Addressing the Immunopathology of Pneumonia-Associated Sepsis

As alluded to in **Box 1**, lung infection may run an uncomplicated course with an appropriate immune response that results in pathogen clearance followed by prompt resolution of inflammation. However, severe infection in susceptible hosts (ie, those with poor resilience) may result in a complex syndrome of immune dysregulation known as sepsis. The pathophysiologic details are beyond the scope of this article and not yet fully established,[196] but two of the key features are uncontrolled, persistent inflammation and a profound state of immunosuppression that affects both innate and adaptive immunity, called immunoparalysis. Therapeutic measures for modulating both aspects have been explored and are discussed here.

Resolution of proinflammatory response
The initiating phase of sepsis involves a hyperinflammatory reaction to microbial PAMPs and DAMPs produced by damaged tissue, followed by activation of complement, endothelial cells (which leads to tissue edema and leukocyte extravasation), neutrophils (which induce damage caused by ROS and proteases), and the coagulation cascade (causing microthrombosis and coagulopathy), all of which interact in potentially amplifying loops that may degenerate into a severe systemic state of inflammation. However, numerous immune mechanisms are in place to control the magnitude and promote the resolution of this potentially devastating process. Proresolution mechanisms include elimination of proinflammatory cytokines, neutrophil apoptosis and efferocytosis, and a switch in macrophage phenotype from inflammatory to reparative (or replacement via monocyte influx).[197] Steroids were discussed earlier, the antiinflammatory properties of which may help to limit the magnitude of inflammatory response in sepsis, but therapeutics designed to stimulate resolution have also been proposed.[197]

Much attention in inflammatory resolution has been focused on the use proresolving mediators, including lipids known as resolvins, lipoxins, and maresins, but most studies to date have been preclinical.[198] However, some intriguing observational data indicate a protective role in CAP for aspirin,[199,200] which is known to generate potent lipoxins[201]; prospective studies are now underway to evaluate for an ameliorative effect in sepsis.[202] Similarly, statins lead to the production of lipoxins,

and established use before presentation is associated with a reduced incidence of CAP (in a retrospective analysis of the JUPITER [Justification for the Use of Statins in Prevention: an Intervention Trial Evaluating Rosuvastatin] trial),[203] and possibly an improvement in mortality. However, conflicting studies and potential confounders such as the so-called healthy user effect must be addressed before drawing definitive conclusions.[204]

Personalized modulation of inflammatory resolution is likely to require metabolomic analysis, first in research studies to establish the differences in lipid milieu between normally resolving pneumonia and protracted disease and then in patients to detect specific molecular deficiencies. Supplementing these patients with synthetic analogues to steer the immune response toward homeostasis may prove a valuable complement to immunosuppressive agents that are intended to dampen its severity.[198]

Reversal of immunosuppression
Within the lung, local immune responses are blunted in the wake of viral and bacterial infection through several mechanisms, including generation of a reparative, antiinflammatory milieu dominated by transforming growth factor beta.[205] However, as pneumonia progresses to sepsis, a profound state of immunosuppression seems to develop after about 3 days, placing patients at high risk of secondary infection, about half of which is respiratory.[196,206] It is during this late stage of sepsis, termed compensatory antiinflammatory response syndrome (CARS), that most deaths occur.[207,208] No clinical trials have yet examined lung-specific interventions to support patients through this vulnerable stage, but there is a substantial body of work on reversing the systemic state of immunosuppression. This article focuses on the use of immunostimulatory cytokines and checkpoint inhibition, but see van der Poll and colleagues[209] for more on the topic.

Granulocyte-macrophage colony–stimulating factor (GM-CSF) promotes granulocyte production, survival, phagocytic function, and extravasation into tissue. It also reverses the downregulation of (human leukocyte antigen, antigen D related (HLA-DR), an important contributor to and biomarker of immunoparalysis in advanced sepsis. The potential efficacy of GM-CSF was shown in a double-blind multicenter trial in which 38 patients with low HLA-DR expression (most of whom presented with pneumonia) were randomized to receive GM-CSF or placebo. The treatment arm showed complete normalization of HLA-DR expression, restored responses to TLR stimulation, improved APACHE (Acute Physiology And

Chronic Health Evaluation) scores, and decreased duration of mechanical ventilation and ICU stay, without significant side effects.[53] This biomarker-guided (ie, theranostic) immunomodulatory approach represents an important example of personalized treatment of pneumonia and a model for future studies. Of note, a related cytokine that similarly stimulates granulocyte production, granulocyte colony–stimulating factor (G-CSF), has been studied in the context of neutropenic pneumonia, but evidence is accumulating to show that the resultant neutrophil reconstitution can precipitate ARDS and therefore G-CSF should be avoided in these patients.[210]

IFNγ, the quintessential T helper 1 (Th1) cytokine, exerts potent stimulatory effects on granulocytes to promote clearance of bacterial and fungal pathogens. Human studies have mostly been limited to case reports and results have been mixed,[211] but administration is generally well tolerated and there is some evidence for efficacy.[212] For instance, Dignani and colleagues[213] described complete resolution of antimicrobial-refractory pulmonary aspergillosis in 3 patients after administration of IFNγ; similar success was seen in 2 cases of invasive aspergillosis and 1 of candidiasis, all involving the lung.[214] In select patients, this may prove a valuable adjunctive therapy for pneumonia; further insights are sure to be generated by an RCT examining its role in the treatment of patients with septic shock (https://clinicaltrials.gov/ct2/show/NCT01649921).

IL-7 predominantly affects adaptive immunity, promoting T cell proliferation, activation, survival, and trafficking to infected tissue. It has shown promise in preclinical models of pneumonia,[215] and is currently the focus of a multicenter clinical trial in septic patients (https://clinicaltrials.gov/ct2/show/NCT02960854).

Checkpoint inhibitors, as applied to sepsis, have been studied mostly in mice, but they may find use in severe pneumonia given the evidence of T-cell exhaustion in a postmortem examination of septic patients (more than half of whom had evidence of lung infection)[216] and evidence for improved pathogen clearance following checkpoint blockade in preclinical models of acute pneumonia.[217,218]

Although some of the trials discussed earlier used a biomarker-based determination of candidates for immunostimulation, selection of patients for therapy may be improved by a more comprehensive immunophenotyping, such as through gene expression signatures or multimarker protein assays, which may improve not only prediction of response but also tailoring of therapy to individuals' specific immune defects. As shown by only 11% of postsepsis deaths being attributable to secondary infection,[206] not all patients require immune stimulation. More sophisticated diagnostics should at the least distinguish patients needing immunosuppression (as discussed in relation to phase III), from those who need stimulation.

Protection and Restoration of Microbiome

The iatrogenic toll of antimicrobials continues to be underestimated, as described in relation to phase III, but nowhere more so than in the gut. In addition to predisposing to CDI, antibiotics select for resistant bacteria and create a state of dysbiosis, which has several harmful consequences. These consequences derive in part from the eradication of commensals, which normally function to protect against outgrowth of pathobionts, a phenomenon termed colonization resistance.[219] Also, through metabolism of dietary fiber, healthy gut microbiota synthesize short-chain fatty acids, which positively influence systemic immune function and maintenance of gut epithelial integrity. Compromise of these mechanisms caused by dysbiosis promotes gut translocation of bacteria and PAMPs, which exacerbates the prolonged, smoldering inflammation of sepsis and in some cases produces frank infection.[220,221]

As explained in relation to phase III, dysbiosis is likely to increase risk of pneumonia. Several microbiome-protective strategies, besides minimizing unnecessary antimicrobial exposure, have been proposed. One creative solution involves coadministration of activated charcoal with antibiotics, which decrease intestinal but not plasma antibiotic levels, thus protecting the gut microbiota.[222] More attention has been given to the literature on oral probiotics, which shows both a trend toward lowering incidence of VAP[223–225] and a significant delay in acquisition of *Pseudomonas aeruginosa* respiratory colonization.[223] Meta-analyses have differed in their conclusions regarding these data,[226,227] but there does seem to be a substantial clinical effect, amounting to an approximate 20% reduction in VAP as estimated by Siempos and Ntaidou.[228] This effect was confirmed as significant by the most recent meta-analysis on the subject.[229] Even stronger data support the use of probiotics in mitigating the risk of CDI in patients receiving antibiotics: a Cochrane analysis showed a number needed to treat of only 12 in patients with a CDI risk greater than 5%.[230] Thus, especially when treating pneumonia in a patient with high risk of CDI, probiotics should be strongly considered.

Prevention of Future Infection

Vaccines have been called the most effective medical intervention ever devised because of their ow cost, ability to prevent disease, and continued efficacy in the presence of drug resistance.[231] They remain the mainstay in the prevention of pneumonia, as exemplified by the highly effective antipneumococcal and antiinfluenza agents. Although in some ways the antithesis of personalized medicine, because they are given to huge populations with minimal stratification, vaccine development and delivery must be improved to decrease the burden of preventable illness and reduce antibiotic use.[232]

With regard to personalized prevention of pneumonia, Evans and colleagues[233–235] have developed a provocative pharmacologic approach wherein inhaled TLR agonists (specifically TLR2/6 and TLR9 ligands) are used to induce a state of tissue resistance; this has been shown to protect mice from both influenza and bacterial pneumonia. Numerous potential applications can be envisaged for such technology, including prophylaxis in patients with hematologic malignancies after myelosuppressive therapy that induces prolonged neutropenia. This prophylactic strategy is currently under investigation as part of a phase I clinical trial (https://clinicaltrials.gov/ct2/show/NCT03097796) and warrants further study.

Sequelae of Pneumonia

Although primarily a lung infection, pneumonia should be considered a systemic illness,[236] with manifestations in numerous extrapulmonary organs, including heart, kidneys, and brain (reviewed by Restrepo and colleagues[237]). As mentioned earlier, premorbid compromise in these systems decreases the patient's physiologic reserve and acute ability to survive infection.

However, there is also an increasing appreciation of the longer-term consequences of pneumonia. In addition to the well-described architectural distortion that may complicate necrotizing pneumonia, as well as the bronchiectasis that may result from repeated infection (exemplified by patients with cystic fibrosis), there is an increased risk of developing obstructive disease in patients who have an episode of pneumonia in early life.[238]

Outside the lung, there is a strong association with cardiovascular events, including an increased 30-day incidence of heart failure ($\sim$15%), arrhythmia ($\sim$5%), and acute coronary syndrome ($\sim$5%).[239] Up to 20% of deaths from CAP are attributable to these complications.[240] Furthermore, although cardiovascular risk is highest immediately after pneumonia, it remains increased for 10 years.[241] The mechanisms underlying increased cardiovascular risk in pneumonia include inflammation-associated endothelial dysfunction and thrombophilia, as well as microbe-specific processes such as the pneumolysin-induced myocyte injury and microabscesses observed in S pneumoniae infection.[242,243]

A strong body of literature suggests that pneumonia can precipitate cognitive decline as well. For instance, one study showed that one year after hospitalization for CAP, one-third of patients over 65 had moderate to severe impairment, and an additional third showed mild impairment.[244] The relationship was shown to be bidirectional, in that premorbid cognitive dysfunction predisposes to pneumonia (likely because of increased risk of aspiration), and pneumonia in turn leads to cognitive impairment.[245] Functional status, quality of life, and mood also decline substantially after an episode of pneumonia.[246,247]

Renal dysfunction frequently complicates sepsis associated with pneumonia by mechanisms relating to systemic inflammation and hemodynamic compromise that are only now becoming clear[248]; however, to our knowledge, the long-term risk of CKD postpneumonia has not been studied. Thirty-day readmission rates are greatly increased after pneumonia (7%–12%),[249,250] as is long-term mortality (40% vs 25% for those hospitalized for other conditions).[251,252] Thus, long-term sequelae both within the lung and without can be severe and represent important opportunities for personalization (eg, treating with aspirin or high-dose statin to prevent major cardiovascular events in patients with vascular risk factors).

SUMMARY

The practical implementation of personalized pneumonia management depends heavily on the clinical setting, which spans from the ambulatory clinic to the academic ICU, where there are vastly different levels of patient acuity and available resources (**Fig. 4**). For instance, ambulatory providers do not have access to advanced diagnostics such as next-generation sequencing on BAL but should also not need them for the management of mild CAP. The focus in that context should be on developing tools that quickly and reliably discriminate between bacterial pneumonia, viral pneumonia, and noninfectious disease, perhaps using qPCR-based host response profiling. Because of the impracticality of waiting for culture data to guide antibiosis in this setting, pathogen characterization will be limited to rapid assays such as viral PCR on upper airway specimens, mass spectrometry on sputum, and/or pathogen-associated biomarkers such as the pneumococcal

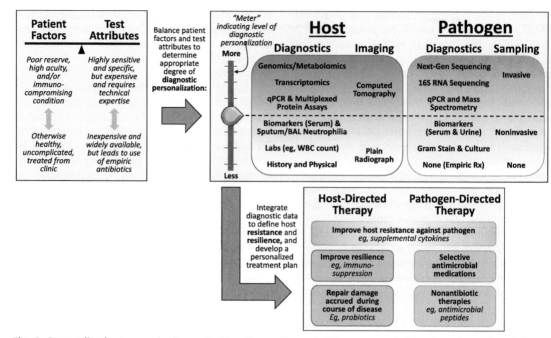

Fig. 4. Personalized pneumonia diagnosis. The diagnostic modalities enumerated in phase I and II and shown here in relative order of cost and availability. Determining the extent of diagnostic work-up (where to set the slider in the upper-right frame) depends on patient factors and test attributes (shown in the left frame). Sicker and higher-risk patients may warrant more comprehensive and expensive testing in order to ensure appropriate antimicrobial coverage and guide immunomodulation. Simpler diagnostics may be appropriate for milder pneumonia, although they put the patient at risk of unnecessary empiric antibiosis, which promotes the spread of resistance and carries numerous potential side effects. As the cost of advanced diagnostics decreases and their availability broadens, the slider should shift upward, bringing the goal of personalized pneumonia management closer to realization. Next-Gen, next-generation; Rx, treatment; WBC, white blood cell.

urine antigen. The principal goal is to identify and treat patients with antimicrobial-sensitive infections and spare those without, thus reducing the massive overuse of antibiotics in the clinic and spread of resistance.

In contrast, for sicker patients in the ICU, more elaborate testing should be considered. For instance, it may be justifiable to perform a several-thousand-dollar host transcriptomic analyses to identify candidates for targeted immunomodulation, because even steroids (a fairly crude form of such therapy) are known to reduce the length of stay in the ICU, the daily costs of which are commensurate with such studies. Furthermore, the use of bacteriologic NGS may be considered in such patients to facilitate institution of highly selective antimicrobials, especially as sequencing costs decrease and antimicrobial susceptibility prediction improves.

Conceptually, a well-designed personalized treatment plan consisting of both antimicrobials and immunomodulation would reduce the hysteresis usually observed during the course of severe pneumonia; that is, the deviation from the resilience curve depicted in **Fig. 5**A, B. This hysteresis

often derives from the immunopathologic consequences of infection, which include ARDS, renal failure, and CARS (the downward curve in **Fig. 5**A). Thus, even when the offending pathogen is cleared, the patient may be left with significant debility and increased risk for secondary infection. Meanwhile, excessive immunosuppression may seem to improve a patient's clinical status but also impairs pathogen clearance and increases susceptibility to infection (see **Fig. 5**B). The ideal therapeutic regimen would therefore involve selective antimicrobials with minimal toxicities to the host, plus tailored immunomodulation that offsets the downward deviation from the curve; the combination should be designed to return patients directly to their premorbid states (**Fig. 5**C).

Ultimately, this may require a multiomic diagnostic platform that deeply characterizes the host, pathogen, and their interaction alongside a comprehensive suite of antimicrobial therapeutics (comprising not only antibiotics but also inhibitors of virulence factors and promoters of host resistance mechanisms) as well as immunomodulators that offset maladaptive host responses to infection and promote

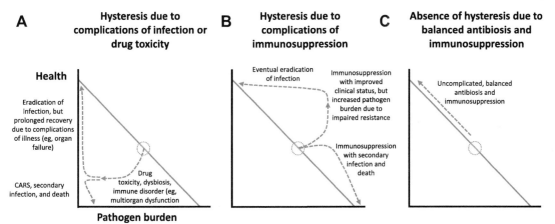

Fig. 5. Hysteresis in treatment and recovery. (*A*) Hysteresis caused by complications of infection or drug toxicity. Administration of antibiotics adds to the potential complications of the infection. Furthermore, failure to offset the immunopathologic consequences of infection can predispose to secondary infection. (*B*) Hysteresis caused by complications of immunosuppression. Immunomodulatory drugs such as steroids offset immunologic disorder but also carry the risk of secondary infection. (*C*) Absence of hysteresis caused by balanced antibiosis and immunomodulation. The ideal combination of antibiotics and adjunctive therapies results in diminished hysteresis, which may be achieved through the use of highly selective antimicrobials, targeted immunosuppression, and minimizing the risks associated with both.

resolution of inflammatory responses. Biomarkers should be developed to guide subsequent cessation of antibiotics. Complementary strategies for preventing secondary infections and restoring microbiomic homeostasis should also be developed. In short, the goal is to not only improve survival from pneumonia but also limit the possible systemic and long-term consequences of infection.

Although a lofty vision, the obstacles to the realization of this goal are less technical than practical. Much of the necessary technology, including host transcriptomics, pathogen NGS, and multiplex protein analyses, already exists. What is needed now is a recognition both within the field and beyond of the clinical burden of pneumonia and the hazards of overuse of antibiotics; this should drive further research into the mechanisms of pneumonia, development of diagnostics and therapeutics, streamlining of technology to reduce costs, and methods for effective clinical implementation.

REFERENCES

1. Ferkol T, Schraufnagel D. The global burden of respiratory disease. Ann Am Thorac Soc 2014;11(3):404–6.

2. Cookson W, Cox MJ, Moffatt MF. New opportunities for managing acute and chronic lung infections. Nat Rev Microbiol 2018;16(2):111–20.

3. World Health Organization. Disease and injury regional estimates, 2000–2011. 2018. Available at: http://www.who.int/healthinfo/global_burden_dise ase/estimates_regional_2000_2011/en/. Accessed April 20, 2018.

4. Albaum MN, Hill LC, Murphy M, et al. Interobserver reliability of the chest radiograph in community-acquired pneumonia. PORT Investigators. Chest 1996;110(2):343–50.

5. Self WH, Courtney DM, McNaughton CD, et al. High discordance of chest x-ray and computed tomography for detection of pulmonary opacities in ED patients: implications for diagnosing pneumonia. Am J Emerg Med 2013; 31(2):401–5.

6. Jain S, Self WH, Wunderink RG, et al. Community-acquired pneumonia requiring hospitalization among U.S. Adults. N Engl J Med 2015;373(5): 415–27.

7. Waters B, Muscedere J. A 2015 update on ventilator-associated pneumonia: new insights on its prevention, diagnosis, and treatment. Curr Infect Dis Rep 2015;17(8):496.

8. Murphy TF. Vaccines for nontypeable *Haemophilus influenzae*: the future is now. Clin Vaccin Immunol 2015;22(5):459–66.

9. Guest JF, Morris A. Community-acquired pneumonia: the annual cost to the National Health Service in the UK. Eur Respir J 1997;10(7): 1530–4.

10. Bush K, Courvalin P, Dantas G, et al. Tackling antibiotic resistance. Nat Rev Microbiol 2011;9(12): 894–6.

11. Blaser MJ. Antibiotic use and its consequences for the normal microbiome. Science 2016;352(6285): 544–5.

12. Zaura E, Brandt BW, Teixeira de Mattos MJ, et al. Same exposure but two radically different responses to antibiotics: resilience of the salivary microbiome versus long-term microbial shifts in feces. MBio 2015;6(6). e01693-15.

13. Lynch SV, Pedersen O. The human intestinal microbiome in health and disease. N Engl J Med 2016; 375(24):2369–79.

14. Sommer F, Anderson JM, Bharti R, et al. The resilience of the intestinal microbiota influences health and disease. Nat Rev Microbiol 2017;15(10): 630–8.

15. Mandell LA, Wunderink RG, Anzueto A, et al. Infectious Diseases Society of America/American Thoracic Society consensus guidelines on the management of community-acquired pneumonia in adults. Clin Infect Dis 2007;44(Suppl 2):S27–72.

16. Kalil AC, Metersky ML, Klompas M, et al. Management of adults with hospital-acquired and ventilator-associated pneumonia: 2016 clinical practice guidelines by the Infectious Diseases Society of America and the American Thoracic Society. Clin Infect Dis 2016;63(5):e61–111.

17. Wunderink RG, Waterer GW. Community-acquired pneumonia. N Engl J Med 2014;370(19):1863.

18. Willis JC, Lord GM. Immune biomarkers: the promises and pitfalls of personalized medicine. Nat Rev Immunol 2015;15(5):323–9.

19. Ayres JS, Schneider DS. Tolerance of infections. Annu Rev Immunol 2012;30:271–94.

20. Schneider DS, Ayres JS. Two ways to survive infection: what resistance and tolerance can teach us about treating infectious diseases. Nat Rev Immunol 2008;8(11):889–95.

21. Kwong JC, Schwartz KL, Campitelli MA. Acute myocardial infarction after laboratory-confirmed influenza infection. N Engl J Med 2018;378(4): 345–53.

22. Quinton LJ, Mizgerd JP. Dynamics of lung defense in pneumonia: resistance, resilience, and remodeling. Annu Rev Physiol 2015;77:407–30.

23. Iwasaki A, Foxman EF, Molony RD. Early local immune defences in the respiratory tract. Nat Rev Immunol 2017;17(1):7–20.

24. Pechous RD. With friends like these: the complex role of neutrophils in the progression of severe pneumonia. Front Cell Infect Microbiol 2017;7: 160.

25. Leiva-Juarez MM, Kolls JK, Evans SE. Lung epithelial cells: therapeutically inducible effectors of antimicrobial defense. Mucosal Immunol 2018;11(1): 21–34.

26. Freifeld AG, Bow EJ, Sepkowitz KA, et al. Clinical practice guideline for the use of antimicrobial agents in neutropenic patients with cancer: 2010 update by the infectious diseases society of America. Clin Infect Dis 2011;52(4):e56–93.

27. Welte T, Dellinger RP, Ebelt H, et al. Concept for a study design in patients with severe community-acquired pneumonia: a randomised controlled trial with a novel IGM-enriched immunoglobulin preparation - the CIGMA study. Respir Med 2015; 109(6):758–67.

28. Ciancanelli MJ, Huang SX, Luthra P, et al. Infectious disease. Life-threatening influenza and impaired interferon amplification in human IRF7 deficiency. Science 2015;348(6233):448–53.

29. Ciancanelli MJ, Abel L, Zhang SY, et al. Host genetics of severe influenza: from mouse Mx1 to human IRF7. Curr Opin Immunol 2016;38:109–20.

30. Brass AL, Huang IC, Benita Y, et al. The IFITM proteins mediate cellular resistance to influenza A H1N1 virus, West Nile virus, and dengue virus. Cell 2009;139(7):1243–54.

31. Allen EK, Randolph AG, Bhangale T, et al. SNP-mediated disruption of CTCF binding at the IFITM3 promoter is associated with risk of severe influenza in humans. Nat Med 2017;23(8):975–83.

32. Everitt AR, Clare S, Pertel T, et al. IFITM3 restricts the morbidity and mortality associated with influenza. Nature 2012;484(7395):519–23.

33. Zhang YH, Zhao Y, Li N, et al. Interferon-induced transmembrane protein-3 genetic variant rs12252-C is associated with severe influenza in Chinese individuals. Nat Commun 2013;4:1418.

34. 1000 Genomes Project Consortium, Abecasis GR, Auton A, Brooks LD, et al. An integrated map of genetic variation from 1,092 human genomes. Nature 2012;491(7422):56–65.

35. To KK, Zhou J, Chan JF, et al. Host genes and influenza pathogenesis in humans: an emerging paradigm. Curr Opin Virol 2015;14:7–15.

36. Marinho FV, Benmerzoug S, Oliveira SC, et al. The emerging roles of STING in bacterial infections. Trends Microbiol 2017;25(11):906–18.

37. Yi G, Brendel VP, Shu C, et al. Single nucleotide polymorphisms of human STING can affect innate immune response to cyclic dinucleotides. PLoS One 2013;8(10):e77846.

38. Ruiz-Moreno JS, Hamann L, Shah JA, et al. The common HAQ STING variant impairs cGAS-dependent antibacterial responses and is associated with susceptibility to Legionnaires' disease in humans. PLoS Pathog 2018;14(1): e1006829.

39. Hawn TR, Verbon A, Lettinga KD, et al. A common dominant TLR5 stop codon polymorphism abolishes flagellin signaling and is associated with susceptibility to legionnaires' disease. J Exp Med 2003;198(10):1563–72.

40. Smelaya TV, Belopolskaya OB, Smirnova SV, et al. Genetic dissection of host immune response in pneumonia development and progression. Sci Rep 2016;6:35021.

41. Hawn TR, Verbon A, Janer M, et al. Toll-like receptor 4 polymorphisms are associated with resistance to Legionnaires' disease. Proc Natl Acad Sci U S A 2005;102(7):2487–9.

42. Rautanen A, Mills TC, Gordon AC, et al. Genome-wide association study of survival from sepsis due to pneumonia: an observational cohort study. Lancet Respir Med 2015;3(1):53–60.

43. Palmenberg AC. Rhinovirus C, asthma, and cell surface expression of virus receptor CDHR3. J Virol 2017;91(7). https://doi.org/10.1128/JVI.00072-17.

44. Bochkov YA, Watters K, Ashraf S, et al. Cadherin-related family member 3, a childhood asthma susceptibility gene product, mediates rhinovirus C binding and replication. Proc Natl Acad Sci U S A 2015;112(17):5485–90.

45. Bonnelykke K, Sleiman P, Nielsen K, et al. A genome-wide association study identifies CDHR3 as a susceptibility locus for early childhood asthma with severe exacerbations. Nat Genet 2014;46(1):51–5.

46. Verhein KC, Vellers HL, Kleeberger SR. Inter-individual variation in health and disease associated with pulmonary infectious agents. Mamm Genome 2018;29(1–2):38–47.

47. Salas A, Pardo-Seco J, Cebey-López M, et al. Whole exome sequencing reveals new candidate genes in host genomic susceptibility to respiratory syncytial virus disease. Sci Rep 2017;7(1): 15888.

48. Jaeger M, Stappers MH, Joosten LA, et al. Genetic variation in pattern recognition receptors: functional consequences and susceptibility to infectious disease. Future Microbiol 2015;10(6): 989–1008.

49. Carvalho A, Cunha C, Pasqualotto AC, et al. Genetic variability of innate immunity impacts human susceptibility to fungal diseases. Int J Infect Dis 2010;14(6):e460–8.

50. Anderson JO, Thundiyil JG, Stolbach A. Clearing the air: a review of the effects of particulate matter air pollution on human health. J Med Toxicol 2012; 8(2):166–75.

51. Prasso JE, Deng JC. Postviral complications: bacterial pneumonia. Clin Chest Med 2017;38(1): 127–38.

52. Meakins JL, Pietsch JB, Bubenick O, et al. Delayed hypersensitivity: indicator of acquired failure of host defenses in sepsis and trauma. Ann Surg 1977;186(3):241–50.

53. Meisel C, Schefold JC, Pschowski R, et al. Granulocyte-macrophage colony-stimulating factor to reverse sepsis-associated immunosuppression: a double-blind, randomized, placebo-controlled multicenter trial. Am J Respir Crit Care Med 2009; 180(7):640–8.

54. Dixon P, Davies P, Hollingworth W, et al. A systematic review of matrix-assisted laser desorption/ionisation time-of-flight mass spectrometry compared to routine microbiological methods for the time taken to identify microbial organisms from positive blood cultures. Eur J Clin Microbiol Infect Dis 2015;34(5):863–76.

55. Bosshard PP. Incubation of fungal cultures: how long is long enough? Mycoses 2011;54(5): e539–45.

56. Torres A, Niederman MS, Chastre J, et al. International ERS/ESICM/ESCMID/ALAT guidelines for the management of hospital-acquired pneumonia and ventilator-associated pneumonia: guidelines for the management of hospital-acquired pneumonia (HAP)/ventilator-associated pneumonia (VAP) of the European Respiratory Society (ERS), European Society of Intensive Care Medicine (ESICM), European Society of Clinical Microbiology and Infectious Diseases (ESCMID) and Asociacion Latinoamericana del Torax (ALAT). Eur Respir J 2017;50(3) [pii:1700582].

57. Fagon JY, Chastre J, Wolff M, et al. Invasive and noninvasive strategies for management of suspected ventilator-associated pneumonia. A randomized trial. Ann Intern Med 2000;132(8):621–30.

58. Canadian Critical Care Trials Group. A randomized trial of diagnostic techniques for ventilator-associated pneumonia. N Engl J Med 2006; 355(25):2619–30.

59. Douglas IS. New diagnostic methods for pneumonia in the ICU. Curr Opin Infect Dis 2016; 29(2),197–204.

60. Lavigne MC. Nonbronchoscopic methods [Nonbronchoscopic bronchoalveolar lavage (BAL), mini-BAL, blinded bronchial sampling, blinded protected specimen brush] to investigate for pulmonary infections, inflammation, and cellular and molecular markers: a narrative review. Clin Pulm Med 2017;24(1):13–25.

61. Caughey G, Wong H, Gamsu G, et al. Nonbronchoscopic bronchoalveolar lavage for the diagnosis for Pneumocystis carinii pneumonia in the acquired immunodeficiency syndrome. Chest 1985;88(5): 659–62.

62. Papazian L, Thomas P, Garbe L, et al. Bronchoscopic or blind sampling techniques for the diagnosis of ventilator-associated pneumonia. Am J Respir Crit Care Med 1995;152(6 Pt 1):1982–91.

63. Humphreys H, Winter R, Baker M, et al. Comparison of bronchoalveolar lavage and catheter lavage to confirm ventilator-associated lower respiratory tract infection. J Med Microbiol 1996; 45(3):226–31.

64. Bello S, Tajada A, Chacón E, et al. "Blind" protected specimen brushing versus bronchoscopic techniques in the aetiolological diagnosis of

ventilator-associated pneumonia. Eur Respir J 1996;9(7):1494–9.

65. Marik PE, Brown WJ. A comparison of bronchoscopic vs blind protected specimen brush sampling in patients with suspected ventilator-associated pneumonia. Chest 1995;108(1):203–7.

66. Tasbakan MS, Gurgun A, Basoglu OK, et al. Comparison of bronchoalveolar lavage and mini-bronchoalveolar lavage in the diagnosis of pneumonia in immunocompromised patients. Respiration 2011;81(3):229–35.

67. Azoulay E, Mokart D, Lambert J, et al. Diagnostic strategy for hematology and oncology patients with acute respiratory failure: randomized controlled trial. Am J Respir Crit Care Med 2010;182(8):1038–46.

68. Jorth P, Staudinger BJ, Wu X, et al. Regional isolation drives bacterial diversification within cystic fibrosis lungs. Cell Host Microbe 2015;18(3):307–19.

69. Erb-Downward JR, Thompson DL, Han MK, et al. Analysis of the lung microbiome in the "healthy" smoker and in COPD. PLoS One 2011;6(2):e16384.

70. Angeletti S. Matrix assisted laser desorption time of flight mass spectrometry (MALDI-TOF MS) in clinical microbiology. J Microbiol Methods 2017;138:20–9.

71. Oviano M, Ramírez CL, Barbeyto LP, et al. Rapid direct detection of carbapenemase-producing Enterobacteriaceae in clinical urine samples by MALDI-TOF MS analysis. J Antimicrob Chemother 2017;72(5):1350–4.

72. Oviano M, Rodríguez-Martínez JM, Pascual Á, et al. Rapid detection of the plasmid-mediated quinolone resistance determinant AAC(6')-Ib-cr in Enterobacteriaceae by MALDI-TOF MS analysis. J Antimicrob Chemother 2017;72(4):1074–80.

73. Griffin PM, Price GR, Schooneveldt JM, et al. Use of matrix-assisted laser desorption ionization-time of flight mass spectrometry to identify vancomycin-resistant enterococci and investigate the epidemiology of an outbreak. J Clin Microbiol 2012;50(9):2918–31.

74. Jung JS, Eberl T, Sparbier K, et al. Rapid detection of antibiotic resistance based on mass spectrometry and stable isotopes. Eur J Clin Microbiol Infect Dis 2014;33(6):949–55.

75. Wunderink RG, Self WH, Anderson EJ, et al. Pneumococcal community-acquired pneumonia detected by serotype-specific urinary antigen detection assays. Clin Infect Dis 2018;66(10):1504–10.

76. Garin N, Marti C. Community-acquired pneumonia: the elusive quest for the best treatment strategy. J Thorac Dis 2016;8(7):E571–4.

77. Houck PM, Bratzler DW, Nsa W, et al. Timing of antibiotic administration and outcomes for Medicare patients hospitalized with community-acquired pneumonia. Arch Intern Med 2004;164(6):637–44.

78. Kemp M, Jensen KH, Dargis R, et al. Routine ribosomal PCR and DNA sequencing for detection and identification of bacteria. Future Microbiol 2010;5(7):1101–7.

79. Woo PC, Lau SK, Teng JL, et al. Then and now: use of 16S rDNA gene sequencing for bacterial identification and discovery of novel bacteria in clinical microbiology laboratories. Clin Microbiol Infect 2008;14(10):908–34.

80. Ellington MJ, Ekelund O, Aarestrup FM, et al. The role of whole genome sequencing in antimicrobial susceptibility testing of bacteria: report from the EUCAST Subcommittee. Clin Microbiol Infect 2017;23(1):2–22.

81. Coll F, Phelan J, Hill-Cawthorne GA, et al. Genome-wide analysis of multi- and extensively drug-resistant Mycobacterium tuberculosis. Nat Genet 2018;50(2):307–16.

82. Nguyen M, Brettin T, Long SW, et al. Developing an in silico minimum inhibitory concentration panel test for Klebsiella pneumoniae. Sci Rep 2018;8(1):421.

83. Li Y, Metcalf BJ, Chochua S, et al. Validation of beta-lactam minimum inhibitory concentration predictions for pneumococcal isolates with newly encountered penicillin binding protein (PBP) sequences. BMC Genomics 2017;18(1):621.

84. Yin Y, Hountras P, Wunderink RG. The microbiome in mechanically ventilated patients. Curr Opin Infect Dis 2017;30(2):208–13.

85. Dickson RP, Erb-Downward JR, Prescott HC, et al. Analysis of culture-dependent versus culture-independent techniques for identification of bacteria in clinically obtained bronchoalveolar lavage fluid. J Clin Microbiol 2014;52(10):3605–13.

86. Kelly BJ, Imai I, Bittinger K, et al. Composition and dynamics of the respiratory tract microbiome in intubated patients. Microbiome 2016;4:7.

87. Byrd AL, Segre JA. Infectious disease. Adapting Koch's postulates. Science 2016;351(6270):224–6.

88. Morschhauser J. Regulation of white-opaque switching in Candida albicans. Med Microbiol Immunol 2010;199(3):165–72.

89. Coates R, Moran J, Horsburgh MJ. Staphylococci: colonizers and pathogens of human skin. Future Microbiol 2014;9(1):75–91.

90. Molyneaux PL, Mallia P, Cox MJ, et al. Outgrowth of the bacterial airway microbiome after rhinovirus exacerbation of chronic obstructive pulmonary disease. Am J Respir Crit Care Med 2013;188(10):1224–31.

91. Dandona P, Nix D, Wilson MF, et al. Procalcitonin increase after endotoxin injection in normal subjects. J Clin Endocrinol Metab 1994;79(6): 1605–8.

92. Christ-Crain M, Stolz D, Bingisser R, et al. Procalcitonin guidance of antibiotic therapy in community-acquired pneumonia: a randomized trial. Am J Respir Crit Care Med 2006;174(1):84–93.

93. Self WH, Balk RA, Grijalva CG, et al. Procalcitonin as a marker of etiology in adults hospitalized with community-acquired pneumonia. Clin Infect Dis 2017;65(2):183–90.

94. Menendez R, Sahuquillo-Arce JM, Reyes S, et al. Cytokine activation patterns and biomarkers are influenced by microorganisms in community-acquired pneumonia. Chest 2012;141(6):1537–45.

95. Pfister R, Kochanek M, Leygeber T, et al. Procalcitonin for diagnosis of bacterial pneumonia in critically ill patients during 2009 H1N1 influenza pandemic: a prospective cohort study, systematic review and individual patient data meta-analysis. Crit Care 2014;18(2):R44.

96. Lelubre C, Anselin S, Zouaoui Boudjeltia K, et al. Interpretation of C-reactive protein concentrations in critically ill patients. Biomed Res Int 2013;2013: 124021.

97. Lisboa T, Seligman R, Diaz E, et al. C-reactive protein correlates with bacterial load and appropriate antibiotic therapy in suspected ventilator-associated pneumonia. Crit Care Med 2008;36(1): 166–71.

98. Paats MS, Bergen IM, Hanselaar WE, et al. Local and systemic cytokine profiles in nonsevere and severe community-acquired pneumonia. Eur Respir J 2013;41(6):1378–85.

99. Liu M, Li H, Xue CX, et al. Differences in inflammatory marker patterns for adult community-acquired pneumonia patients induced by different pathogens. Clin Respir J 2018;12(3):974–85.

100. Siljan WW, Holter JC, Nymo SH, et al. Cytokine responses, microbial aetiology and short-term outcome in community-acquired pneumonia. Eur J Clin Invest 2018;48(1). https://doi.org/10.1111/eci.12865.

101. Stolz D, Stulz A, Müller B, et al. BAL neutrophils, serum procalcitonin, and C-reactive protein to predict bacterial infection in the immunocompromised host. Chest 2007;132(2):504–14.

102. Choi SH, Hong SB, Hong HL, et al. Usefulness of cellular analysis of bronchoalveolar lavage fluid for predicting the etiology of pneumonia in critically ill patients. PLoS One 2014;9(5):e97346.

103. Jenner RG, Young RA. Insights into host responses against pathogens from transcriptional profiling. Nat Rev Microbiol 2005;3(4):281–94.

104. Ramilo O, Allman W, Chung W, et al. Gene expression patterns in blood leukocytes discriminate patients with acute infections. Blood 2007;109(5): 2066–77.

105. Zaas AK, Chen M, Varkey J, et al. Gene expression signatures diagnose influenza and other symptomatic respiratory viral infections in humans. Cell Host Microbe 2009;6(3):207–17.

106. Parnell GP, McLean AS, Booth DR, et al. A distinct influenza infection signature in the blood transcriptome of patients with severe community-acquired pneumonia. Crit Care 2012; 16(4):R157.

107. Zaas AK, Burke T, Chen M, et al. A host-based RT-PCR gene expression signature to identify acute respiratory viral infection. Sci Transl Med 2013; 5(203):203ra126.

108. Landry ML, Foxman EF. Antiviral response in the nasopharynx identifies patients with respiratory virus infection. J Infect Dis 2018;217(6): 897–905.

109. Tang BM, Shojaei M, Parnell GP, et al. A novel immune biomarker IFI27 discriminates between influenza and bacteria in patients with suspected respiratory infection. Eur Respir J 2017;49(6) [pii: 1602098].

110. Tsalik EL, Henao R, Nichols M, et al. Host gene expression classifiers diagnose acute respiratory illness etiology. Sci Transl Med 2016;8(322): 322ra11.

111. Tsalik EL, McClain M, Zaas AK. Moving toward prime time: host signatures for diagnosis of respiratory infections. J Infect Dis 2015;212(2):173–5.

112. Burnham KL, Davenport EE, Radhakrishnan J, et al. Shared and distinct aspects of the sepsis transcriptomic response to fecal peritonitis and pneumonia. Am J Respir Crit Care Med 2017; 196(3):328–39.

113. Morley D, Torres A, Cillóniz C, et al. Predictors of treatment failure and clinical stability in patients with community acquired pneumonia. Ann Transl Med 2017;5(22):443.

114. Menendez R, Martínez R, Reyes S, et al. Biomarkers improve mortality prediction by prognostic scales in community-acquired pneumonia. Thorax 2009;64(7):587–91.

115. Andrijevic I, Matijasevic J, Andrijevic L, et al. Interleukin-6 and procalcitonin as biomarkers in mortality prediction of hospitalized patients with community acquired pneumonia. Ann Thorac Med 2014;9(3):162–7.

116. Bacci MR, Leme RC, Zing NP, et al. IL-6 and TNF-alpha serum levels are associated with early death in community-acquired pneumonia patients. Braz J Med Biol Res 2015;48(5):427–32.

117. Kruger S, Ewig S, Marre R, et al. Procalcitonin predicts patients at low risk of death from community-acquired pneumonia across all CRB-65 classes. Eur Respir J 2008;31(2):349–55.

118. van Vught LA, Endeman H, Meijvis SC, et al. The effect of age on the systemic inflammatory response in patients with community-acquired pneumonia. Clin Microbiol Infect 2014;20(11):1183–8.

119. Yende S, D'Angelo G, Kellum JA, et al. Inflammatory markers at hospital discharge predict subsequent mortality after pneumonia and sepsis. Am J Respir Crit Care Med 2008;177(11):1242–7.

120. Fernandez-Botran R, Uriarte SM, Arnold FW, et al. Contrasting inflammatory responses in severe and non-severe community-acquired pneumonia. Inflammation 2014;37(4):1158–66.

121. Oshansky CM, Gartland AJ, Wong SS, et al. Mucosal immune responses predict clinical outcomes during influenza infection independently of age and viral load. Am J Respir Crit Care Med 2014;189(4):449–62.

122. Peiris JS, Yu WC, Leung CW, et al. Re-emergence of fatal human influenza A subtype H5N1 disease. Lancet 2004;363(9409):617–9.

123. de Jong MD, Simmons CP, Thanh TT, et al. Fatal outcome of human influenza A (H5N1) is associated with high viral load and hypercytokinemia. Nat Med 2006;12(10):1203–7.

124. Chung LP, Waterer GW. Genetic predisposition to respiratory infection and sepsis. Crit Rev Clin Lab Sci 2011;48(5–6):250–68.

125. Reilly JP, Meyer NJ, Christie JD. Genetics in the prevention and treatment of sepsis. In: Ward NS, Levy MM, editors. Sepsis: definitions, pathophysiology and the challenge of bedside management. Cham (Switzerland): Humana Press; 2017. p. 237–64.

126. Zhou J, To KK, Dong H, et al. A functional variation in CD55 increases the severity of 2009 pandemic H1N1 influenza A virus infection. J Infect Dis 2012;206(4):495–503.

127. Davenport EE, Burnham KL, Radhakrishnan J, et al. Genomic landscape of the individual host response and outcomes in sepsis: a prospective cohort study. Lancet Respir Med 2016;4(4):259–71.

128. Laxminarayan R, Duse A, Wattal C, et al. Antibiotic resistance-the need for global solutions. Lancet Infect Dis 2013;13(12):1057–98.

129. US Centers for Disease Control and Prevention. Antibiotic resistance threats in the United States. 2013. Available from: http://www.cdc.gov/drugresistance/pdf/ar-threats-2013-508.pdf. Accessed April 15, 2018.

130. Elliott E, Brink AJ, van Greune J, et al. In vivo development of ertapenem resistance in a patient with pneumonia caused by Klebsiella pneumoniae with an extended-spectrum beta-lactamase. Clin Infect Dis 2006;42(11):e95–8.

131. Holmes AH, Moore LS, Sundsfjord A, et al. Understanding the mechanisms and drivers of antimicrobial resistance. Lancet 2016;387(10014):176–87.

132. WHO. Antimicrobial resistance: global report of surveillance. Geneva (Switzerland): WHO; 2014. p. 1–256.

133. O'Neill, J. Tackling drug-resistant infections globally: final report and recommendations. (The Review On Antimicrobial Resistance). 2016. Available at: https://amr-review.org/sites/default/files/160518_Final paper_with cover.pdf. Accessed April 16, 2018.

134. Hensgens MP, Goorhuis A, van Kinschot CM, et al. Clostridium difficile infection in an endemic setting in The Netherlands. Eur J Clin Microbiol Infect Dis 2011;30(4):587–93.

135. Mehta RL, Pascual MT, Soroko S, et al. Spectrum of acute renal failure in the intensive care unit: the PICARD experience. Kidney Int 2004;66(4):1613–21.

136. Perazella MA. Drug use and nephrotoxicity in the intensive care unit. Kidney Int 2012;81(12):1172–8.

137. Kalghatgi S, Spina CS, Costello JC, et al. Bactericidal antibiotics induce mitochondrial dysfunction and oxidative damage in mammalian cells. Sci Transl Med 2013;5(192):192ra85.

138. Lessa FC, Winston LG, McDonald LC, Emerging Infections Program C. difficile Surveillance Team. Burden of Clostridium difficile infection in the United States. N Engl J Med 2015;372(9):825–34.

139. McAleer JP, Kolls JK. Contributions of the intestinal microbiome in lung immunity. Eur J Immunol 2018;48(1):39–49.

140. Schuijt TJ, Lankelma JM, Scicluna BP, et al. The gut microbiota plays a protective role in the host defence against pneumococcal pneumonia. Gut 2016;65(4):575–83.

141. Gauguet S, D'Ortona S, Ahnger-Pier K, et al. Intestinal microbiota of mice influences resistance to Staphylococcus aureus pneumonia. Infect Immun 2015;83(10):4003–14.

142. Abt MC, Osborne LC, Monticelli LA, et al. Commensal bacteria calibrate the activation threshold of innate antiviral immunity. Immunity 2012;37(1):158–70.

143. Budden KF, Gellatly SL, Wood DL, et al. Emerging pathogenic links between microbiota and the gut-lung axis. Nat Rev Microbiol 2017;15(1):55–63.

144. Ichinohe T, Pang IK, Kumamoto Y, et al. Microbiota regulates immune defense against respiratory tract influenza A virus infection. Proc Natl Acad Sci U S A 2011;108(13):5354–9.

145. Hakansson AP, Orihuela CJ, Bogaert D. Bacterial-host interactions: physiology and pathophysiology of respiratory infection. Physiol Rev 2018;98(2):781–811.

146. Salk HM, Simon WL, Lambert ND, et al. Taxa of the nasal microbiome are associated with influenza-specific IgA response to live attenuated influenza vaccine. PLoS One 2016;11(9):e0162803.

147. Garnacho-Montero J, Gutiérrez-Pizarraya A, Escoresca-Ortega A, et al. De-escalation of empirical therapy is associated with lower mortality in patients with severe sepsis and septic shock. Intensive Care Med 2014;40(1):32–40.

148. Osanlou O, Pirmohamed M, Daly AK. Pharmacogenetics of Adverse Drug Reactions. Adv Pharmacol 2018;83:155–90.

149. Baietto L, Corcione S, Pacini G, et al. A 30-years review on pharmacokinetics of antibiotics: is the right time for pharmacogenetics? Curr Drug Metab 2014;15(6):581–98.

150. Wald-Dickler N, Holtom P, Spellberg B. Busting the myth of "Static vs. Cidal": a systemic literature review. Clin Infect Dis 2018;66(9):1470–4.

151. Karlstrom A, Boyd KL, English BK, et al. Treatment with protein synthesis inhibitors improves outcomes of secondary bacterial pneumonia after influenza. J Infect Dis 2009;199(3):311–9.

152. Karlstrom A, Heston SM, Boyd KL, et al. Toll-like receptor 2 mediates fatal immunopathology in mice during treatment of secondary pneumococcal pneumonia following influenza. J Infect Dis 2011; 204(9):1358–66.

153. Brown LA, Mitchell AM, Mitchell TJ. Streptococcus pneumoniae and lytic antibiotic therapy: are we adding insult to injury during invasive pneumococcal disease and sepsis? J Med Microbiol 2017;66:1253–6.

154. Kupferschmidt K. Resistance fighters. Science 2016;352(6287):758–61.

155. Day T, Read AF. Does high-dose antimicrobial chemotherapy prevent the evolution of resistance? PLoS Comput Biol 2016;12(1):e1004689.

156. Pena-Miller R, Laehnemann D, Jansen G, et al. When the most potent combination of antibiotics selects for the greatest bacterial load: the smile-frown transition. PLoS Biol 2013;11(4): e1001540.

157. Roberts JA, Kruger P, Paterson DL, et al. Antibiotic resistance–what's dosing got to do with it? Crit Care Med 2008;36(8):2433–40.

158. Andersson DI, Hughes D. Microbiological effects of sublethal levels of antibiotics. Nat Rev Microbiol 2014;12(7):465–78.

159. Schuetz P, Wirz Y, Sager R, et al. Effect of procalcitonin-guided antibiotic treatment on mortality in acute respiratory infections: a patient level meta-analysis. Lancet Infect Dis 2018;18(1): 95–107.

160. Pertel PE, Bernardo P, Fogarty C, et al. Effects of prior effective therapy on the efficacy of daptomycin and ceftriaxone for the treatment of community-acquired pneumonia. Clin Infect Dis 2008;46(8):1142–51.

161. Baker CM, Ferrari MJ, Shea K. Beyond dose: pulsed antibiotic treatment schedules can maintain individual benefit while reducing resistance. Sci Rep 2018;8(1):5866.

162. Neofytos D, Railkar R, Mullane KM, et al. Correlation between circulating fungal biomarkers and clinical outcome in invasive aspergillosis. PLoS One 2015;10(6):e0129022.

163. Uranga A, España PP, Bilbao A, et al. Duration of antibiotic treatment in community-acquired pneumonia: a multicenter randomized clinical trial. JAMA Intern Med 2016;176(9):1257–65.

164. Choi SH, Hong SB, Ko GB, et al. Viral infection in patients with severe pneumonia requiring intensive care unit admission. Am J Respir Crit Care Med 2012;186(4):325–32.

165. Luyt CE, Combes A, Deback C, et al. Herpes simplex virus lung infection in patients undergoing prolonged mechanical ventilation. Am J Respir Crit Care Med 2007;175(9):935–42.

166. Papazian L, Hraiech S, Lehingue S, et al. Cytomegalovirus reactivation in ICU patients. Intensive Care Med 2016;42(1):28–37.

167. Waghmare A, Englund JA, Boeckh M. How I treat respiratory viral infections in the setting of intensive chemotherapy or hematopoietic cell transplantation. Blood 2016;127(22):2682–92.

168. Shah JN, Chemaly RF. Management of RSV infections in adult recipients of hematopoietic stem cell transplantation. Blood 2011;117(10): 2755–63.

169. Gorcea CM, Tholouli E, Turner A, et al. Effective use of oral ribavirin for respiratory syncytial viral infections in allogeneic haematopoietic stem cell transplant recipients. J Hosp Infect 2017;95(2): 214–7.

170. Trang TP, Whalen M, Hilts-Horeczko A, et al. Comparative effectiveness of aerosolized versus oral ribavirin for the treatment of respiratory syncytial virus infections: a single-center retrospective cohort study and review of the literature. Transpl Infect Dis 2018;20(2):e12844.

171. de la Fuente-Nunez C, Silva ON, Lu TK, et al. Antimicrobial peptides: role in human disease and potential as immunotherapies. Pharmacol Ther 2017; 178:132–40.

172. Yang H, Yu J, Wei H. Engineered bacteriophage lysins as novel anti-infectives. Front Microbiol 2014; 5:542.

173. Corti D, Cameroni E, Guarino B, et al. Tackling influenza with broadly neutralizing antibodies. Curr Opin Virol 2017;24:60–9.

174. Anderson R, Feldman C. Pneumolysin as a potential therapeutic target in severe pneumococcal disease. J Infect 2017;74(6):527–44.

175. Czaplewski L, Bax R, Clokie M, et al. Alternatives to antibiotics–a pipeline portfolio review. Lancet Infect Dis 2016;16(2):239–51.

176. Bodier-Montagutelli E, Morello E, L'Hostis G, et al. Inhaled phage therapy: a promising and challenging approach to treat bacterial respiratory infections. Expert Opin Drug Deliv 2017;14(8): 959–72.

177. Kaufmann SHE, Dorhoi A, Hotchkiss RS, et al. Host-directed therapies for bacterial and viral infections. Nat Rev Drug Discov 2018;17(1):35–56.

178. Armstrong-James D, Brown GD, Netea MG, et al. Immunotherapeutic approaches to treatment of fungal diseases. Lancet Infect Dis 2017;17(12): e393–402.

179. Salzer HJ, Wassilew N, Köhler N, et al. Personalized medicine for chronic respiratory infectious diseases: tuberculosis, nontuberculous mycobacterial pulmonary diseases, and chronic pulmonary aspergillosis. Respiration 2016;92(4): 199–214.

180. Trojan T, Collins R, Khan DA. Safety and efficacy of treatment using interleukin-2 in a patient with idiopathic CD4(+) lymphopenia and *Mycobacterium avium-intracellulare*. Clin Exp Immunol 2009; 156(3):440–5.

181. Ntoumenopoulos G, Presneill JJ, McElholum M, et al. Chest physiotherapy for the prevention of ventilator-associated pneumonia. Intensive Care Med 2002;28(7):850–6.

182. Rose L, Adhikari NK, Leasa D, et al. Cough augmentation techniques for extubation or weaning critically ill patients from mechanical ventilation. Cochrane Database Syst Rev 2017;(1):CD011833.

183. Nakagawa NK, Franchini ML, Driusso P, et al. Mucociliary clearance is impaired in acutely ill patients. Chest 2005;128(4):2772–7.

184. Konrad F, Schreiber T, Brecht-Kraus D, et al. Mucociliary transport in ICU patients. Chest 1994;105(1): 237–41.

185. Van Goor F, Hadida S, Grootenhuis PD, et al. Rescue of CF airway epithelial cell function in vitro by a CFTR potentiator, VX-770. Proc Natl Acad Sci U S A 2009;106(44):18825–30.

186. Solomon GM, Fu L, Rowe SM, et al. The therapeutic potential of CFTR modulators for COPD and other airway diseases. Curr Opin Pharmacol 2017;34: 132–9.

187. Sligl WI, Asadi L, Eurich DT, et al. Macrolides and mortality in critically ill patients with community-acquired pneumonia: a systematic review and meta-analysis. Crit Care Med 2014;42(2):420–32.

188. Tauber SC, Nau R. Immunomodulatory properties of antibiotics. Curr Mol Pharmacol 2008;1(1): 68–79.

189. Kutty G, Davis AS, Ferreyra GA, et al. β-Glucans are masked but contribute to pulmonary inflammation during pneumocystis pneumonia. J Infect Dis 2016;214(5):782–91.

190. Torres A, Sibila O, Ferrer M, et al. Effect of corticosteroids on treatment failure among hospitalized patients with severe community-acquired pneumonia and high inflammatory response: a randomized clinical trial. JAMA 2015;313(7):677–86.

191. Blum CA, Nigro N, Briel M, et al. Adjunct prednisone therapy for patients with community-acquired pneumonia: a multicentre, double-blind, randomised, placebo-controlled trial. Lancet 2015;385(9977):1511–8.

192. Joosten LA, Abdollahi-Roodsaz S, Dinarello CA, et al. Toll-like receptors and chronic inflammation in rheumatic diseases: new developments. Nat Rev Rheumatol 2016;12(6):344–57.

193. Opal SM, Laterre PF, Francois B, et al. Effect of eritoran, an antagonist of MD2-TLR4, on mortality in patients with severe sepsis: the ACCESS randomized trial. JAMA 2013;309(11):1154–62.

194. Lynn M, Rossignol DP, Wheeler JL, et al. Blocking of responses to endotoxin by E5564 in healthy volunteers with experimental endotoxemia. J Infect Dis 2003;187(4):631–9.

195. Lima CX, Souza DG, Amaral FA, et al. Therapeutic effects of treatment with anti-TLR2 and Anti-TLR4 monoclonal antibodies in polymicrobial sepsis. PLoS One 2015;10(7):e0132336.

196. Hotchkiss RS, Moldawer LL, Opal SM, et al. Sepsis and septic shock. Nat Rev Dis Primers 2016;2: 16045.

197. Fullerton JN, Gilroy DW. Resolution of inflammation: a new therapeutic frontier. Nat Rev Drug Discov 2016;15(8):551–67.

198. Serhan CN. Treating inflammation and infection in the 21st century: new hints from decoding resolution mediators and mechanisms. FASEB J 2017; 31(4):1273–88.

199. Falcone M, Russo A, Cangemi R, et al. Lower mortality rate in elderly patients with community-onset pneumonia on treatment with aspirin. J Am Heart Assoc 2015;4(1):e001595.

200. Falcone M, Russo A, Farcomeni A, et al. Septic shock from community-onset pneumonia: is there a role for aspirin plus macrolides combination? Intensive Care Med 2016;42(2):301–2.

201. Spite M, Serhan CN. Novel lipid mediators promote resolution of acute inflammation: impact of aspirin and statins. Circ Res 2010;107(10):1170–84.

202. Eisen DP, Moore EM, Leder K, et al. AspiriN to Inhibit SEPSIS (ANTISEPSIS) randomised controlled trial protocol. BMJ Open 2017;7(1): e013636.

203. Novack V, MacFadyen J, Malhotra A, et al. The effect of rosuvastatin on incident pneumonia: results from the JUPITER trial. CMAJ 2012;184(7): E367–72.

204. Batais MA, Khan AR, Bin Abdulhak AA. The use of statins and risk of community-acquired pneumonia. Curr Infect Dis Rep 2017;19(8):26.

205. Roquilly A, McWilliam HEG, Jacqueline C, et al. Local modulation of antigen-presenting cell development after resolution of pneumonia induces long-term susceptibility to secondary infections. Immunity 2017;47(1):135–147 e5.

206. van Vught LA, Klein Klouwenberg PM, Spitoni C, et al. Incidence, risk factors, and attributable mortality of secondary infections in the intensive care unit after admission for sepsis. JAMA 2016; 315(14):1469–79.

207. Hotchkiss RS, Karl IE. The pathophysiology and treatment of sepsis. N Engl J Med 2003;348(2): 138–50.

208. Hotchkiss RS, Monneret G, Payen D. Sepsis-induced immunosuppression: from cellular dysfunctions to immunotherapy. Nat Rev Immunol 2013;13(12):862–74.

209. van der Poll T, van de Veerdonk FL, Scicluna BP, et al. The immunopathology of sepsis and potential therapeutic targets. Nat Rev Immunol 2017;17(7): 407–20.

210. Karlin L, Darmon M, Thiéry G, et al. Respiratory status deterioration during G-CSF-induced neutropenia recovery. Bone Marrow Transplant 2005;36(3): 245–50.

211. Delsing CE, Gresnigt MS, Leentjens J, et al. Interferon-gamma as adjunctive immunotherapy for invasive fungal infections: a case series. BMC Infect Dis 2014;14:166.

212. A controlled trial of interferon gamma to prevent infection in chronic granulomatous disease. The International Chronic Granulomatous Disease Cooperative Study Group. N Engl J Med 1991;324(8): 509–16.

213. Dignani MC, Rex JH, Chan KW, et al. Immunomodulation with interferon-gamma and colony-stimulating factors for refractory fungal infections in patients with leukemia. Cancer 2005;104(1): 199–204.

214. Armstrong-James D, Teo IA, Shrivastava S, et al. Exogenous interferon-gamma immunotherapy for invasive fungal infections in kidney transplant patients. Am J Transplant 2010;10(8):1796–803.

215. Shindo Y, Fuchs AG, Davis CG, et al. Interleukin 7 immunotherapy improves host immunity and survival in a two-hit model of Pseudomonas aeruginosa pneumonia. J Leukoc Biol 2017;101(2): 543–54.

216. Boomer JS, To K, Chang KC, et al. Immunosuppression in patients who die of sepsis and multiple organ failure. JAMA 2011;306(23):2594–605.

217. Rutigliano JA, Sharma S, Morris MY, et al. Highly pathological influenza A virus infection is associated with augmented expression of PD-1 by functionally compromised virus-specific CD8+ T cells. J Virol 2014;88(3):1636–51.

218. Jensen IJ, Sjaastad FV, Griffith TS, et al. Sepsis-induced T cell immunoparalysis: the ins and outs of impaired T Cell immunity. J Immunol 2018; 200(5):1543–53.

219. Buffie CG, Pamer EG. Microbiota-mediated colonization resistance against intestinal pathogens. Nat Rev Immunol 2013;13(11):790–801.

220. Kitsios GD, Morowitz MJ, Dickson RP, et al. Dysbiosis in the intensive care unit: microbiome science coming to the bedside. J Crit Care 2017;38:84–91.

221. Meng M, Klingensmith NJ, Coopersmith CM. New insights into the gut as the driver of critical illness and organ failure. Curr Opin Crit Care 2017;23(2): 143–8.

222. de Gunzburg J, Ghozlane A, Ducher A, et al. Protection of the human gut microbiome from antibiotics. J Infect Dis 2018;217(4):628–36.

223. Forestier C, Guelon D, Cluytens V, et al. Oral probiotic and prevention of Pseudomonas aeruginosa infections: a randomized, double-blind, placebo-controlled pilot study in intensive care unit patients. Crit Care 2008;12(3):R69.

224. Randomized controlled study of probiotics containing Lactobacillus casei (Shirota strain) for prevention of ventilator-associated pneumonia. J Med Assoc Thai 2015;98(3):253–9.

225. Hua F, Xie H, Worthington HV, et al. Oral hygiene care for critically ill patients to prevent ventilator-associated pneumonia. Cochrane Database Syst Rev 2016;(10):CD008367.

226. Liu KX, Zhu YG, Zhang J, et al. Probiotics' effects on the incidence of nosocomial pneumonia in critically ill patients: a systematic review and meta-analysis. Crit Care 2012;16(3):R109.

227. Gu WJ, Wei CY, Yin RX. Lack of efficacy of probiotics in preventing ventilator-associated pneumonia probiotics for ventilator-associated pneumonia: a systematic review and meta-analysis of randomized controlled trials. Chest 2012;142(4):859–68.

228. Siempos II, Ntaidou TK. Probiotics for prevention of ventilator-associated pneumonia. Chest 2013; 143(4):1185–6.

229. Manzanares W, Lemieux M, Langlois PL, et al. Probiotic and synbiotic therapy in critical illness: a systematic review and meta-analysis. Crit Care 2016; 19:262.

230. Goldenberg JZ, Yap C, Lytvyn L, et al. Probiotics for the prevention of Clostridium difficile-associated diarrhea in adults and children. Cochrane Database Syst Rev 2017;(12):CD006095.

231. Ehreth J. The value of vaccination: a global perspective. Vaccine 2003;21(27–30):4105–17.

232. Laxminarayan R, Matsoso P, Pant S, et al. Access to effective antimicrobials: a worldwide challenge. Lancet 2016;387(10014):168–75.

233. Cleaver JO, You D, Michaud DR, et al. Lung epithelial cells are essential effectors of inducible resistance to pneumonia. Mucosal Immunol 2014;7(1): 78–88.

234. Duggan JM, You D, Cleaver JO, et al. Synergistic interactions of TLR2/6 and TLR9 induce a high level of resistance to lung infection in mice. J Immunol 2011;186(10):5916–26.

235. Leiva-Juarez MM, Ware HH, Kulkarni VV, et al. Inducible epithelial resistance protects mice against leukemia-associated pneumonia. Blood 2016;128(7):982–92.

236. Feldman C, Anderson R. Pneumonia as a systemic illness. Curr Opin Pulm Med 2018;24(3):237–43.

237. Restrepo MI, Reyes LF, Anzueto A. Complication of community-acquired pneumonia (including cardiac complications). Semin Respir Crit Care Med 2016;37(6):897–904.

238. Edmond K, Scott S, Korczak V, et al. Long term sequelae from childhood pneumonia; systematic review and meta-analysis. PLoS One 2012;7(2): e31239.

239. Corrales-Medina VF, Suh KN, Rose G, et al. Cardiac complications in patients with community-acquired pneumonia: a systematic review and meta-analysis of observational studies. PLoS Med 2011;8(6):e1001048.

240. Corrales-Medina VF, Alvarez KN, Weissfeld LA, et al. Association between hospitalization for pneumonia and subsequent risk of cardiovascular disease. JAMA 2015;313(3):264–74.

241. Rae N, Finch S, Chalmers JD. Cardiovascular disease as a complication of community-acquired pneumonia. Curr Opin Pulm Med 2016;22(3):212–8.

242. Brown AO, Mann B, Gao G, et al. *Streptococcus pneumoniae* translocates into the myocardium and forms unique microlesions that disrupt cardiac function. PLoS Pathog 2014;10(9):e1004383.

243. Alhamdi Y, Neill DR, Abrams ST, et al. Circulating pneumolysin is a potent inducer of cardiac injury during pneumococcal infection. PLoS Pathog 2015;11(5):e1004836.

244. Girard TD, Self WH, Edwards KM, et al. Long-term cognitive impairment after hospitalization for community-acquired pneumonia: a prospective cohort study. J Gen Intern Med 2018;33(6):929–35.

245. Shah FA, Pike F, Alvarez K, et al. Bidirectional relationship between cognitive function and pneumonia. Am J Respir Crit Care Med 2013;188(5): 586–92.

246. Dalager-Pedersen M, Thomsen RW, Schønheyder HC, et al. Functional status and quality of life after community-acquired bacteraemia: a matched cohort study. Clin Microbiol Infect 2016; 22(1):78.e1-8.

247. Davydow DS, Hough CL, Levine DA, et al. Functional disability, cognitive impairment, and depression after hospitalization for pneumonia. Am J Med 2013;126(7):615–624 e5.

248. Kellum JA, Prowle JR. Paradigms of acute kidney injury in the intensive care setting. Nat Rev Nephrol 2018;14(4):217–30.

249. Jasti H, Mortensen EM, Obrosky DS, et al. Causes and risk factors for rehospitalization of patients hospitalized with community-acquired pneumonia. Clin Infect Dis 2008;46(4):550–6.

250. Capelastegui A, España Yandiola PP, Quintana JM, et al. Predictors of short-term rehospitalization following discharge of patients hospitalized with community-acquired pneumonia. Chest 2009; 136(4):1079–85.

251. Kaplan V, Angus DC, Griffin MF, et al. Hospitalized community-acquired pneumonia in the elderly: age- and sex-related patterns of care and outcome in the United States. Am J Respir Crit Care Med 2002;165(6):766–72.

252. Mortensen EM, Metersky ML. Long-term mortality after pneumonia. Semin Respir Crit Care Med 2012;33(3):319–24.

UNITED STATES POSTAL SERVICE ®

Statement of Ownership, Management, and Circulation
(All Periodicals Publications Except Requester Publications)

1. Publication Title	2. Publication Number	3. Filing Date
CLINICS IN CHEST MEDICINE	000 - 765	9/18/2018

4. Issue Frequency	5. Number of Issues Published Annually	6. Annual Subscription Price
MAR, JUN, SEP, DEC	4	$366.00

7. Complete Mailing Address of Known Office of Publication (Not printer) (Street, city, county, state, and ZIP+4®)

ELSEVIER INC.
230 Park Avenue, Suite 800
New York, NY 10169

Contact Person
STEPHEN R. BUSHING

Telephone (Include area code)
215-239-3688

8. Complete Mailing Address of Headquarters or General Business Office of Publisher (Not printer)

ELSEVIER INC.
230 Park Avenue, Suite 800
New York, NY 10169

9. Full Names and Complete Mailing Addresses of Publisher, Editor, and Managing Editor (Do not leave blank)

Publisher (Name and complete mailing address)

TAYLOR E BALL, ELSEVIER INC.
1600 JOHN F KENNEDY BLVD. SUITE 1800
PHILADELPHIA, PA 19103-2899

Editor (Name and complete mailing address)

COLLEEN DIETZLER, ELSEVIER INC.
1600 JOHN F KENNEDY BLVD. SUITE 1800
PHILADELPHIA, PA 19103-2899

Managing Editor (Name and complete mailing address)

PATRICK MANLEY, ELSEVIER INC.
1600 JOHN F KENNEDY BLVD. SUITE 1800
PHILADELPHIA, PA 19103-2899

10. Owner (Do not leave blank. If the publication is owned by a corporation, give the name and address of the corporation immediately followed by the names and addresses of all stockholders owning or holding 1 percent or more of the total amount of stock. If not owned by a corporation, give the names and addresses of the individual owners. If owned by a partnership or other unincorporated firm, give its name and address as well as those of each individual owner. If the publication is published by a nonprofit organization, give its name and address.)

Full Name	Complete Mailing Address
WHOLLY OWNED SUBSIDIARY OF REED/ELSEVIER, US HOLDINGS	1600 JOHN F KENNEDY BLVD. SUITE 1800 PHILADELPHIA, PA 19103-2899

11. Known Bondholders, Mortgagees, and Other Security Holders Owning or Holding 1 Percent or More of Total Amount of Bonds, Mortgages, or Other Securities. If none, check box ► ☐ None

Full Name	Complete Mailing Address
N/A	

12. Tax Status (For completion by nonprofit organizations authorized to mail at nonprofit rates) (Check one)
The purpose, function, and nonprofit status of this organization and the exempt status for federal income tax purposes:

☒ Has Not Changed During Preceding 12 Months
☐ Has Changed During Preceding 12 Months (Publisher must submit explanation of change with this statement)

PS Form **3526**, July 2014 (Page 1 of 4 (see instructions page 4)) PSN: 7530-01-000-9931 PRIVACY NOTICE: See our privacy policy on www.usps.com.

---

13. Publication Title		14. Issue Date for Circulation Data Below
CLINICS IN CHEST MEDICINE		JUNE 2018

15. Extent and Nature of Circulation		Average No. Copies Each Issue During Preceding 12 Months	No. Copies of Single Issue Published Nearest to Filing Date
a. Total Number of Copies (Net press run)		400	514
b. Paid Circulation (By Mail and Outside the Mail)	(1) Mailed Outside-County Paid Subscriptions Stated on PS Form 3541 (Include paid distribution above nominal rate, advertiser's proof copies, and exchange copies)	234	278
	(2) Mailed In-County Paid Subscriptions Stated on PS Form 3541 (Include paid distribution above nominal rate, advertiser's proof copies, and exchange copies)	0	0
	(3) Paid Distribution Outside the Mails Including Sales Through Dealers and Carriers, Street Vendors, Counter Sales, and Other Paid Distribution Outside USPS®	108	149
	(4) Paid Distribution by Other Classes of Mail Through the USPS (e.g., First-Class Mail®)	0	0
c. Total Paid Distribution (Sum of 15b (1), (2), (3), and (4))		342	427
d. Free or Nominal Rate Distribution (By Mail and Outside the Mail)	(1) Free or Nominal Rate Outside-County Copies included on PS Form 3541	45	70
	(2) Free or Nominal Rate In-County Copies included on PS Form 3541	0	0
	(3) Free or Nominal Rate Copies Mailed at Other Classes Through the USPS (e.g., First-Class Mail)	0	0
	(4) Free or Nominal Rate Distribution Outside the Mail (Carriers or other means)	45	70
e. Total Free or Nominal Rate Distribution (Sum of 15d (1), (2), (3) and (4))		45	70
f. Total Distribution (Sum of 15c and 15e)		387	497
g. Copies not Distributed (See Instructions to Publishers #4 (page #3))		13	17
h. Total (Sum of 15f and g)		400	514
i. Percent Paid (15c divided by 15f times 100)		88.37%	85.92%

* If you are claiming electronic copies, go to line 16 on page 3. If you are not claiming electronic copies, skip to line 17 on page 3.

16. Electronic Copy Circulation		Average No. Copies Each Issue During Preceding 12 Months	No. Copies of Single Issue Published Nearest to Filing Date
a. Paid Electronic Copies	►	0	0
b. Total Paid Print Copies (Line 15c) + Paid Electronic Copies (Line 16a)	►	342	427
c. Total Print Distribution (Line 15f) + Paid Electronic Copies (Line 16a)	►	387	497
d. Percent Paid (Both Print & Electronic Copies) (16b divided by 16c × 100)	►	88.37%	85.92%

☒ I certify that 50% of all my distributed copies (electronic and print) are paid above a nominal price.

17. Publication of Statement of Ownership

☒ If the publication is a general publication, publication of this statement is required. Will be printed in the **DECEMBER 2018** issue of this publication.

☐ Publication not required.

18. Signature and Title of Editor, Publisher, Business Manager, or Owner

STEPHEN R. BUSHING INVENTORY DISTRIBUTION CONTROL MANAGER

Stephen R. Bushing Date 9/18/2018

I certify that all information furnished on this form is true and complete. I understand that anyone who furnishes false or misleading information on this form or who omits material or information requested on the form may be subject to criminal sanctions (including fines and imprisonment) and/or civil sanctions (including civil penalties).

PS Form **3526**, July 2014 (Page 3 of 4) PRIVACY NOTICE: See our privacy policy on www.usps.com

Moving?

Make sure your subscription moves with you!

To notify us of your new address, find your **Clinics Account Number** (located on your mailing label above your name), and contact customer service at:

Email: journalscustomerservice-usa@elsevier.com

800-654-2452 (subscribers in the U.S. & Canada)
314-447-8871 (subscribers outside of the U.S. & Canada)

Fax number: 314-447-8029

Elsevier Health Sciences Division
Subscription Customer Service
3251 Riverport Lane
Maryland Heights, MO 63043

ELSEVIER

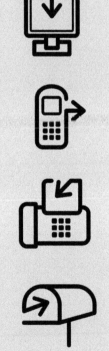